SPORT, RECOVERY, AND PERFORMANCE

Sport, Recovery, and Performance is a unique multi-disciplinary collection which examines both the psychological and physiological dimensions to recover from sport. Including contributions from medicine, neuroscience, psychology, and sport science, the book expertly explores the implications for applied and strategic interventions to both retain and stabilise performance, and promote health and well-being.

Including chapters written by leading experts, the book represents an important milestone in this evolving field of study. It covers issues around measuring recovery, the impact of overtraining on sleep and mental health, and addresses topics such as the impact of travel on performance. The book informs not only how managing recovery can improve performance, but also offers insights in how recovery can sustain athletes' physical and mental health.

Citing research from a range of individual and team sports, as well as extreme situations and the workplace, this is an important book that will be widely read across sport sciences.

Prof. Dr Michael Kellmann is Head of Unit of Sport Psychology at the Faculty of Sport Science at Ruhr University Bochum, Germany. He is also Honorary Professor in the School of Human Movement and Nutrition Sciences at the University of Queensland, Australia.

Prof. Dr Jürgen Beckmann is Chair of Sport Psychology at the Department of Sport and Health Sciences at Technical University of Munich, Germany. He was president of the German Society for Sport Psychology (asp), editor in chief of the *German Journal of Sport Psychology*, and on the editorial board of several international journals (currently *Frontiers in Psychology*).

'Fifteen years after the publication of *Enhancing Recovery* it is time for another resource that brings together cutting-edge research on the importance of recovery for athletic performance and health. Michael Kellmann and Jürgen Beckmann have gathered the world's leading scholars from both psychology and physiology in a joint perspective on recovery research and its practical application. This book's interdisciplinarity is unique and an advancement that many other research areas could profit from. I recommend this book to anyone who wants to learn from the best on how to improve the performance and health of athletes by enhancing their recovery.'

—**Dr. Anne-Marie Elbe**, *President of FEPSAC*
(European Federation of Sport Psychology)

SPORT, RECOVERY, AND PERFORMANCE

Interdisciplinary Insights

Edited by Michael Kellmann
and Jürgen Beckmann

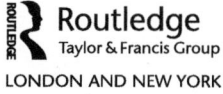

First published 2018
by Routledge
2 Park Square, Milton Park, Abingdon, Oxon OX14 4RN

and by Routledge
711 Third Avenue, New York, NY 10017

Routledge is an imprint of the Taylor & Francis Group, an informa business

© 2018 selection and editorial matter, Michael Kellmann and Jürgen Beckmann; individual chapters, the contributors

The right of Michael Kellmann and Jürgen Beckmann to be identified as the authors of the editorial material, and of the authors for their individual chapters, has been asserted in accordance with sections 77 and 78 of the Copyright, Designs and Patents Act 1988.

All rights reserved. No part of this book may be reprinted or reproduced or utilised in any form or by any electronic, mechanical, or other means, now known or hereafter invented, including photocopying and recording, or in any information storage or retrieval system, without permission in writing from the publishers.

Trademark notice: Product or corporate names may be trademarks or registered trademarks, and are used only for identification and explanation without intent to infringe.

British Library Cataloguing-in-Publication Data
A catalogue record for this book is available from the British Library

Library of Congress Cataloging-in-Publication Data
A catalog record for this book has been requested

ISBN: 978-1-138-28776-1 (hbk)
ISBN: 978-1-138-28777-8 (pbk)
ISBN: 978-1-315-26814-9 (ebk)

Typeset in Bembo
by Apex CoVantage, LLC

CONTENTS

List of contributors viii
Acknowledgements and preface xi

PART I
Conceptualizing the problem 1

1 Monitoring the recovery-stress state in athletes 3
  Jahan Heidari, Sarah Kölling, Maximilian Pelka, and Michael Kellmann

2 Developing athlete monitoring systems: Theoretical basis and practical applications 19
  Aaron J. Coutts, Stephen Crowcroft, and Tom Kempton

3 Perceptions and practises of recovery modalities in elite team athletes 33
  Ranel Venter and Roné Grobbelaar

PART II
Psychophysiological determinants of underrecovery 49

4 Overtraining – what do we know? 51
  Romain Meeusen and Kevin De Pauw

5 Recovery-stress balance and psychobiosocial states
   monitoring of road cyclists   63
   *Claudio Robazza, Fabio Forzini, Selenia di Fronso, and
   Maurizio Bertollo*

6 Psychophysiological features of soccer players' recovery-stress
   balance during the in-season competitive phase   74
   *Maurizio Bertollo, Fabio Yuzo Nakamura, Laura Bortoli,
   and Claudio Robazza*

7 Managing the training load of overreached athletes:
   Insights from the detraining and tapering literature   87
   Laurent Bosquet, Nicolas Berryman, and Iñigo Mujika

8 Recovery-stress balance and injury risk in team sports   108
   Michel Brink and Koen Lemmink

9 Stress, underrecovery, and health problems in athletes   119
   Raphael Frank, Insa Nixdorf, and Jürgen Beckmann

10 Quantification of training and competition loads in
   endurance sports: A key to recovery-stress balance
   and performance   132
   Avish P. Sharma and Iñigo Mujika

PART III
The impact of sleep on recovery   **149**

11 The role of sleep in maximising performance in elite athletes   151
   Johnpaul Caia, Vincent G. Kelly, and Shona L. Halson

12 Sleep, dreams, and athletic performance   168
   Daniel Erlacher and Felix Ehrlenspiel

13 Domestic and international travel: Implications for
   performance and recovery in team-sport athletes   183
   Rob Duffield and Peter M. Fowler

PART IV
Transfer to related areas   **199**

14 What do sport coaches know about recovery?   201
   Christine Nash and John Sproule

15 Stress and recovery in extreme situations   221
    Michel Nicolas, Marvin Gaudino, and Philippe Vacher

16 Stress and recovery in applied settings: Long working
    hours, recovery, and breaks   233
    K. Wolfgang Kallus and Kerstin Gaisbachgrabner

17 Psychological relaxation techniques to enhance
    recovery in sports   247
    Michael Kellmann, Maximilian Pelka, and Jürgen Beckmann

18 Sport, recovery, and performance: A concluding summary   260
    Michael Kellmann and Jürgen Beckmann

Index   *267*

CONTRIBUTORS

Beckmann, Jürgen, Technical University of Munich, Germany

Berryman, Nicolas, Bishop's University, Canada, and National Institute of Sport of Québec, Canada

Bertollo, Maurizio, University G. d'Annunzio, Italy, and University of Suffolk, UK

Bortoli, Laura, University G. d'Annunzio, Italy

Bosquet, Laurent, University of Poitiers, France, and University of Montréal, Canada

Brink, Michel, University of Groningen, Netherlands

Caia, Johnpaul, The University of Queensland, Australia

Coutts, Aaron J., University of Technology Sydney, Australia

Crowcroft, Stephen, University of Technology Sydney, Australia, and New South Wales Institute of Sport, Australia

De Pauw, Kevin, Vrije Universiteit Brussel, Belgium

di Fronso, Selenia, University G. d'Annunzio, Italy

Duffield, Rob, University of Technology Sydney, Australia

Ehrlenspiel, Felix, Technical University of Munich, Germany

Erlacher, Daniel, University of Bern, Switzerland

Forzini, Fabio, University of Trieste, Italy

Fowler, Peter M., Aspetar Orthopaedic and Sports Medicine Hospital, Qatar

Frank, Raphael, Technical University of Munich, Germany

Gaisbachgrabner, Kerstin, University of Graz, Austria

Gaudino, Marvin, University of Burgundy, France

Grobbelaar, Roné, Stellenbosch University, South Africa

Halson, Shona L., Australian Institute of Sport, Australia

Heidari, Jahan, Ruhr University Bochum, Germany

Kallus, K. Wolfgang, University of Graz, Austria

Kellmann, Michael, Ruhr University Bochum, Germany, and The University of Queensland, Australia

Kelly, Vincent G., The University of Queensland, Australia

Kempton, Tom, University of Technology Sydney, Australia, and Carlton Football Club, Australia

Kölling, Sarah, Ruhr University Bochum, Germany, and Stellenbosch University, South Africa

Lemmink, Koen, University of Groningen, Netherlands

Meeusen, Romain, Vrije Universiteit Brussel, Belgium, and James Cook University, Australia

Mujika, Iñigo, University of the Basque Country, Spain, and Finis Terrae University, Chile

Nakamura, Fabio Yuzo, University of Londrina, Brasil

Nash, Christine, University of Edinburgh, UK

Nicolas, Michel, University of Burgundy, France

Nixdorf, Insa, Technical University of Munich, Germany

Pelka, Maximilian, Ruhr University Bochum, Germany

Robazza, Claudio, University G. d'Annunzio, Italy

Sharma, Avish P., Australian Institute of Sport, Australia and University of Canberra, Australia

Sproule, John, University of Edinburgh, UK

Vacher, Philippe, University of Burgundy, France

Venter, Ranel, Stellenbosch University, South Africa

ACKNOWLEDGEMENTS AND PREFACE

Acknowledgements

This book is based on a conference on *Recovery and Performance* held at Technical University Munich (TUM) Science and Study Center Raitenhaslach (Germany), from September 21–23, 2016. We gratefully acknowledge the financial support received from TUM and the German Science Foundation (DFG). Moreover, we would like to express special thanks to Frau Weiand and staff at the Center for assistance with organisation on-site and outstanding hospitality, Petra Sollnberger for coordinating the participation of the colleagues from all over the world and providing invaluable and extremely reliable administrative support, as well as Simon Blaschke for all the additional jazz including participants' safe transport.

Preface

Publications in medicine, psychology, and sport sciences on stress and coping with stress are abundant. However, the approaches are largely limited because they are constricted to certain types of biological and psychological mechanisms and in line with that they are hardly ever interdisciplinary. Recovery can be considered an overarching concept that demands an interdisciplinary perspective. This was exactly what incited us to invite colleagues from various scientific disciplines working in various countries on recovery processes to convene for an exchange of ideas, results, and the development of a joint perspective. We are very glad that Routledge shared our enthusiasm for publishing the productive outcomes of this convention.

Beckmann, J., & Kellmann, M. (2018). Acknowledgements and preface. In M. Kellmann & J. Beckmann (Eds.), *Sport, Recovery, and Performance: Interdisciplinary Insights* (pp. xi–xiii). Abingdon: Routledge.

Only recently the importance of recovery for performance and health was fully realised. Regeneration research primarily focuses on somatic processes. Especially, research on overtraining has demonstrated that this limited perspective is insufficient for a genuine conceptualisation of the problem of overtraining and recovering from it. Recovery processes such as sleep, autonomous heart rate abatement, post-stress changes in blood circulation and metabolism, hormonal changes, and most of all, autonomous recovery activities, are not or only a partial part of the regeneration concept. From our perspective recovery is a general concept that integrates regeneration, and in addition to physical recovery, there are psychological and cognitive recovery processes involved. Physiological stress and performance decrements are accompanied by significant psychological alterations from sleep disturbance to depressive behaviour. Accordingly, an interdisciplinary approach with a multi-dimensional assessment of recovery is essential to adequately fulfil this highly complex process.

During the last two decades the significance of recovery for performance processes as well as health issues has been realised. Developing research on recovery in several scientific disciplines provided multifaceted empirical evidence for the significance of its different aspects of recovery in these domains. The symposium on *Recovery and Performance* we organised in 2016 initiated interdisciplinary discussion of several disciplines in recovery research and served as a kick off for interdisciplinary international research on recovery and performance (Picture 1). This discussion is reflected in the chapters of the present book. Basic research issues are one major focus but theory-practise transfer is also addressed constituting another

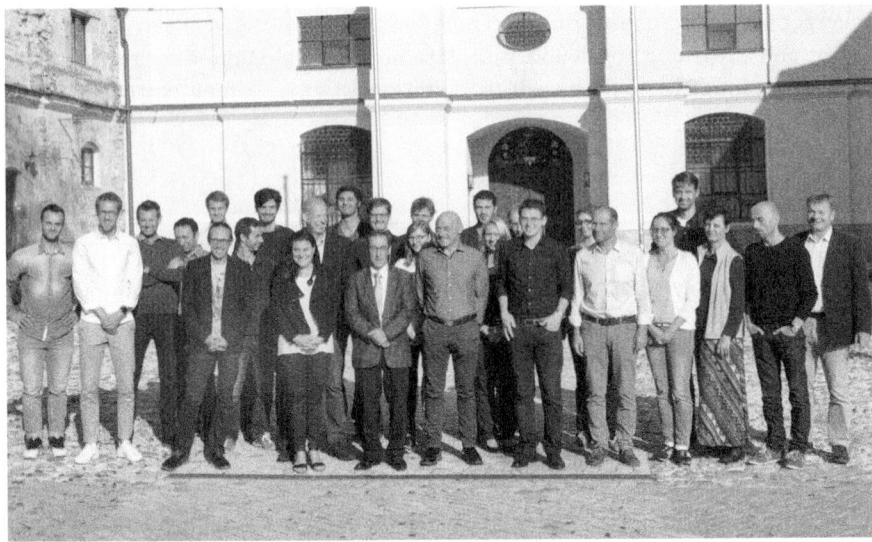

PICTURE 1 Participants of the Symposium *Recovery and Performance* held at Technical University Munich (TUM) Science and Study Center Raitenhaslach (Germany), from September 21–23, 2016.

main goal. Based upon the contemporary models of recovery and performance in different scientific disciplines such as medicine, neuroscience, psychology, and sport science implications for applied and strategic interventions to retain and to stabilise performance ability are suggested and discussed.

The contributors to this book have a range of backgrounds, experiences, and viewpoints. They all agree that the development of a concise interdisciplinary model of recovery would be a major step ahead in finding solutions resulting from a lack of or inadequate recovery in the societal extremely relevant areas of performance and health. The authors firmly believe that the book can serve as a mediator for an emerging interdisciplinary or even transdisciplinary perspective on recovery and performance.

Bringing together some of the world's leading experts, this multi-disciplinary collection examines both the psychological and physiological dimensions to recover from stress in sport and other areas of performance. Featuring chapters on overtraining, sleep, the relationship to injury, as well as the role of stress, the book illustrates how performance, both in individual and team sports, can be better managed through understanding the recovery process. Also including chapters discussing the impact of travel on performance, as well as guidance on measurement and training, this is an important book for students and scholars across sports science as well as any coach interested in the latest research.

Jürgen Beckmann & Michael Kellmann

PART I
Conceptualizing the problem

1
MONITORING THE RECOVERY-STRESS STATE IN ATHLETES

Jahan Heidari, Sarah Kölling, Maximilian Pelka, and Michael Kellmann

Introduction

Elite athletes form an unique sample of individuals with regard to their needs and abilities compared to the general population. In the following, an example of a prototypical year of a NFL (National Football League)-player is provided. The report is based on personal experiences by the authors and illustrations by Weinfuss (2014), who vividly described the physical and mental challenges NFL-players are confronted with during both season and offseason. The exemplary description of a season of an elite athlete should introduce the overall topic of monitoring stress and recovery which will be discussed in this chapter and throughout the book. Typical daily life situations and events of a NFL-player are delineated, indicating potential starting points for appropriate and effective monitoring in sports settings.

> **NFL-player, 5th season (with reference to Weinfuss, 2014):**
>
> *As a NFL player, your season ideally lasts from July until the beginning of February, if you make the playoffs and proceed to the Super Bowl. During these seven months, you are exposed to a stressful and tough schedule, involving meetings, practice, weekly games, and off-the-field responsibilities. Apart from the intense physical demands you are constantly confronted with, also mental strains exist requiring your resources.*

Heidari, J., Kölling, S., Pelka, M., & Kellmann, M. (2018). Monitoring the recovery–stress state in athletes. In M. Kellmann & J. Beckmann (Eds.), *Sport, Recovery and Performance: Interdisciplinary Insights* (pp. 3–18). Abingdon: Routledge.

> *It is a fast-paced life, leaving almost no room for detachment and cognitive processing of all the stimuli and experiences you have to deal with. Your focus and concentration are exclusively directed towards winning the next game in order to attain the overall goal: To win the Super Bowl. In the course of the season, family and social contacts come short and do not receive the attention they deserve, as travelling time, game preparation and tactical meetings consume a considerable amount of time. Unwinding takes place predominantly on a physical level, for example via stretching activities, massages, and ice baths after a weekend's game day. A regular week would then continue with the preparation for the next opponent, consisting of video analyses of games and specific plays. This theoretical information also needs to be addressed on the field during practice. Additionally, each position meets with the respective coach to obtain explicit input relevant for their own performance. On top, strength training sessions are implemented up to four times per week to prevent injuries and prepare for the physical challenges in the life of a NFL-player. But in the end, it was all worth it when you reach the ultimate goal, to win a Super Bowl. The longer the season lasts, the more you experience minor injuries due to an exhaustive season and the necessity to provide your mind and body with an extensive recovery period increases constantly.*
>
> *At first glance, the offseason appears to be the long-desired and welcomed break allowing for comprehensive physical and mental recovery. But many of us fear the abrupt change from a structured and packed schedule to a daily routine without football-related obligations. Players frequently report a habituation process to the offseason life, which is accompanied by mental detachment from the season-specific rhythm and in particular, an adjustment to the family-related rhythm. We need to find our place in the daily routine of the family while recovering from the physical complaints that have accumulated over the season. After two to four weeks, this offseason 'stress' may be increased by slowly resuming offseason training in order to keep the physical fitness and prepare for the next season. For a football player, recovery represents a delicate and juggling act, consisting of both physical and mental strategies to be placed at the right time in a reasonable dose. In the end, the NFL is a business, which does not allow weaknesses and exceptions from your schedule in order to obtain your physical and mental balance.*

The scenario describes the course of a typical year for a professional football player competing at the highest level. Regardless of sports type, strict schedules resembling those of NFL-players are on the agenda of elite athletes. In general, competitive athletes are constantly confronted with considerable physical and psychological strains, which may stem from training routines, pressure to perform, or self-inflicted expectations (Drew, Cook, & Finch, 2016; Markser, 2011). According to the scenario, athletes may consider this potpourri of sport-specific challenges and influences as stressful, which may result in a disturbance of the balance between stress and recovery. Nevertheless, an inference with the organismic equilibrium via challenging external and internal stimuli cannot be generalised as a genuinely negative event (Lazarus, 1999). For professional athletes with noble goals (e.g., Super Bowl, Champions League), certain stressors can be contemplated as adequately challenging, such as tactical or strength training sessions. They enable athletes to perform on a higher level in crucial situations, for example in the final minutes of a playoff game. Hence, it is the concept of distress which is characterised as an aversive, adverse state in which stimuli are perceived as stressors exceeding the personal coping resources.

Referring to the aforementioned NFL example, the susceptibility of players to potential stressors, such as media presence or training sessions, may vary significantly. While one player perceives the media as motivating and performance enhancing, another athlete might feel hampered by the environmental expectations and the pressure to perform. Notably, not only interindividual differences may be present, but each athlete experiences certain situations as varyingly stressful depending on his psychological resilience, which is modified by competitive, organisational, and personal factors (Sarkar & Fletcher, 2014).

The recovery-stress state

In response to these multi-faceted stressors, ensuring comprehensive recovery has emerged as essential strategy to establish a functional health condition and guarantee a continuous ability to perform in elite sports (Kellmann, 2002b; Kellmann & Kallus, 2016). Recovery can be defined as:

> *an inter- and intraindividual multilevel (e.g., psychological, physiological, social) process in time for the re-establishment of personal resources and their full functional capacity. Recovery includes a broad range of physiological processes like sleep, motivated behavior (like eating and drinking) and goal-oriented components (like relaxation or meeting friends). Recovery activities can be passive or active and in many instances recovery is achieved indirectly by activities, which stimulate recovery processes like active sports.*
> (Kallus, 2016, p. 42)

The basic concept of recovery consists of the idea that resources need to be restored to regain a homeostatic and biorhythmic balance. Essentially, recovery depends on a reduction of, a change of, or a break from stress and comprises a gradual and cumulative process that is dependent on previous activities or events (Kellmann, 2002b). A challenging event such as a NFL playoff game between two division rivals might exhibit considerable psychological and physical stress on the players and requires extensive recovery depending on the specific needs of each athlete. Peak performance is only achievable if athletes are recovered appropriately after exposition to demanding activities by optimally balancing stress with adequate recovery throughout a longer period of time, for instance an entire season of a NFL-player

(Kellmann, 2010). Potential recovery strategies can be divided into active, passive, and pro-active methods (Kellmann, 2002b). Active recovery involves moderate exercise during the recovery process to eliminate the results of fatigue through a target-oriented physical activity (e.g., a cool-down programme directly after a match or on the following morning). A passive approach could consist of sauna, massages, or just sitting or lying quietly. Thereby, physiological reactions to physiological stimuli such as heat, cold, or pressure to restore pre-task performance states are initiated and are accompanied by psychological adaptations. In case recovery includes a purposeful, self-initiated, and self-determined action, it can be characterised as pro-active recovery (e.g., dynamic stretching or systematically breathing for just a few minutes during a half-time break). In addition, recovery is tightly linked to environmental circumstances. Exemplarily, athletes are frequently obliged to give interviews after demanding matches causing a postponement of the recovery process. A delay of only 10–15 minutes may result in disturbed or reduced recovery which negatively affects the homeostatic equilibrium (Reilly & Ekblom, 2005). Research in football (Fullagar et al., 2016), rowing (Kölling et al., 2016), strength training (Raeder et al., 2016), and cycling (Hammes et al., 2016) highlights the importance of the recovery process regarding injury and training monitoring in a variety of sports.

Consequences of a recovery-stress imbalance

In case demands become overwhelming and sufficient recovery is not applied, a return to a state of physiological and psychological homeostasis with a balanced recovery-stress state cannot be realised (Goldstein, 2009). This transition from a stable recovery-stress state to an imbalance of stress and recovery can be characterised as a gradual process, with stress and recovery representing intertwined and interdependent constructs. According to Kellmann (2002b), the complexity of fine-tuning recovery and stress can only be obtained when considering all factors that influence performance, such as training (e.g., extent, intensity, training techniques, periodisation), lifestyle (e.g., sleep, nutrition, recreational activities), state of health (e.g., cold, infections), or environment (e.g., family, team members, school/university). A lack of awareness of the importance of the recovery-stress balance may lead to dysfunctional behaviour, such as inappropriate time management, excessive training and workloads, or ineffective priorities. A continuous exposition to this potpourri of dysfunctional demands may overwhelm the resources of athletes, ultimately causing hazardous health conditions such as underrecovery, the overtraining syndrome or even the burnout syndrome (Gustafsson, Hassmén, Kenttä, & Johansson, 2008; Meeusen et al., 2013). A constant downward spiral illustrates the relationship between these three states. At the outset, underrecovery establishes and serves as the antecedent of overtraining and burnout in terms of individual well-being, performance decrements, and influence on short- and long-term health development (Kellmann, 2002b).

Underrecovery is defined as an imbalance of recovery periods and daily life demands of an athlete (Kellmann, 2002b). If athletes reach the state of chronic underrecovery, short periods of rest or spontaneous recovery interventions appear to be ineffective. Longer rest periods (from several weeks to months) including professional help from medical doctors or psychologists are required for a re-establishment of the recovery-stress equilibrium. With additional training load, recovery demands increase proportionally. However, a short-term planned episode of recovery (e.g., a day off following a strenuous practise session) stimulates long-term restorative effects. On the contrary, an increase of training load and intensity over a longer time accompanied by inadequate or inappropriate recovery may end in long-term underrecovery followed by overtraining (Kellmann, 2010; Roose, de Vries, Schmikli, Backx, & van Doornen, 2009). At each stage, recovery can work as a regulatory mechanism. In principle, it is understood that the higher an athlete's stress level, the higher the demands for recovery to reach an individual's optimal recovery-stress state. Therefore, an exposition to high stress does not necessarily imply negative consequences as long as recovery demands are met accordingly (Kellmann, 2002b). These interconnections between stress and recovery reflect the central idea of the 'scissor model' established by Kellmann (2002b). Problematically, a lack of potent coping strategies in combination with chronic stress can lead to overtraining as an inevitable consequence (Gustafsson et al., 2008). Overtraining can be contemplated as the result of too much training and stress together with insufficient recovery (Meeusen et al., 2013). Therefore, underrecovery can be classified as a longer-lasting pre-condition to the overtraining syndrome. Overtraining has been primarily associated with physiological stress and represents a particular characteristic of sports. On the contrary, the burnout syndrome considers psychological factors to a greater extent (Gustafsson, Kenttä, & Hassmén, 2011) and is prevalent in various performance areas and disciplines (Leiter, Bakker, & Maslach, 2014; Maslach, Schaufeli, & Leiter, 2001). A sports-related integrated framework was developed by Gustafsson and colleagues (2011) for the purpose of directing future research in the sports domain. Burnout denotes a negative emotional reaction to sports participation and is defined by the three central attributes of exhaustion, cynicism, and inefficacy (Maslach et al., 2001). While it is known that overtrained athletes are still capable of maintaining their performance motivation to continue with training, a burned-out athlete will commonly lack the motivation to pursue his/her activity (Fry, Morton, & Keast, 1991). Similarly, burnout has been conceptualised as an exhaustive psychophysiological response to massive chronic stress that develops gradually (Gustafsson, Kenttä, Hassmen, Lundqvist, & Durand-Bush, 2007). Burnout has also been shown to provoke affective, cognitive, motivational, and behavioural consequences with chronic emotional and physical exhaustion as key components (Goodger, Gorely, Lavallee, & Harwood, 2007). A summary of the central characteristics and differences between underrecovery, overtraining, and burnout is provided in Table 1.1. Negative health-related outcomes due to augmented stress and reduced recovery are not limited to underrecovery, overtraining, or burnout. Health issues may also manifest in injuries, back pain, or psychiatric disorders (Glick, Stillman, Reardon, & Ritvo, 2012; Heidari et al., 2016; van der Does, Brink, Otter, Visscher, & Lemmink, 2017). The descriptions in the football

TABLE 1.1 Central characteristics of underrecovery, overtraining, and burnout.

Concept	Symptoms	Consequences	Interventions
Underrecovery	*Physiological:* Physical complaints; increased muscle soreness	*Short term:* Tiredness; exhaustion; lethargy; decreased motivation; negative cognitions	*Short term:* Systematic application of relaxation/ recovery techniques in early stages of underrecovery
	Psychological: Reduced stress tolerance; sleep disturbances; lack of energy; phases of emotional disturbances	*Long term:* Performance decrements; health issues; overtraining; burnout	*Long term:* Rest periods (days to weeks); periods of lower training intensity; individualised, proactive recovery activities
Overtraining	*Physiological:* Chronic muscle or joint pain; elevated resting heart rate; increased physical fatigue	*Short term:* Tiredness; exhaustion; concentration deficits; apathy towards training	*Short term:* Lack of effective short-term interventions
	Psychological: Increased cognitive fatigue; irritability; lack of enthusiasm/ ambition; personality/mood changes	*Long term:* Hormonal changes; injuries, illnesses, and infections; performance collapse	*Long term:* Acquisition of coping strategies; restoration of energy reserves; rest periods (weeks to months)
Burnout	*Physiological:* Physical exhaustion; immunodeficiency	*Short term:* Injuries, illnesses, and infections; break from sports participation	*Short term:* Lack of effective short-term interventions
	Psychological: Emotional exhaustion; reduced sense of personal accomplishment; sport devaluation	*Long term:* Withdrawal from sports participation	*Long term:* Consultation of specialist (e.g., psychologist) extensive break from sport-related activities

Note. The transition from underrecovery to a state of overtraining and burnout is a gradual and interdependent process, resulting in an overlap of symptoms and consequences. Whereas physical symptoms are more pronounced in overtraining, burnout is predominantly marked by psychological issues. These central characteristics were extracted from several different scientific sources (Gustafsson et al., 2011; Kellmann, 2002b; Kellmann & Altfeld, 2014; Meeusen et al., 2013).

scenario correspond to scientific findings reporting a trend to experience under-recovery towards the end of a season, which is accompanied by a higher proneness to injuries (Faude, Kellmann, Ammann, Schnittker, & Meyer, 2011; Koutedakis & Sharp, 1998). These tendencies pronounce the necessity to recover and unwind not only in the course of a season, but during the offseason as well. In case of the NFL, an immediate change between a meticulously structured season and an offseason without any football-related obligations occurs, which requires resources for the adaption process. In addition, the ideal, individualised timing for starting with the offseason training needs to be identified and should be performed in a reasonable and synchronised manner.

For this purpose, monitoring instruments can serve as a useful tool in order to establish the ideal intensity, timing, and frequency of exercises, thereby allowing for a personalised schedule depending on the individual recovery-stress balance. Monitoring recovery processes and stress levels has gained significance in professional sports in the recent years in order to prevent potential detrimental consequences and to optimise performance (Saw, Main, & Gastin, 2016). The issue of systematic monitoring in elite sports will be discussed from both a scientific and practical point of view.

Monitoring the recovery-stress state in athletes

Regular monitoring encompasses the assessment of training and competition loads as well as the consequences on an individual level. Therefore, both objective and subjective standardised instruments have to be considered to guarantee for a comprehensive monitoring of athletic performance (Bourdon et al., 2017; Halson, 2014; Meeusen et al., 2013).

Performance can be interpreted as a measurable indicator, as it directly represents the athlete's performance capability and readiness to compete optimally. Selected surrogate performance parameters such as countermovement jumps, multiple rebound jumps (Raeder et al., 2016; Wiewelhove et al., 2015), or the Lamberts and Lambert submaximal cycle test (Hammes et al., 2016; Lamberts, Swart, Noakes, & Lambert, 2011) can be implemented into training processes without disturbing routines. Furthermore, physiological and biochemical parameters can be considered as markers of maladaptation. Performance requirements can be determined, e.g., via the maximal oxygen uptake or the lactate threshold. A critical health status can be detected via blood measures, such as nutrient deficiency as well as inflammatory or hormonal parameters which facilitate training or intervention prescriptions (Saw, Main, et al., 2016). However, high costs and the time lag between measurement and laboratory report exclude the applicability on a daily basis. Moreover, no agreement on the best or most practical parameter is present (Halson, 2014; Saw et al., 2016). It appears to be a difficult task to clearly distinct normal physiological variations from clear signs of maladaptation in response to intensive training stimuli (Freitas, Nakamura, Miloski, Samulski, & Bara-Filho, 2014; Gleeson, 2002). This might be explained by intra-individual and inter-individual variability regarding exercise characteristics, circadian rhythms as well as nutrition and hydration status (Saw, Main, et al., 2016). Recent research promotes an individualised approach by generating intra-individual reference ranges for monitoring muscle recovery. As physiological variables, creatine kinase and urea were selected. Based on these individualised cut-off values, a classification into recovered and non-recovered athletes can be performed (Hecksteden et al., in press).

Furthermore, the subjective perception represents an important perspective for the monitoring process (Kellmann, 2010; Meeusen et al., 2013; Saw, Main, & Gastin, 2015b). A recent systematic review highlighted the superiority of subjective measures compared to objective procedures in terms of consistency and sensitivity in reflecting acute and chronic training loads (Saw et al., 2016). These findings specifically referred to the monitoring of perceived stress and recovery as well as mood disturbances. Currently, several questionnaires exist which are used in both sports science research and sports practise. These can be distinguished based on three aspects: (a) target group of athletes; (b) assessment of single or multiple constructs; and (c) focus on stressors or resulting symptoms (Saw et al., 2016). Grove and colleagues (2014) assumed that athlete-specific measures evaluating multiple constructs may better reflect performance capacities of athletes. A selection of the most common tools will be discussed briefly in this section, whereas further details and recommendations are provided by Saw, Kellmann, Main, and Gastin (2017).

Rating of Perceived Exertion

Borg (1998) developed a one-dimensional scale to assess perceived exertion in response to a specific training load (*Rating of Perceived Exertion*; RPE). Training intensity is rated on a scale ranging from 6 (*very, very light*) to 20 (*very, very hard*). Scherr and colleagues (2013) have shown that stress intensities can be depicted independently from the type of stress, age, and gender. This scale has been developed further to rate the global intensity of a training session (Foster, 1998; Foster et al., 2001). Thirty minutes after the training session, athletes rate the perceived intensity on a scale from 0 (*rest*) to 10 (*maximal*). The individual training load is then calculated by multiplying the score with the training duration (Impellizzeri, Rampinini, Coutts, Sassi, & Marcora, 2004). Thus, it is a useful tool to evaluate each training session and to receive an overview of inter-individual differences within one team. Although these two scales constitute very economic and sport-specific instruments, they focus on the stressors (i.e., training stimuli) and disregard their consequences (i.e., symptoms). Excessive training may also lead to psychological signs of maladaptation such as mood disturbances, which cannot be assessed with the RPE (Meeusen et al., 2013).

Profile of Mood States

One of the most common questionnaires in overtraining research is the Profile of Mood States (POMS; McNair, Lorr, & Droppleman, 1992), which has been applied in abundant studies (Armstrong & Van Heest, 2002; Bresciani et al., 2011; LeUnes & Burger, 2000; Umeda et al., 2008). Depending on the research question or monitoring purpose, the answer mode can be adapted from 'How have you been feeling the past week including today' to 'How do you feel right now' (Terry & Lane, 2000). Via the assessment of six mood dimensions (i.e., *Tension, Depression, Anger, Vigour, Fatigue, Confusion*), an 'iceberg-profile' can be generated, with high values of *Vigour* being considered as favourable (Andreato et al., 2014). According to a meta-analysis by Beedie, Terry, and Lane (2000), data of the POMS can be used to predict short-term performance. This questionnaire represents a useful tool to detect mood disturbances during or following intensified training, before competitions and for long-term monitoring. For instance, Raglin (1993) has shown that disturbed mood is associated with intensified training, while reductions of the workload lead to mood improvements. Although the POMS covers mood multi-dimensionally, it focuses on negative mood states whereas the measurement of positive mood is limited to the scale *Vigour*. Thus, it underestimates the recovery aspect (Kellmann, 2002a; Mäetsu, Jürimäe, & Jürimäe, 2005).

Recovery-Stress Questionnaire for Athletes

In order to obtain an overview of sport-specific as well as external factors (e.g., social activities) affecting the overall recovery-stress state of an athlete, the *Recovery-Stress Questionnaire for Athletes* (RESTQ-Sport; Kellmann & Kallus, 2001, 2016) provides a thorough evaluation. A total of 19 scales assess general stress (*General Stress, Emotional Stress, Social Stress, Conflicts/Pressure, Fatigue, Lack of Energy, Physical Complaints*) and general recovery (*Success, Social Recovery, Physical Recovery, General Well-being, Sleep Quality*) as well as sport-specific stress (*Disturbed Breaks, Emotional Exhaustion, Injury*) and sport-specific recovery (*Being in Shape, Personal Accomplishment, Self-Efficacy, Self-Regulation*) facets which can be depicted in a profile to describe the recovery-stress balance encompassing a time frame of the previous three days and nights. The applicability of the RESTQ-Sport as monitoring instrument as well as indicator of (chronic) nonfunctional overreaching or (chronic) underrecovery, respectively, has been established in several publications (Bresciani et al., 2011; Brink, Visscher, Coutts, & Lemmink, 2012; Laux, Krumm, Diers, & Flor, 2015; Meister, Faude, Amman, Schnittker, & Meyer, 2013; Otter, Brink, van der Does, & Lemmink, 2016). As it consists of 76 items, monitoring intervals should be determined in consultation with the athlete to guarantee compliance. This might be enhanced by implementing the recently developed, abbreviated version comprising only 36 items with 12 scales (Kellmann & Kallus, 2016).

The Acute Recovery and Stress Scale and the Short Recovery and Stress Scale

The *Acute Recovery and Stress Scale* (ARSS) entails an adjective list with 32 items covering eight scales of physical, mental, emotional and overall recovery and stress

(Kellmann, Kölling, & Hitzschke, 2016; Nässi, Ferrauti, Meyer, Pfeiffer, & Kellmann, 2017). It could be demonstrated that the ARSS constitutes a very sensitive tool to detect changes regarding the acute recovery-stress state in training camps and short microcycles (Hammes et al., 2016; Kölling et al., 2015). Moreover, the ARSS was modified to a short version consisting of only eight scales (i.e., *Physical Performance Capability*, *Mental Performance Capability*, *Emotional Balance*, *Overall Recovery*, *Muscular Stress*, *Lack of Activation*, *Negative Emotional State*, *Overall Stress*). The *Short Recovery and Stress Scale* (SRSS) is suitable for multiple measurements within short intervals, e.g., in experimental settings to assess recovery strategies (Pelka et al., 2017; Wiewelhove et al., 2016) as well as for long-term monitoring (Kölling et al., 2016). Before applying the SRSS, it is suggested to introduce the ARSS as it provides a more detailed picture of the current recovery-stress state (Kellmann et al., 2016). Thus, a combined implementation with regular SRSS assessment and occasional ARSS measurements can be considered.

Conclusion and recommendations for practise

As the effectiveness of self-report measures depends on the compliance and diligence of the athletes, it is of great importance to guarantee confidential and appropriate implementation and evaluation of athletes' data. Due to predictable items and the athlete's possible desire to provide favourable answers, positive and trustful athlete-staff relationships form the basis for successful monitoring with subjective measures (Kellmann & Beckmann, 2003; Saw et al., 2015b). Guidelines for the applicability of the presented subjective measures are suggested in Table 1.2.

Established monitoring routines based on self-report measures might enhance communication between coaches and athletes as well as within the coaching staff (Saw et al., 2015b). In larger training groups and teams, feedback on the individual's current state following straining competitions or practises is available quickly and gathered in an economic manner. By this means, position- and person-specific, individualised training regimens can be designed according to the psychophysiological state following a competition or exercise. Referring to the NFL, a quarterback might require profound cognitive recovery after a game, whereas recovery for the running back should rather focus on physical aspects due to the diverging tasks these positions require. Similarly, this can be applied to all team sports with regard to position-specific interventions. Additionally, context-specific monitoring should be taken into account. Stress for elite athletes may not only emerge from sport-specific stressors, but also from personal or social factors. These aspects can also be addressed with subjective instruments and can be evaluated via a coach-athlete dialogue. However, it should be kept in mind that subjective measures are accompanied by several drawbacks and demonstrate limitations. Hence, a combination with physiological assessments should be implemented to obtain a detailed picture of individual performance states over time. This information may serve as a starting point to initiate a structured counselling process with an athlete or group of athletes. Together with a sport psychologist, athletes with recovery deficits could

TABLE 1.2 Overview of subjective monitoring instruments in sports.

Instrument	Dimension(s)	Time frame	Single training session	Daily	Weekly	Microcycle	Mesocycle	Macrocycle	Training camp	1-day Competition	Championships/ Tournament	Irregular occasions[a]
RPE	1 stress dimension (perceived exertion)	Now	✓	✓	☑	☑	☑	☑	✓	✓	×	×
Session-RPE	1 stress dimension (overall exertion of training)	30 min after training	✓	✓	☑	☑	☑	☑	✓	✓	×	×
ARSS	4 recovery & 4 stress scales (physical, mental, emotional, overall)	Now	✓	✓	✓	✓	✓	✓	✓	✓	✓	✓
SRSS	4 recovery & 4 stress items (physical, mental, emotional, overall)	Now	✓	✓	✓	✓	✓	✓	✓	✓	✓	✓
RESTQ-Sport-76	7 general & 3 sport-specific stress scales, 5 general & 4 sport-specific recovery scales	3 days/nights	×	×	✓	✓	✓	✓	✓		✓	✓
RESTQ-Sport-36	3 general & 3 sport-specific stress scales, 3 general & 3 sport-specific recovery scales	3 days/nights	×	×	✓	✓	✓	✓	✓		✓	✓
POMS	6 mood states (tension, depression, anger, vigour, fatigue, confusion)	Now/1 week	✓	✓	✓	✓	✓	✓	✓	✓	✓	✓

Note. ✓ = Applicable ☑ = Applicable with restrictions × = Not applicable

RPE = Rating of Perceived Exertion; ARSS = Acute Recovery and Stress Scale; SRSS = Short Recovery and Stress Scale; RESTQ-Sport = Recovery-Stress Questionnaire for Athletes; POMS = Profile of Mood States; [a] = e.g., pre- and/or post-specific events such as holidays, injuries, or illnesses.

elaborate their individual recovery strategy or program. First, a suitable recovery strategy should be learned and practised before it may be applied systematically. Second, a schedule of when to integrate psychological recovery techniques in the training process or daily routines needs to be established. Constant feedback and exchange of ideas between athlete and coach should also represent an integral element during the entire process. Naturally, a comprehensive evaluation of physiological and psychological parameters and subsequent information about potential recovery strategies requires time and financial resources and should be executed at selected time points (e.g., after preseason, after the season). Nevertheless, the burden on the athletes should be kept to a minimum. Frequency and type of monitoring tools depend on the specific conditions of the sport, age of the athletes, time of the season, etc. In general, change sensitive measures can be applied daily or twice-daily, whereas more stable constructs and comprehensive measures should be applied as required, e.g., weekly, monthly or infrequently (Saw, Main, & Gastin, 2015a). The progress in research has led to a plethora of possibilities to analyse, monitor, and improve athletic performance. On the downside, the constant exposition to performance tests and the awareness of continuous observation may result in an overstressing of athletes. The monitoring of stress may then become a stressor itself, thereby exhibiting adverse effects. Essentially, the individual needs, strengths, weaknesses, and personality characteristics need to be considered when establishing effective monitoring in the athletic population.

References

Andreato, L. V., de Moraes, S. M. F., Del Conti Esteves, J. V., Miranda, M. L., Pastório, J. J., Pastório, E. J., . . . Franchini, E. (2014). Psychological, physiological, performance and perceptive responses to Brazilian jiu-jitsu combats. *Kinesiology*, *46*(1), 44–52.

Armstrong, L. E., & Van Heest, J. L. (2002). The unknown mechanism of the overtraining syndrome. Clues from depression and psychoneuroimmunology. *Sports Medicine*, *32*, 185–209.

Beedie, C. J., Terry, P. C., & Lane, A. M. (2000). Profile of Mood States and atheltic performance: Two meta-analyses. *Journal of Applied Sport Psychology*, *12*, 49–68.

Borg, G. (1998). *Borg's Perceived Exertion and Pain Scale*. Champaign, IL: Human Kinetics.

Bourdon, P. C., Cardinale, M., Murray, A., Gastin, P., Kellmann, M., Varley, M. C., Gabbett, T. J., Coutts, A. J., Burgess, D. J., Gregson, W., & Cable, N. T. (2017). Monitoring athlete training loads: Consensus statement. *International Journal of Sports Physiology and Performance*, *12*(Suppl. 2), S2161–S2170.

Bresciani, G., Cuevas, M. J., Molinero, O., Almar, M., Suay, F., Salvador, A., . . . Gonzáles-Gallego, J. (2011). Signs of overload after an intensified training. *International Journal of Sports Medicine*, *32*, 338–343.

Brink, M. S., Visscher, C., Coutts, A. J., & Lemmink, K. A. M. (2012). Changes in perceived stress and recovery in overreached young elite soccer players. *Scandinavian Journal of Medicine & Science in Sports*, *22*, 285–292.

Drew, M. K., Cook, J., & Finch, C. F. (2016). Sports-related workload and injury risk: Simply knowing the risks will not prevent injuries. *British Journal of Sports Medicine*, *50*, 1306–1308.

Faude, O., Kellmann, M., Ammann, T., Schnittker, R., & Meyer, T. (2011). Seasonal changes in stress indicators in high level football. *International Journal of Sports Medicine*, *32*(4), 259–265.

Foster, C. (1998). Monitoring training in athletes with reference to overtraining syndrome. *Medicine and Science in Sports and Exercise*, *30*, 1164–1168.

Foster, C., Florhaug, J. A., Franklin, J., Gottschall, L., Hrovatin, L. A., Parker, S., . . . Dodge, C. (2001). A new approach to monitoring exercise training. *Journal of Strength and Conditioning Research*, *15*, 109–115.

Freitas, V. H., Nakamura, F. Y., Miloski, B., Samulski, D., & Bara-Filho, M. G. (2014). Sensitivity of physiological and psychological markers to training load intensification in volleyball players. *Journal of Sports Science and Medicine*, *13*, 571–579.

Fry, R. W., Morton, A. R., & Keast, D. (1991). Overtraining in athletes. *Sports Medicine*, *12*(1), 32–65.

Fullagar, H. H. K., Duffield, R., Skorski, S., White, D., Bloomfield, J., Kölling, S., & Meyer, T. (2016). Sleep, travel and recovery responses of national footballers during and following long-haul international air travel. *International Journal of Sports Physiology and Performance*, *11*, 86–95.

Gleeson, M. (2002). Biochemical and immunological markers of over-training. *Journal of Sports Science and Medicine*, *1*(2), 31–41.

Glick, I. D., Stillman, M. A., Reardon, C. L., & Ritvo, E. C. (2012). Managing psychiatric issues in elite athletes. *The Journal of Clinical Psychiatry*, *73*(5), 640–644.

Goldstein, D. S. (2009). Sympathetic noradrenergic adrenomedullary hormonal systems in stress and distress. In G. Fink (Ed.), *Stress science: Neuroendocrinology* (pp. 399–405). Oxford, UK: Elsevier.

Goodger, K., Gorely, T., Lavallee, D., & Harwood, C. (2007). Burnout in sport: A systematic review. *The Sport Psychologist*, *21*(2), 127–151.

Grove, J. R., Main, L. C., Partridge, K., Bishop, D. J., Russell, S., Shepherdson, A., & Ferguson, L. (2014). Training distress and performance readiness: Laboratory and field validation of a brief self-report measure. *Scandinavian Journal of Medicine and Science in Sports*, *24*, e83-e90.

Gustafsson, H., Hassmén, P., Kenttä, G., & Johansson, M. (2008). A qualitative analysis of burnout in elite Swedish athletes. *Psychology of Sport and Exercise*, *9*, 800–816.

Gustafsson, H., Kenttä, G., & Hassmén, P. (2011). Athlete burnout: An integrated model and future research directions. *International Review of Sport and Exercise Psychology*, *4*(1), 3–24.

Gustafsson, H., Kenttä, G., Hassmén, P., Lundqvist, C., & Durand-Bush, N. (2007). The process of burnout: A multiple case study of three elite endurance athletes. *International Journal of Sport Psychology*, *38*(4), 388–416.

Halson, S. L. (2014). Monitoring training load to understand fatigue in athletes. *Sports Medicine*, *44*(2), 139–147.

Hammes, D., Skorski, S., Schwindling, S., Ferrauti, A., Pfeiffer, M., Kellmann, M., & Meyer, T. (2016). Can the Lamberts and Lambert submaximal cycle test (LSCT) indicate fatigue and recovery in trained cyclists? *International Journal of Sports Physiology and Performance*, *11*, 328–336.

Hecksteden, A., Pitsch, W., Rossˇ, J., Pfeiffer, M., Kellmann, M., Ferrauti, A., & Meyer, T. (in press). A new method to individualize monitoring of muscle recovery in athletes. *International Journal of Sports Physiology and Performance*. doi:10.1123/ijspp.2016-0120

Heidari, J., Mierswa, T., Kleinert, J., Ott, I., Levenig, C., Hasenbring, M., & Kellmann, M. (2016). Parameters of low back pain chronicity among athletes: Associations with physical and mental stress. *Physical Therapy in Sport*, *21*, 31–37.

Impellizzeri, F. M., Rampinini, E., Coutts, A. J., Sassi, A., & Marcora, S. M. (2004). Use of RPE-based training load in soccer. *Medicine and Science in Sports and Exercise, 36,* 1042–1047.

Kallus, K. W. (2016). Stress and recovery: An overview. In K. W. Kallus & M. Kellmann (Eds.), *The Recovery-Stress Questionnaires: User manual* (pp. 27–48). Frankfurt: Pearson Assessment.

Kellmann, M. (2002a). Psychological assessment of underrecovery. In M. Kellmann (Ed.), *Enhancing recovery: Preventing underperformance in athletes* (pp. 37–55). Champaign, IL: Human Kinetics.

Kellmann, M. (2002b). Underrecovery and overtraining: Different concepts – similar impact? In M. Kellmann (Ed.), *Enhancing recovery: Preventing underperformance in athletes* (pp. 3–24). Champaign, IL: Human Kinetics.

Kellmann, M. (2010). Preventing overtraining in athletes in high-intensity sports and stress/recovery monitoring. *Scandinavian Journal of Medicine & Science in Sports, 20,* 95–102.

Kellmann, M., & Altfeld, S. (2014). Underrecovery syndrome. In R. C. Eklund & G. Tenenbaum (Eds.), *Encyclopedia of sport and exercise psychology* (Vol. 2, pp. 773–775). New York, NY: Sage.

Kellmann, M., & Beckmann, J. (2003). Research and intervention in sport psychology: New perspectives on an inherent conflict. *International Journal of Sport and Exercise Psychology, 1,* 13–26.

Kellmann, M., & Kallus, K. W. (2001). *Recovery-Stress Questionnaire for Athletes: User manual.* Champaign, IL: Human Kinetics.

Kellmann, M., & Kallus, K. W. (2016). Recovery-Stress Questionnaire for Athletes. In K. W. Kallus & M. Kellmann (Eds.), *The Recovery-Stress Questionnaires: User manual* (pp. 86–131). Frankfurt: Pearson Assessment.

Kellmann, M., Kölling, S., & Hitzschke, B. (2016). *Das Akutmaß und die Kurzskala zur Erfassung von Erholung und Beanspruchung im Sport – Manual* [The Acute Measure and the Short Scale of Recovery and Stress for Sports – Manual]. Hellenthal: Sportverlag Strauß.

Kölling, S., Hitzschke, B., Holst, T., Ferrauti, A., Meyer, T., Pfeiffer, M., & Kellmann, M. (2015). Validity of the Acute Recovery and Stress Scale – training monitoring of the German junior national field hockey team. *International Journal of Sports Science and Coaching, 10,* 529–542.

Kölling, S., Steinacker, J. M., Endler, S., Ferrauti, A., Meyer, T., & Kellmann, M. (2016). The longer the better: Sleep-wake patterns during preparation of the World Rowing Junior Championships. *Chronobiology International, 33*(1), 73–84.

Koutedakis, Y., & Sharp, C. (1998). Seasonal variations of injury and overtraining in elite athletes. *Clinical Journal of Sport Medicine, 8*(1), 18–21.

Lamberts, R. P., Swart, J., Noakes, T. D., & Lambert, M. I. (2011). A novel submaximal cycle test to monitor fatigue and predict cycling performance. *British Journal of Sports Medicine, 45,* 797–804.

Laux, P., Krumm, B., Diers, M., & Flor, H. (2015). Recovery-stress balance and injury risk in professional football players: A prospective study. *Journal of Sports Sciences, 33,* 2140–2148.

Lazarus, R. S. (1999). *Stress and emotion: A new synthesis.* New York City, NY: Springer.

Leiter, M. P., Bakker, A. B., & Maslach, C. (2014). The contemporary context of job burnout. In M. P. Leiter, A. B. Bakker, & C. Maslach (Eds.), *Burnout at work: A psychological perspective* (pp. 1–9). New York, NY: Psychology Press.

LeUnes, A., & Burger, J. (2000). Profile of Mood States research in sport and exercise psychology: Past, present, and future. *Journal of Applied Sport Psychology, 12,* 5–15.

Mäetsu, J., Jürimäe, J., & Jürimäe, T. (2005). Monitoring of performance and training in rowing. *Sports Medicine, 35,* 597–617.

Markser, V. Z. (2011). Sport psychiatry and psychotherapy: Mental strains and disorders in professional sports. Challenge and answer to societal changes. *European Archives of Psychiatry and Clinical Neuroscience, 261*, 182–185.

Maslach, C., Schaufeli, W. B., & Leiter, M. P. (2001). Job burnout. *Annual Review of Psychology, 52*(1), 397–422.

McNair, D. M., Lorr, M., & Droppleman, L. F. (1992). *Revised manual for the Profile of Mood States*. San Diego, CA: Educational and Industrial Testing Service.

Meeusen, R., Duclos, M., Foster, C., Fry, A., Glesson, M., Nieman, D., . . . Urhausen, A. (2013). Prevention, diagnosis and treatment of the overtraining syndrome: Joint consensus statement of the European College of Sport Science (ECSS) and the American College of Sports Medicine (ACSM). *Medicine and Science in Sports and Exercise, 45*, 186–205.

Meister, S., Faude, O., Amman, T., Schnittker, R., & Meyer, T. (2013). Indicators for high physical strain and overload in elite football players. *Scandinavian Journal of Medicine & Science in Sports, 23*, 156–163.

Nässi, A., Ferrauti, A., Meyer, T., Pfeiffer, M., & Kellmann, M. (2017). Development of two short measures for recovery and stress in sport. *European Journal of Sport Science, 17*(7), 894–903.

Otter, R. T. A., Brink, M. S., van der Does, H. T. D., & Lemmink, K. A. P. M. (2016). Monitoring perceived stress and recovery in relation to cycling performance in female athletes. *International Journal of Sports Medicine, 37*, 12–18.

Pelka, M., Kölling, S., Ferrauti, A., Meyer, T., Pfeiffer, M., & Kellmann, M. (2017). Acute effects of psychological relaxation techniques between two physical tasks. *Journal of Sports Sciences, 35*(3), 216–223.

Raeder, C., Wiewelhove, T., Álvaro de Paula Simola, R., Kellmann, M., Meyer, T., Pfeiffer, M., & Ferrauti, A. (2016). Assessment of fatigue and recovery in male and female athletes following six days of intensified strength training. *Journal of Strength and Conditioning Research, 30*, 3412–3427.

Raglin, J. S. (1993). Overtraining and staleness: Psychometric monitoring of endurance athletes. In R. B. Singer, M. Murphey, & L. K. Tennant (Eds.), *Handbook of research on sport psychology* (pp. 840–850). New York, NY: Palgrave Macmillan.

Reilly, T., & Ekblom, B. (2005). The use of recovery methods post-exercise. *Journal of Sports Sciences, 23*(6), 619–627.

Roose, J., de Vries, W. R., Schmikli, S. L., Backx, F. J. G., & van Doornen, L. J. P. (2009). Evaluation and opportunities in overtraining approaches. *Research Quarterly for Exercise & Sport, 80*(4), 756–764.

Sarkar, M., & Fletcher, D. (2014). Psychological resilience in sport performers: A review of stressors and protective factors. *Journal of Sports Sciences, 32*, 1419–1434.

Saw, A. E., Kellmann, M., Main, L. C., & Gastin, P. B. (2017). Athlete self-report measures in research an practice: Considerations for the discerning reader and fastidious practitioner. *International Journal of Sports Physiology and Performance, 12*(Suppl. 2), S2127–S2135.

Saw, A. E., Main, L. C., & Gastin, P. B. (2015a). Monitoring athletes through self-report: Factors influencing implementation. *Journal of Sports Science and Medicine, 14*, 137–146.

Saw, A. E., Main, L. C., & Gastin, P. B. (2015b). Role of self-report measure in athlete preparation. *Journal of Strength and Conditioning Research, 29*, 685–691.

Saw, A. E., Main, L. C., & Gastin, P. B. (2016). Monitoring the athlete training response: Subjective self-report measures trump commonly used objective measures: A systematic review. *British Journal of Sports Medicine, 50*(5), 281–291.

Scherr, J., Wolfarth, B., Christle, J. W., Pressler, A., Wagenpfeil, S., & Halle, M. (2013). Associations between Borg's Rating of Perceived Exertion and physiological measures of exercise intensity. *European Journal of Applied Physiology, 113*, 147–155.

Terry, P. C., & Lane, A. M. (2000). Normative values for the Profile of Mood States for use with athletic samples. *Journal of Applied Sport Psychology, 12*, 93–109.

Umeda, T., Suzuka, K., Takahashi, I., Yamamoto, Y., Tanabe, M., Kojima, A., . . . Sugawara, N. (2008). Effects of intense exercise on the physiological and mental condition of female university judoists during a training camp. *Journal of Sports Science, 26*, 897–904.

van der Does, H. T., Brink, M. S., Otter, R. T., Visscher, C., & Lemmink, K. A. (2017). Injury risk is increased by changes in perceived recovery of team sport players. *Clinical Journal of Sport Medicine, 27*, 46–51.

Weinfuss, J. (2014). *Recovery both physical and mental.* Retrieved November 8, 2016, from www.espn.com/nfl/story/_/id/10396406/hot-read-recovering-nfl-season-physical-mental

Wiewelhove, T., Raeder, C., Meyer, T., Kellmann, M., Pfeiffer, M., & Ferrauti, A. (2015). Markers for routine assessment of fatigue and recovery in male and female team sport athletes during high-intensity interval training. *PLoS One, 10*(10), e0139801.

Wiewelhove, T., Raeder, C., Meyer, T., Kellmann, M., Pfeiffer, M., & Ferrauti, A. (2016). Effect of repeated active recovery during a high-intensity interval training shock microcycle on markers of fatigue. *International Journal of Sports Physiology and Performance, 11*, 1060–1066.

2
DEVELOPING ATHLETE MONITORING SYSTEMS

Theoretical basis and practical applications

Aaron J. Coutts, Stephen Crowcroft, and Tom Kempton

Introduction

Athlete monitoring is now common practise in high-performance sport. Fundamentally, athlete monitoring involves quantifying the athletes training load and their responses to that training. The main reasons for monitoring athletes are that it can provide information to refine the training process, increase athlete performance readiness and reduce risk of injury and illness. Through a systematic approach to athlete monitoring an improved understanding of the complex relationships between training, performance, and injury can be obtained. The purpose of this chapter is to examine the training theory that underpins athlete monitoring and discuss the key components of an athlete monitoring system. Additionally, a discussion of methods used to analyse and interpret these data will also be provided.

Theoretical basis of athlete monitoring

The main aim of athletic training is to provide a stimulus that is effective in improving physical performance. For positive adaptations to occur, a careful balance between training dose and recovery is required (Matveyev, 1981). At the simplest level, the performance responses can be explained by the fitness-fatigue model. The fitness-fatigue model is a simple approach to quantify a dose-response relationship of training load to fitness, fatigue, and performance. Original work from Banister, Calvert, Savage, and Bach (1975), used a systems theory to analyse the response of

Coutts, A. J., Crowcroft, S., & Kempton, T. (2018). Developing athlete monitoring systems: Theoretical basis and practical applications. In M. Kellmann & J. Beckmann (Eds.), *Sport, Recovery, and Performance: Interdisciplinary Insights* (pp. 19–32). Abingdon: Routledge.

physical training from a function (see equation 2.1), that comprises both a fitness response to improve performance and a fatigue response that decreases performance.

Modelled Performance = (fitness from training model) − K (fatigue from training model)

Equation 2.1: Banisters original systems theory approach to analyse training. K = The constant that adjusts for the magnitude of the fatigue effect relative to the fitness effect.

The fitness-fatigue model can be used to understand the training-recovery cycle to single and/or multiple bouts of exercise. Figure 2.1A shows the theoretical fitness and fatigue response to a single training bout, whilst Figure 2.1B shows the modelled responses to a series of bouts (i.e., a training program). Figure 2.1B clearly shows that during periods of intensified training, where increased training loads are undertaken in the absence of appropriate recovery, that fatigue is increased having a negative influence upon performance.

Whilst the training-recovery cycle appears simple, there are a myriad of complex psychobiological adaptations that occur which make it difficult to predict the fitness and fatigue effects of training for individual athletes. As a result, it is now common that sport scientists examine these dose-response relationships on a regular basis to guide decisions on training content for individual athletes. Furthermore, despite a growing body of applied work in high-performance sport, there is still a relatively poor understanding of the most appropriate tools and methods that can be used to assess how individuals are coping with training. It is most likely that there are no single criterion measures of training load, fitness and fatigue that can be applied to all athletes. Therefore, we recommend that a multi-dimensional athlete monitoring system that is based on the fitness-fatigue model. It is important that such systems be developed whilst accounting for the cultural and logistical limitations that are commonly encountered in high-performance sport (i.e., select input measures feasible to the athlete/sport). Regardless of the environment, the essential components

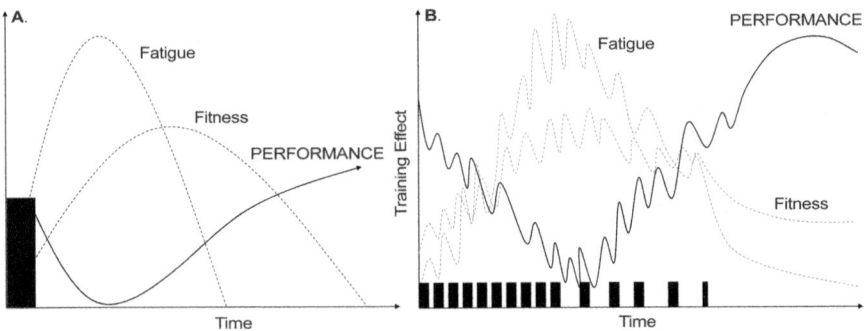

FIGURE 2.1 The modelled fitness and fatigue responses to (A) a single bout; and (B) a sequence of training bouts.

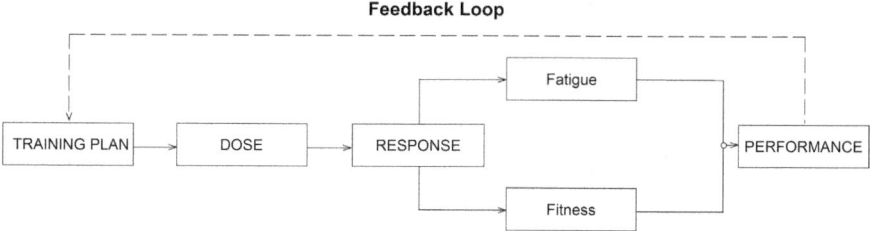

FIGURE 2.2 Conceptual model for developing athlete monitoring systems.

of this system should include quantifying training load measures for each athlete and their fitness and fatigue responses to that training. Figure 2.2 provides a conceptual model for how the various aspects of training load, fitness and fatigue can fit into an iterative monitoring system that can apply to most athletes.

Fundamental components of an athlete monitoring system

Training load

Training load is the input variable in a training system that coaches and scientists most commonly manipulate to elicit the desired training response. As such, quantifying and monitoring training load should form the foundation of any athlete monitoring system. The following sections provide an overview of various constructs of training load and how they may be integrated into athlete monitoring.

Physical training is typically quantified with reference to the type, frequency, duration, and intensity of each exercise bout. Traditionally, training load has been described as a measure of *external load* (e.g., work or speed and distance covered) (Impellizzeri, Rampinini, & Marcora, 2005). Recently, microtechnologies such as global positioning system (GPS) and micro electrical mechanical system (MEMS) components have allowed for increasingly detailed information on the external loads completed by the athlete (Malone, Lovell, Varley, & Coutts, 2017). These advances have led to the widespread use of external load measures for quantifying training in both endurance and team sports. Indeed, these devices now provide detailed information on various aspects of external load such as distance travelled above specified speeds, the number of accelerations/decelerations as well as the body loads experienced in three dimensions. With the data available from the microsensors in these devices it is also possible to count discrete activities such as collisions, tackles, changes of direction, and/or twisting activities (Gastin, McLean, Spittle, & Breed, 2013; Hulin, Gabbett, Johnston, & Jenkins, 2017; Keaney, Withers, Parker-Simmons, Gastin, & Netto, 2016). Collectively, these data can provide detailed information to scientists and coaches on the loads completed by athletes. However, despite the large amount of information provided there are cases where the associated cost, time-intensive data analysis, and measurement precision issues has limited the effective use of such devices (Coutts, 2014).

Importantly, the external load measures provided from these devices may not accurately depict the psychophysiological stress imposed on individual athletes, as other factors such as current fitness level or training environment may play a role. Accordingly, it is the relative psychophysiological stress imposed on the athlete known as the *internal training load* that provides the signal for adaptation (Viru & Viru, 2000). The relationship between internal and external training load measures and training outcome is shown in Figure 2.3.

Many researchers have attempted to develop practical methods for quantifying internal training load that incorporates both training duration and individual training intensity. Historically, heart rate (HR) has been the most common method for assessing internal load. However, with intermittent activity – which is common to many sports – HR may not reflect both the aerobic and anaerobic contributions to energy provision, or accurately compare stress from different modes of training (e.g., skills training vs. resistance training) (Coutts, Rampinini, Marcora, Castagna, & Impellizzeri, 2009). Fortunately, Carl Foster developed the session-RPE method as a global rating of session intensity (Foster, Daines, Hector, Snyder, & Welsh, 1996; Foster et al., 2001). The session-RPE method of monitoring training load in team

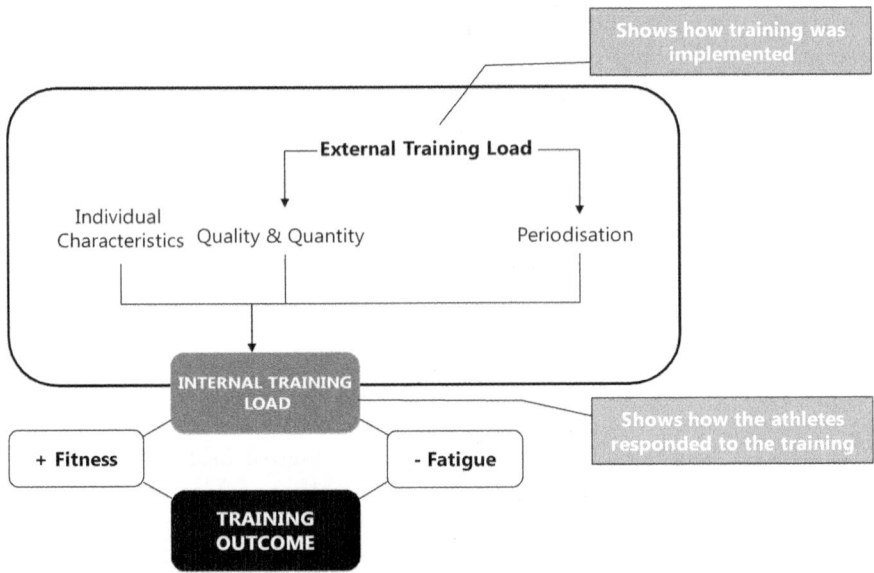

FIGURE 2.3 The relationship between internal and external training load on training outcomes.

Adapted from Impellizzeri, Rampinini, et al. (2005).

players requires each athlete to provide a rating of perceived exertion (RPE) for each exercise session along with a measure of training time (Foster et al., 2001). To calculate a measure of session intensity, athletes are asked a simple question '*How intense was your workout?*' (usually within 30 minutes of finishing their workout). A single value representing the magnitude of training load for each session is then calculated by the multiplication of training intensity – determined from Borg's RPE scales (Borg, 1998) – by the training session duration. Compared to alternative measures of internal load (i.e., HR or blood lactate measures) the session-RPE method enables coaches to combine training load from different training modalities in the same units for an accurate reflection of total training load.

There are now numerous measures, or constructs, of training load that can be measured and used in athlete monitoring. The various constructs of external and internal load should be used by scientists and coaches for different purposes. The external load is used to prescribe and quantify training the stimulus and the internal load used to measure how the athletes respond to the training dose. Whilst each of these measures helps to understand the training process for athletes, the value of load monitoring is increased when these measures are contextualised against each other and against the athlete's fitness and fatigue responses to training.

Fitness

Measuring changes in fitness is a fundamental component of an athlete monitoring system that can be used to interpret if the prescribed training has been appropriate for individual athletes. Without regular fitness measures, it is difficult to accurately determine if athletes are adapting to training, and/or if the athlete's fitness status has been adequately developed. Anecdotally, it is often questioned after poor performance if the result was due to lack of fitness or other physical capacities. Assessing fitness has been a difficult task for applied sport scientists as most gold standard assessment procedures require expensive laboratory equipment, maximal effort exercise, and interruptions to the training program.

Criteria for a fitness test that can be included in a monitoring system are that it should be valid and reliable, able to accurately reflect training status, cost effective, and easy to implement with minimal disruption to normal training. Accordingly, recent focus has aimed to develop non-fatiguing fitness tests that assess physiological responses (i.e., HR, blood lactate and RPE) to standardised submaximal work (Buchheit, 2014, 2015; Buchheit et al., 2013; Buchheit, Simpson, Al Haddad, Bourdon, & Mendez-Villanueva, 2011; Crowcroft et al., 2015; Impellizzeri, Mognoni, Sassi, & Rampinini, 2005; Lamberts, Swart, Noakes, & Lambert, 2010). This research has resulted in the development of simple field tests assessing HR responses to standard bouts of exercise to monitor athletes acute and chronic fitness adaptations to training (Buchheit, 2014).

Resting HR, HR response to exercise (HR_{ex}), and HR recovery (HRR) following exercise are simple measures that can be collected from athletes in the training setting – and have been reported to have some utility for assessing athlete fitness. For example, as HR is closely related to oxygen uptake during continuous exercise, a lower HR_{ex} provides a good marker of an athlete's aerobic fitness level that can be collected from a brief standardised submaximal exercise bout. However, since recent research has shown that lower submaximal HR can also be associated with overreaching (Aubry et al., 2015), it is critical that HR responses be interpreted in the context of other factors such as the training load, fatigue status and non-training stressors.

The main practical utility of HR measures is that they are non-invasive and time efficient, relatively cheap, and can be routinely applied to many athletes. However, despite its common implementation in the field, HR monitoring is still not accepted as a gold standard fitness test. This is likely due to the lack of consistency in methods of application and/or interpretation of changes in these variables. Nonetheless, despite these limitations, simple HR measures may provide useful insight into the fitness-related changes to training – especially if they are interpreted in the context of other important aspects such as training load and athlete fatigue status.

Fatigue

Athlete fatigue is a difficult concept to define, thus making its precise measurement problematic. Due to its multifactorial genesis, there is no commonly agreed on definition of fatigue. However, it is generally accepted that athlete fatigue is a psychobiological state associated with an inability to complete a physical task that was once achievable within a recent time frame and is usually associated with altered perceptions of effort, along with feelings of tiredness and/or exhaustion. Whilst the physiological and psychological mechanisms underlying subjective fatigue are not yet fully understood, there is consensus that measurements of subjective fatigue are an essential aspect of athlete monitoring.

There are many psychometric tools that can be used to assess various aspects of subjective fatigue, including the Profile of Mood States (McNair, Lorr, & Droppleman, 1971), Daily Analysis of Life Demands for Athletes (Rushall, 1990), Total Quality of Recovery (Kenttä & Hassmén, 1998), Recovery-Stress Questionnaire for Athletes (Kellmann & Kallus, 2016), Acute Recovery and Stress Scale (Kellmann, Kölling, & Hitzschke, 2016), and the Short Recovery and Stress Scale (Kellmann et al., 2016). Many of these tools are extensive and take longer than a few minutes to complete which limits their use for routinely monitoring athletes. Therefore, short customised questionnaires which can be administered on a regular basis have become common place (Taylor, Chapman, Cronin, Newton, & Gill, 2012). Notably, it has recently been shown that various customised single-item psychometric measures – such as perceptions of fatigue, mood, soreness, and fatigue – have greater sensitivity to acute and chronic training loads than commonly used objective measures (Saw, Main, & Gastin, 2016). For example, recent studies from professional rugby league (McLean, Coutts, Kelly, McGuigan, & Cormack, 2010), soccer (Thorpe, Atkinson, Drust, & Gregson, 2017; Thorpe et al., 2015), and Australian football (Buchheit et al., 2013) have shown that these custom-designed psychometric scales are sensitive to daily, within-weekly, and seasonal changes in training load. Additionally, there are now recommendations for steps that can be taken in order to minimise sources of error when implementing these short custom-designed psychometric scales in practise (Saw, Kellmann, Main, & Gastin, 2017).

Whilst longer questionnaires that include multidimensional assessment of factors surrounding fatigue (and recovery) status of athletes have strong empirical support, in the practical setting, specific single item questionnaires may be attractive as they are time efficient and offer ease of interpretation (Bowling, 2005). While there appears to be support for the use of short or single item questionnaires for assessing subjective fatigue, future research is still required to assess the efficacy of using single item scales compared to the validated but longer multidimensional tools (Saw et al., 2017).

Other components

Various biochemical markers have also been suggested as useful components of athlete monitoring systems (Urhausen & Kindermann, 1992). Specifically, markers of muscle damage, hormonal, and immune measures have shown to respond to changes in training intensity and dose and have been associated with overreaching in a variety of athletes (Coutts, Reaburn, Piva, & Rowsell, 2007; Halson et al., 2002). However, due to logistical issues such as drawing blood or obtaining saliva samples from athletes, along with the costs and time for analysis, these measures are not usually suitable for daily monitoring. Nonetheless, these measures may be useful for investigating athletes already showing signs or symptoms of overtraining.

Regular musculoskeletal assessments such as range of motion, muscle strength imbalances, and clinical assessments have been used to identify injury risk factors and therefore are often incorporated into athlete monitoring systems. However, whilst a complete review of these tools is beyond the scope of this chapter, we recommend that these be included if they are implemented by skilled clinicians who understand the noise in these tests and the importance of standardised test procedures. The benefit of using these measures in monitoring is that they can assist in understanding how individual athletes may be coping with training and can be used to monitor and manage an individual athlete's musculoskeletal health.

Analysing data

Whilst it is essential for athlete monitoring systems to have strong proof of concept for its design and consist of valid and reliable measures; the effectiveness of the system is dependent on how well the data can be used to inform coaching and training decisions. In high-performance sport, decisions around manipulating training need to be relayed to the coach within a brief period prior to training commencing. Traditionally, a heavy reliance has been placed upon identifying trends in monitoring data visually; however, with the development of integrated monitoring systems there is a need for stronger evidence to highlight the likelihood of a particular outcome (i.e., injury, illness or change in performance) (Taylor et al., 2012). Therefore, the purpose of the following section is to address several key concepts used to develop evidence informed monitoring systems to assist in decision-making around training prescription.

Contextualising training load

Understanding the non-linear individual athlete dose-response relationships between training on performance, fitness and fatigue is a major challenge in athlete monitoring. There are an increasing number of scientific reports using various analysis methods of monitoring data to suggest readiness to perform, the likelihood of illness or injury risk and methods to estimate performance outcomes (Foster et al., 1996; Gabbett, 2016; Wallace, Slattery, & Coutts, 2014). The following section will aim to describe some of the commonly used methods to contextualise training load data.

The fitness-fatigue model is a simple approach to quantify a dose-response relationship of training load to performance. Although this method has previously been used to predict performance, fitness, and fatigue measures, the overly simplistic nature of what is a complex non-linear dose-response relationship in highly trained athletes limits its efficacy when applied in practise. Indeed, large variability in the predicted compared to actual responses (i.e., performance, fitness, and fatigue) from these models has identified limitations in the application of this model in the development of training plans for elite athletes (Hellard et al., 2006). This may be due to the many different constructs that influence performance outcomes which may be over simplified in these mathematical models. Furthermore, this approach assumes a single measure can quantify sports performance. As such, the application of this approach may be limited in sports where performance is dependent upon a combination of physical, technical, and tactical skills (as these structures cannot be integrated into a single measure). Nonetheless, the benefit of using the fitness-fatigue model is that it provides a theoretical foundation for planning future training and it may assist in reducing training errors.

The acute-to-chronic workload ratio (ACWR) is similar to the fitness-fatigue model where, fitness is comparable to that of chronic workload (e.g., 28 days rolling average workload) and fatigue is comparable to an acute workload (e.g., 7 days rolling average workload). Although initial use of this model was to plan and predict performance, recently this simplified approach with rolling averages has been suggested as an approach to monitor injury risk, particularly within team sports (Gabbett, 2016). Indeed, there is a large body of evidence that has reported large spikes in acute workloads are associated to a substantial increase in injury risk. However, there has been some questioning from the use of a simple rolling average approach, which fails to account for the decaying nature of both fitness and fatigue over time. An alternative exponentially weighted moving average (EWMA) approach which a higher weighting to the more recent training loads completed by the athlete has been suggested as a more effective measure of training balance. Indeed, a recent comparison of these two approaches has shown that the EWMA is more sensitive to identify the increased injury risk, particularly during periods of high acute workloads (Murray, Gabbett, Townshend, & Blanch, 2017).

Contextualising the training response with monitoring tools

The purpose of monitoring an athlete's training response is to assess if an athlete is tolerating the demands of training. Whilst many observational studies have shown monitoring tools are responsive to changes in training load, injury, and illness, the magnitude of change from baseline values required to influence performance outcomes is not yet fully understood. Currently, few studies have attempted to determine the 'meaningful change' required for a monitoring variable to have an impact upon important training outcomes. The following section will aim to address some of the considerations around inferring outcomes from athlete monitoring variables.

Smallest meaningful change

For any monitoring variable to be practically useful, sport scientists must first understand the 'true' or meaningful change required for it to be an important practical consideration (i.e., level of change in a variable that is beyond its normal day-to-day variation). When quantifying the smallest meaningful change in performance, an approach based upon Cohen's effect size principle is recommended. The measure is calculated as a change in performance outcome that is greater or less than 0.2 (small effect) multiplied the between/or individual athlete co-efficient of variance (CV). However, as many monitoring variables (e.g., physiological or perceptual measures) are indirectly related to changes in performance, using a larger fraction of CV may be more appropriate (e.g., 0.5, or 1 x CV) (Buchheit, 2014). The fraction of the CV selected to identify a meaningful change is highly dependent upon the sport (i.e., the nature of the performance requirements), the type of training being completed, and how the monitoring variables are collected. For example the CV of the same subjective wellness questionnaire have ranged from ~5% in highly trained swimmers to between 12–32% in Australian football players (Crowcroft, McCleave, Slattery, & Coutts, 2017; Gastin, Meyer, & Robinson, 2013). These findings demonstrate that monitoring tools need to be assessed relevant to the sport or way they are being implemented (Saw et al., 2017). Additionally, it is also important to assess the specificity and sensitivity of measures to the likelihood of important outcome measures (i.e., performance, injury, illness etc.) (Buchheit, 2014).

Highlighting 'red flags' with sensitivity and specificity

A simple reporting method used to demonstrate a change in monitoring variables is through a traffic light alert system to identify 'red flags' (potential risks to inhibit training quality, elevated risk of injury or illness) (Robertson, Bartlett, & Gastin,

2017). When managing many athletes, this method may be useful as a 'lead generator' for sport science or coaching staff to start a discussion as to how the athlete is tolerating training demands. However, very few scientific reports have attempted to assess the efficacy of an alert system to highlight the increased likelihood of an outcome when monitoring the training response.

A common analytical approach used to assess if monitoring variables are effective to identify an outcome (e.g., performance change, injury, or illness), is to compare the accuracy of a monitoring cut off value against a binary outcome (e.g., Did performance improve? – yes or no). These values can then be applied to quantify the accuracy and optimal cut-off values to inform decision makers of the likelihood of an outcome (Fawcett, 2006). For example, Buchheit, Rabbani, and Beigi (2014) compared the use of an intra-individual CV and the between athlete standard deviation as different cut-off values to assess change in HR and RPE following a standard warm up to changes in running performance. This analysis identified that variations in HR outside of the intra-individual CV could improve the predictive accuracy in highlighting individual performance change. However, developments on this analysis has since shown that the use of any single monitoring variable has poor discriminatory ability to highlight performance changes (Crowcroft et al., 2017). As such the need for a multi-dimensional monitoring system could be required to improve the diagnostic accuracy of athlete monitoring systems.

Developing multi-dimensional monitoring systems

The interpretation of any monitoring variable must be interpreted in the context of the athletes' training phase and training load. Several studies have identified the importance of contextualising physiological and perceptual measures with training load, particularly during intensified training periods (Aubry et al., 2015; Bellenger et al., 2016; Hug et al., 2014). A framework derived from these studies identified that attenuated performance would see a noticeable shift in physiological measures and a large negative change in subjective measures during increased training load. However, the same change in the absence of negative subjective measures may indicate positive training adaptations and a likely improvement in performance. These findings highlight the need to contextualise changes in training load, fitness, and fatigue measures with each other to gain a comprehensive understanding of how athletes are responding to training.

To overcome some of the limitations in interpreting data from multi-dimensional monitoring systems (i.e., predicting outcome measures), advanced data analytic techniques such as neural networks or machine learning have been proposed. Indeed, a case study reported a high prediction accuracy of the performance of an elite swimmer using a neural network model using training monitoring data (Edelmann-Nusser, Hohmann, & Henneberg, 2002). However, since these modelling techniques require large data sets over extended periods to 'train' the predictive accuracy its practical usefulness may be limited. Furthermore, due to the 'black box' functioning where the outcomes don't explicitly explain causal relationships of each input variable to the outcomes, some have urged caution in blindly adopting neural networks to model athlete training responses (Hellard et al., 2006). Therefore, while the use of advanced modelling techniques may provide an attractive analysis method for predicting performance outcomes from athlete monitoring data, the practical utility in the daily training environment are not yet established.

Conclusion and recommendations for practise

Athlete monitoring systems are now common place in high-performance sports. The goal of these systems is to monitor how individual athletes are responding to training. Due to the perceived benefits of these systems, many high-performance organisations make significant financial and human resource investments in this area. Whilst there is no criterion structure, an athlete monitoring system should be based on sound theoretical foundation, developed to resources available, and fit the culture of organisation. Fundamental measures that should be incorporated in these systems include quantifying training load, fitness, and fatigue. Following this, correct interpretation of the data requires that all changes be contextualised in relation to the actual training load completed by the athlete, whilst accounting for the magnitude of change required for practical importance in monitoring the training response. In practise, these measures may be used to inform coaches and sport science staff on all aspects of an athlete status (i.e., fitness, injury risk, readiness to perform, well-being etc.). When these systems are implemented effectively, important feedback can then be provided to athletes and coaches that assist in improving the training process and result in enhanced readiness to perform and reduced injury risk.

References

Aubry, A., Hausswirth, C., Louis, J., Coutts, A. J., Buchheit, M., & Le Meur, Y. (2015). The development of functional overreaching is associated with a faster heart rate recovery in endurance athletes. *PLoS One, 10*(10), e0139754.

Banister, E. W., Calvert, T. W., Savage, M. V., & Bach, T. (1975). A systems model of training for athletic performance. *Australian Journal of Sports Medicine and Exercise Science, 7*, 57–61.

Bellenger, C. R., Karavirta, L., Thomson, R. L., Robertson, E. Y., Davison, K., & Buckley, J. D. (2016). Contextualising parasympathetic hyperactivity in functionally overreached athletes with perceptions of training tolerance. *International Journal of Sports Physiology and Performance, 11*(5), 685–692.

Borg, G. (1998). *Borg's Perceived Exertion and Pain Scales*. Champaign, IL: Human Kinetics.

Bowling, A. (2005). Just one question: If one question works, why ask several? *Journal of Epidemiology and Community Health, 59*, 342–345.

Buchheit, M. (2014). Monitoring training status with HR measures: Do all roads lead to Rome? *Frontiers of Physiology, 5*(73). doi:10.3389/fphys.2014.00073

Buchheit, M. (2015). Sensitivity of monthly heart rate and psychometric measures for monitoring physical performance in highly trained young handball players. *International Journal of Sports Medicine, 36*(5), 351–356.

Buchheit, M., Rabbani, A., & Beigi, H. T. (2014). Predicting changes in high-intensity intermittent running performance with acute responses to short jump rope workouts in children. *Journal of Sports Science and Medicine*, *13*, 476–482.

Buchheit, M., Racinais, S., Bilsborough, J. C., Bourdon, P. C., Voss, S. C., Hocking, J., . . . Coutts, A. J. (2013). Monitoring fitness, fatigue and running performance during a preseason training camp in elite football players. *Journal of Science and Medicine in Sport*, *16*(6), 550–555.

Buchheit, M., Simpson, M. B., Al Haddad, H., Bourdon, P. C., & Mendez-Villanueva, A. (2011). Monitoring changes in physical performance with heart rate measures in young soccer players. *European Journal of Applied Physiology*, *112*, 711–723.

Coutts, A. J. (2014). In the age of technology, Occam's razor still applies. *International Journal of Sports Physiology and Performance*, *9*(5), 741.

Coutts, A. J., Rampinini, E., Marcora, S. M., Castagna, C., & Impellizzeri, F. M. (2009). Heart rate and blood lactate correlates of perceived exertion during small-sided soccer games. *Journal of Science and Medicine in Sport*, *12*(1), 79–84.

Coutts, A. J., Reaburn, P., Piva, T. J., & Rowsell, G. J. (2007). Monitoring for overreaching in rugby league players. *European Journal of Applied Physiology*, *99*(3), 313–324.

Crowcroft, S., Duffield, R., McCleave, E., Slattery, K., Wallace, L. K., & Coutts, A. J. (2015). Monitoring training to assess changes in fitness and fatigue: The effects of training in heat and hypoxia. *Scandinavian Journal of Medicine and Science in Sport*, *25*(Suppl. 1), 287–295.

Crowcroft, S., McCleave, E., Slattery, K., & Coutts, A. J. (2017). Assessing the measurement sensitivity and diagnostic characteristics of athlete monitoring tools in national swimmers. *International Journal of Sports Physiology and Performance*, *12*(Suppl 2), S2295–S2100.

Edelmann-Nusser, J., Hohmann, A., & Henneberg, B. (2002). Modeling and prediction of competitive performance in swimming upon neural networks. *European Journal of Sport Science*, *2*(2), 1–10.

Fawcett, T. (2006). An introduction to ROC analysis. *Pattern Recognition Letters*, *27*(8), 861–874.

Foster, C., Daines, E., Hector, L., Snyder, A. C., & Welsh, R. (1996). Athletic performance in relation to training load. *Wisconsin Medical Journal*, *95*, 370–374.

Foster, C., Florhaug, J. A., Franklin, J., Gottschall, L., Hrovatin, L. A., Parker, S., . . . Dodge, C. (2001). A new approach to monitoring exercise training. *Journal of Strength and Conditioning Research*, *15*(1), 109–115.

Gabbett, T. J. (2016). The training-injury prevention paradox: Should athletes be training smarter and harder? *British Journal of Sports Medicine*, *50*(5), 273–280.

Gastin, P. B., McLean, O., Spittle, M., & Breed, R. V. (2013). Quantification of tackling demands in professional Australian football using integrated wearable athlete tracking technology. *Journal of Science and Medicine in Sport*, *16*(6), 589–593.

Gastin, P. B., Meyer, D., & Robinson, D. (2013). Perceptions of wellness to monitor adaptive responses to training and competition in elite Australian football. *Journal of Strength and Conditioning Research*, *27*(9), 2518–2526.

Halson, S. L., Bridge, M. W., Meeusen, R., Busschaert, B., Gleeson, M., Jones, D. A., & Jeukendrup, A. E. (2002). Time course of performance changes and fatigue markers during intensified training in cyclists. *Journal of Applied Physiology*, *93*(3), 947–956.

Hellard, P., Avalos, M., Lacoste, L., Barale, F., Chatard, J. C., & Millet, G. P. (2006). Assessing the limitations of the Banister model in monitoring training. *Journal of Sports Sciences*, *24*(5), 509–520.

Hug, B., Heyer, L., Naef, N., Buchheit, M., Wehrlin, J. P., & Millet, G. P. (2014). Tapering for marathon and cardiac autonomic function. *International Journal of Sports Medicine*, *35*(8), 676–683.

Hulin, B. T., Gabbett, T. J., Johnston, R. D., & Jenkins, D. G. (2017). Wearable microtechnology can accurately identify collision events during professional rugby league match-play. *Journal of Science and Medicine in Sport, 20,* 638–642.

Impellizzeri, F. M., Mognoni, P., Sassi, A., & Rampinini, E. (2005). Validity of a submaximal running test to evaluate aerobic fitness changes in soccer players. In T. Reilly, J. Cabri, & D. Araujo (Eds.), *Science and football V* (pp. 105–111). London, UK: Routledge.

Impellizzeri, F. M., Rampinini, E., & Marcora, S. M. (2005). Physiological assessment of aerobic training in soccer. *Journal of Sports Sciences, 23*(6), 583–592.

Keaney, E., Withers, S., Parker-Simmons, S., Gastin, P., & Netto, K. J. (2016). The training load of aerial skiing. *International Journal of Performance Analysis in Sport, 16,* 726–736.

Kellmann, M., & Kallus, K. W. (2016). The Recovery-Stress Questionnaire for Athletes. In K. W. Kallus & M. Kellmann (Eds.), *The Recovery-Stress Questionnaires: User manual* (pp. 86–131). Frankfurt am Main: Pearson Assessment.

Kellmann, M., Kölling, S., & Hitzschke, B. (2016). *Das Akutmaß und die Kurzskala zur Erfassung von Erholung und Beanspruchung im Sport – Manual* [The Acute Measure and the Short Scale of Recovery and Stress for Sports – Manual]. Hellenthal: Sportverlag Strauß.

Kenttä, G., & Hassmén, P. (1998). Overtraining and recovery: A conceptual model. *Sports Medicine, 26*(1), 1–17.

Lamberts, R. P., Swart, J., Noakes, T. D., & Lambert, M. I. (2010). A novel submaximal cycle test to monitor fatigue and predict cycling performance. *British Journal of Sports Medicine, 45,* 797–804.

Malone, J. J., Lovell, R., Varley, M. C., & Coutts, A. J. (2017). Unpacking the black box: Applications and considerations for using GPS devices in sport. *International Journal of Sports Physiology and Performance, 12*(Suppl 2), S218–S226.

Matveyev, L. (1981). *Fundamentals of sports training.* Moscow, Russia: Progress Publishers.

McLean, B. D., Coutts, A. J., Kelly, V., McGuigan, M. R., & Cormack, S. J. (2010). Neuromuscular, endocrine, and perceptual fatigue responses during different length between-match microcycles in professional rugby league players. *International Journal of Sports Physiology and Performance, 5*(3), 367–383.

McNair, D. M., Lorr, M., & Droppleman, L. F. (1971). *EITS Profile for Mood States.* San Diego: Educational and Industrial Testing Service.

Murray, N. B., Gabbett, T. J., Townshend, A. D., & Blanch, P. (2017). Calculating acute:chronic workload ratios using exponentially weighted moving averages provides a more sensitive indicator of injury likelihood than rolling averages. *British Journal of Sports Medicine, 51,* 749–754.

Robertson, S., Bartlett, J. D., & Gastin, P. B. (2017). Red, amber or green? Athlete monitoring in team sport: The need for decision support systems. *International Journal of Sports Physiology and Performance, 12*(Suppl. 2), S2273–S2279.

Rushall, B. S. (1990). A tool for measuring stress tolerance in elite athletes. *Journal of Applied Sport Psychology, 2*(1), 51–66.

Saw, A. E., Kellmann, M., Main, L. C., & Gastin, P. B. (2017). Athlete self-report measures in research and practice: Recommendations for the discerning reader and fastidious practitioner. *International Journal of Sports Physiology and Performance, 12*(Suppl 2), S2127–S2135.

Saw, A. E., Main, L. C., & Gastin, P. B. (2016). Monitoring the athlete training response: Subjective self-reported measures trump commonly used objective measures: A systematic review. *British Journal of Sports Medicine, 50*(5), 281–291.

Taylor, K., Chapman, D. W., Cronin, J. B., Newton, M. J., & Gill, N. (2012). Fatigue monitoring in high performance sport: A survey of current trends. *Journal of Australian Strength and Conditioning, 20*(1), 12–23.

Thorpe, R. T., Atkinson, G., Drust, B., & Gregson, W. (2017). Monitoring fatigue status in elite team sport athletes: Implications for practice. *International Journal of Sports Physiology and Performance, 12*(Suppl. 2), S2227–S2234.

Thorpe, R. T., Strudwick, A. J., Buchheit, M., Atkinson, G., Drust, B., & Gregson, W. (2015). Monitoring fatigue during the in-season competitive phase in elite soccer players. *International Journal of Sports Physiology and Performance, 10*(8), 958–964. doi:10.1123/ijspp.2015-0004

Urhausen, A., & Kindermann, W. (1992). Biochemical monitoring of training. *Clinical Journal of Sports Medicine, 2*(1), 52–61.

Viru, A., & Viru, M. (2000). Nature of training effects. In W. E. Garret & D. T. Kirkendall (Eds.), *Exercise and sport science* (pp. 67–95). Philadelphia: Lippincott Williams and Wilkins.

Wallace, L. K., Slattery, K. M., & Coutts, A. J. (2014). A comparison of methods for quantifying training load: Relationships between modelled and actual training responses. *European Journal of Applied Physiology, 114*(1), 11–20.

3
PERCEPTIONS AND PRACTISES OF RECOVERY MODALITIES IN ELITE TEAM ATHLETES

Ranel Venter and Roné Grobbelaar

Introduction

Most elite athletes (individual and team) participate in demanding training and competition schedules. Team players from many top clubs may have additional commitments such as inter-provincial league matches and tournaments, other cup matches, or represent their country in international competitions. Apart from these commitments, elite athletes are also exposed to pressure from personal relationships, media demands, sponsor needs, international travel, more public interest, e-communications, and social media (Botterill & Wilson, 2002; Keilani et al., 2016) compared to amateur players.

In recent years, it has been acknowledged by elite athletes (Kenttä & Hassmén, 2002) and coaches that emphasis should shift from a focus on predominantly physical training to include an understanding of the importance of the 'spaces between training' (McGee, 2000). Emphasising the importance of recovery during these 'spaces', Botterill and Wilson (2002, pp. 153–154) wrote:

> With education and awareness of rest and recovery strategies, they (athletes) will know when to push themselves and realize that it is appropriate to push as long as the necessary rest and recovery efforts are being made. Though athletes will continue to push themselves, they will also give themselves permission to take the necessary rest and recovery measures in order for optimal quality training and performance enhancement to occur. A self-aware athlete will not only know when to increase or implement the recovery techniques, but also know which recovery strategies will be most useful at that particular time in life and training. Clearly athletes – indeed, all people – need to

Venter, R., & Grobbelaar, R. (2018). Perceptions and practises of recovery modalities in elite team athletes. In M. Kellmann & J. Beckmann (Eds.), *Sport, Recovery, and Performance: Interdisciplinary Insights* (pp. 33–48). Abingdon: Routledge.

recover physically, mentally, and emotionally. At times even social and spiritual recovery needs to be facilitated.

Lambert and Borresen (2006) suggested that inadequate recovery is a training error impeding athletes from producing peak performances. During periods where the training or competition schedule is particularly congested, recovery time might be insufficient to restore homeostasis in athletes and as a result, may expose them to chronic fatigue, potential underperformance, and injury (Kellmann, 2010; Nédélec et al., 2012).

The athlete is described as a "psychosociophysiological entity" (Kenttä & Hassmén, 2002, p. 58) and recovery strategies should assist to re-establish psychological, physiological, emotional, social, and behavioural components in order to allow athletes to utilise these resources again (Kellmann & Kallus, 2001; Nédélec et al., 2012). As an athlete can experience fatigue in most of these aforementioned components, recovery strategies should address metabolic, neuronal, psychological, and environmental stressors in athletes (Calder, 2000; Nédélec et al., 2013). Although athletes do not always have the knowledge and experience, they should be informed and included in choosing appropriate modalities they are comfortable with, which address their recovery needs, and which are suitable for their specific situation (Kellmann, 2002; Moreno, Ramos-Castro, Rodas, Tarragó, & Capdevila, 2015). Considering that a recovery strategy is effective, Jeffreys (2005) stated that by including athletes in the decision making process for an appropriate integrated recovery programme, compliance to the recovery strategy will be facilitated.

Recovery modalities

Although a diversity of recovery modalities has been reported throughout sports literature, there is a lack of information about recovery modalities team athletes are using, as well as their perceptions of the importance of various recovery modalities. Recovery modalities frequently available to the athletes were grouped by Venter, Potgieter, and Barnard (2010) into four general categories, namely, natural strategies, physical and physiological strategies, psychosociological strategies, as well as complementary/alternative medicine strategies, although the supposed effects of various modalities could overlap between various systems.

Natural strategies

Natural strategies are seen as modalities that do not require any special devices, such as sleep, nutrition (Halson, 2008), active recovery (Bompa, 2009), stretching (Sands et al., 2013), and spending time in nature (Lee et al., 2011), seen as restorative environments (Bodin & Hartig, 2003; Scopelliti & Giuliani, 2004). Considering these requirements that can easily be obtained, it should be relatively easy for players from all levels of participation to apply natural strategies for recovery.

Although sleep can be regarded as a lifestyle factor, there is general consensus on the importance of sleep quality and nutrition for athletes' well-being, sport performance, recovery, and being effective in counteracting the fatigue mechanisms (Bird, 2013; Fullagar et al., 2015). In a study by Venter (2014) which involved 890 team athletes from field hockey, netball, rugby, and soccer, sleep as recovery modality was rated as important by all players from all sport codes, regardless of gender, type of sport or level of participation.

Sleep is a critical recovery modality for optimal performance. Hanton, Fletcher, and Coughlan (2005) reported that disturbed sleep patterns were mentioned as a major environmental stressor by elite team players. Environmental, logistical, and training-related factors, such as traveling or training/competing at night, can easily disrupt athletes' normal sleep-wake cycles (Fullagar et al., 2015). Athletes are often required to wake up early for morning training sessions and thereby lose sleep or disrupt their normal sleeping patterns and thus their quantity of sleep. High-intensity training and the associated muscle soreness and physical discomfort also disrupt sleep. Consequently, it is clear that both sleep quantity and quality can be easily disturbed by factors out of the athletes' control. When traveling, anxiety due to different surroundings and environments can be a major contributor to pre-sleep cognitive arousal (Carney & Waters, 2006), while a strange setting, noise and light (Venter et al., 2010), as well as extreme temperatures (Öhrström & Skånberg, 2004) can negatively affect the onset and quality of sleep.

A number of players reported that they experience problems waking-up in the morning, which could indicate sleep deprivation (Venter et al., 2010). Despite the frequent suggestions to athletes to incorporate daytime naps as part of their recovery period (Reilly & Edwards, 2007), Venter (2014) reported that daytime naps were not perceived as important in soccer, hockey, netball, or rugby players. Players often increase the amount of hours they sleep over weekends, possibly to address their lack of sleep from weekdays (Venter et al., 2010). However, going to bed early, taking daytime naps or sleeping more over weekend are not always possible due to other lifestyle commitments (Sargent, Halson, & Roach, 2014) and also is greatly affected by the type of sport and level of participation.

Athletes are often advised to gradually recover from high-intensity exercise through a cool-down period (Harris & Elbourn, 2002). An active cool-down is used after training by team players from different sports to varying degrees. Venter and colleagues (2010) reported that compared to hockey, rugby and netball players, soccer players used an active cool-down most frequent; whereas rugby players used it at least. From these teams, national-level players used an active cool-down after training significantly more than the provincial-level players. Even though stretching and slow jogging are most often used by these players, walking, rowing, and self-massage was also mentioned as being used as part of their active cool-down (Venter et al., 2010).

All participants included in the study by Van Wyk and Lambert (2009) reported stretching as a strategy that effectively aids recovery. The use of stretching was easily supported by biokineticists and fitness coaches; however, not always by physiotherapists and doctors (Van Wyk & Lambert, 2009). Reports from Van Wyk and Lambert (2009) showed that 74% of athletes used stretching after matches because it was rated as an effective strategy to relieve muscle soreness, in order, by physical therapists, fitness coaches, physiotherapists, and doctors.

Halson (2011) stated that the role of active recovery in reducing lactate concentrations after exercise may be important for athletes. Furthermore, active recovery is anecdotally reported to be one of the most common forms of recovery utilised by the majority of athletes. Considering the use of active cool-down after training compared to after a match, rugby players used an active cool-down more frequently after training than after matches, while field hockey, netball, and soccer players used an active cool-down more frequently after matches than after training (Venter et al., 2010). It might be that, due to the fact that rugby is a contact sport, players felt sorer after a match than after a training session. Players might therefore not regard an active cool-down as important or suitable to their specific post-match situation and needs (Venter et al., 2010). However, an active cool-down was only rated by netball and soccer players amongst the most important recovery modalities; whereas rugby players rated an active cool down as least important, compared to the other groups (Venter, 2014). Taken together, when given the choice, athletes would rather spend more energy and time on reducing inflammation and pain during the recovery period than spending more energy on active recovery (Bahnert, Norton, & Lock, 2013). This is an important note to coaches when they design recovery strategies.

Fluid replacement was rated as an important recovery strategy by all players from all team sport codes, regardless of gender, type of sport or level of participation (Venter, 2014). As could be expected, international level players regarded fluid replacement significantly more important than national-level players (Venter, 2014), possibly due to higher intensities during sometimes longer matches. Amongst the soccer, rugby, netball, and hockey players investigated by Venter and colleagues (2010), it was shown that 44% of the players from the total group never had a strategy for rehydration after training sessions, 15% of the players sometimes had a strategy, 22% regularly had a strategy, and 19% stated that they always had a rehydration strategy (Venter et al., 2010). It should be noted that the content or quality of the hydration strategies were not evaluated or reported on.

Although fluid replacement was rated amongst the most important recovery modalities by all groups, aspects relating to refuelling (e.g., eat shortly after training/match, snacks after training/match) did not follow the same pattern (Venter, 2014). Hockey, netball, rugby, and soccer are characterised by high-intensity intermittent exercises in most positions, which reduce muscle glycogen stores (Williams, 2007). Rugby specifically is a game with physical impact, causing muscle damage (Mashiko, Umeda, Nakaji, & Sugawara, 2004) and it could therefore be concluded that rugby players perceived the role of supplements as important in addressing their needs with regards to muscle repair. Moreover, Van Wyk and Lambert (2009) reported that rugby players are advised by medical support staff to use supplements for recovery purposes. Venter and colleagues (2010) reported that, out of the 890 team players, 48% of the players never had a strategy, 14% sometimes had a strategy,

20% regularly had a strategy, and 18% of the players always had a strategy for refuelling after training.

Comparable with rehydration, a difference existed between national- and club-level players in terms of a strategy for refuelling after training, with national-level players using refuelling more frequent than club-level players (Venter et al., 2010), possibly due to the difference in management structures and physical requirements during matches and training. International level players rated snacks (type of snacks not reported) after a match as significantly more important than club-level players (Venter, 2014). A possible reason for this is that athletes might experience bowel discomfort if they eat solid foods shortly after exercise (Holway & Spriet, 2011) and might therefore rather make use of liquid supplements (Venter, 2014). This is especially true for players competing at lower levels where they might be uninformed on proper refuelling strategies, as shown by national-level players who applied refuelling strategies more often, who might have more education with regards to the importance of post-exercise refuelling, as well as more exposure and access to post-exercise snacks (Venter, 2014). National-level players might also experience a greater need for rehydrating and refuelling due to the intensity of competition, as well as their managing staff possibly providing more support to players. It should be noted that Venter and colleagues (2010) and Venter (2014) reported on team players from one country, with results not necessarily generalisable to all sports and different cultural areas.

Physical and physiological strategies

It has been suggested that more emphasis is often placed on recovery modalities relating to physical and physiological recovery than on psychological, emotional, and social aspects of recovery (Kellmann, 2010). From literature it is evident that a vast number of modalities relating to physical and physiological recovery are being evaluated and suggested for use by athletes. These modalities include, amongst others, cryotherapy, ice packs and ice bags, cryocuffs, cooling jackets, cold water or ice water immersion, cold whirlpools, cryochambers, thermotherapy (warm water immersion and whirlpools, saunas), contrast water therapy (massage, foam rolling, compression therapies, neuromuscular electrical stimulation), whole-body vibration and hyperbaric oxygen therapy, and a combination of these modalities (Bieuzen, Bleakley, & Costello, 2013; Carrasco, Sañudo, De Hoyo, Pradas, & Da Silva, 2011; Hamid, Nawawi, Abdullah, & Latif, 2013; Hohenauer, Clarys, Baeyens, & Clijsen, 2016; Hohenauer, Taeymans, Baeyens, Clarys, & Clijsen, 2015; Leeder, Gissane, Van Someren, Gregson, & Howatson, 2012; Malone, Blake, & Caulfield, 2014; Pearcey et al., 2015; Selfe et al., 2014; Venter et al., 2010). From this, water immersion has received most attention in literature.

Cold water immersion (CWI) to prevent *delayed onset muscle soreness* (DOMS) (Cheung, Hume, & Maxwell, 2003) in the sporting environment remains one of the most widely used recovery modalities in clinical practise (Sellwood, Brukner, Williams, Nicol, & Hinman, 2007). Cheung and colleagues (2003) defined DOMS as a type I muscle strain injury that presents with tenderness of stiffness to palpation and movement. From reports investigated by Van Wyk and Lambert (2009), 34% of professionals rated CWI as an 'effective' and 36% rated it as 'extremely effective' recovery strategy. In the study by Venter and colleagues (2010), players indicated that they used cryotherapy to varying degrees after training. Rugby players used cryotherapy more after training sessions than players from hockey, netball, and soccer sport codes. Due to the physical nature of rugby that causes muscle damage, it could be concluded that rugby players perceived the role of an ice bath as important in addressing their needs in regard to muscle repair (Venter, 2014). Rugby players may, due to the fact that rugby is a professional sport in South Africa, have better access to facilities where they can use cryotherapy after training and matches, as well as being advised by medical staff to use ice baths (Van Wyk & Lambert, 2009).

Level of participation (club, national, international) often influences the use of cryotherapy on a regular basis. Nevertheless, cryotherapy is used more often after matches than after training sessions by club, national, and international players (Venter et al., 2010). Provincial- and national-level players used cryotherapy significantly more frequent than club-level players after training sessions and matches (Venter et al., 2010). Moreover, it is suggested that these players do not use cryotherapy on a regular basis, but rather only in specific instances, like at a training camp or at a tournament (Venter et al., 2010). Berdejo-del-Fresno and Laupheimer (2015) reported significant differences between recovery behaviours of elite futsal players when attending a national training camp compared to training at their own clubs.

When given the choice, a relatively high percentage of players make use of CWI because of the increased perception of recovery (Bahnert et al., 2013). A recent review showed that CWI can reduce the subjective assessment of pain by 16% (Leeder et al., 2012). Athletes often show improved performance when they believe they received a beneficial recovery strategy (Stanley, Buchheit, & Peake, 2012). As athletes believe and expect improvement in DOMS following CWI, the subjective measurement of muscle soreness is improved (Leeder et al., 2012) and can be linked to improved perceptions of relaxation by athletes (Stanley et al., 2012). The use of CWI is, however, not always practical due to unavailability at competition and training venues, although portable bins have become more available to athletes recently. Logistically it requires constant monitoring of temperature (Hohenauer et al., 2016).

Athletes believe that CWI is a beneficial recovery strategy due to enhanced feeling of recovery, reduced perception of fatigue and improved subjective assessment of muscle soreness. Therefore, athletes generally expect improved recovery from exercise after CWI (Broatch, Petersen, & Bishop, 2014) compared to active and passive recovery, as well as with the use of compression garments and supplementation (Halson, 2011). At an elite level, coaches, sport scientists and medical staff decide on the most applicable recovering modality after training, depending on the phase or specific microcycle in the training year (Elias, Wyckelsma, Varley, McKenna, & Aughey, 2013).

It is possible that heightened subjective interpretation of discomfort during a physical activity, together with the expectation of having muscle soreness after training and the significant pain experienced during immersion, may improve or worsen subjective assessments of recovery (Sellwood et al., 2007), especially between genders (Venter, 2014). Considering that extreme cryotherapy can induce a significant painful stimulus and that both physiological and psychological factors influences the experience of pain, the effectiveness thereof may differ between genders (Sellwood et al., 2007).

The study done by Venter and colleagues (2010) on rugby, soccer, hockey, and netball players showed that the majority (68%) of players never use contrast water therapy (CWT) after training and 65% indicated that they never use it after matches, showing that it is not as frequently used as CWI in this specific sample. A study comparing different recovery modalities showed that CWT lowered subjective measures of muscle soreness significantly more than passive recovery; however, no differences were found when CWT was compared to CWI, active recovery, stretching or the use of compression garments (Bieuzen et al., 2013). Conflicting results showed that an athlete's beliefs in the benefits of CWI may stem from the stimulus itself. Athletes believe and expect that the discomfort associated with CWI makes it a more beneficial recovery strategy, as shown by improved mental and physical readiness for exercise, decreased fatigue, lower pain levels (Broatch et al., 2014), and feeling more awake (Bieuzen et al., 2013) which collectively relates to enhanced recovery.

A study investigating the placebo effect of water immersion showed that athletes could be led to believe that a placebo was effective in promoting recovery from high-intensity exercise. The researchers concluded that acute benefits of cold water immersion could be partly related to the placebo effect (Broatch et al., 2014). Consequently, athletes that trust their coaching team can be deceived into utilizing recovery methods that have more psychological than physiological benefits. These findings highlight that water therapy for recovery may have a greater psychological than physiological impact. When athletes are, however, given the choice, a high percentage frequently uses other physical recovery strategies such as compression garments and massages (Bahnert et al., 2013), which can have both physiological and psychological benefits.

Hockey, netball, and soccer players mentioned that massage was used after matches, while rugby players indicated that massage was used more on non-training days (Venter et al., 2010). Massage has shown to enhance recovery through psychological mechanisms that include decreased pain sensation and fatigue (Broatch et al., 2014). National-level players used massage more than club- and provincial-level players after training sessions and on non-training days. However, massage was not a popular mode of recovery (Venter et al., 2010).

Psychosociological recovery modalities

Psychological techniques are suggested to counteract distress, increase motivation, decrease anxiety, enhance the ability to cope with stressors, improve a sense of well-being and to reduce training and/or life stress, to ultimately improve recovery and have a positive influence on performance outcomes (Fuller & Paccagnella, 2004; Keilani et al., 2016). Recently, Pelka and colleagues (2017) showed that systematic breathing led to better sprint performances during a recovery session of 25 minutes, compared to yoga and progressive muscle relaxation.

Considering that psychological and mental stress can impact physiological responses, athletes' belief in the effectiveness of a recovery strategy can influence the subsequent responses to the strategy used and also related to the performance (Cook & Beaven, 2013). Psychological strategies that are often used by athletes include communication to significant others, debriefing, progressive muscle relaxation, imagery, meditation, autogenic training, prayer, music and sound, breathing exercises, mood lifting activities, and restricted environment stimulation therapy (flotation) (Eliakim, Bodner, Meckel, Nemet, & Eliakim, 2013; Solberg et al., 2000).

In a recent study by Keilani and colleagues (2016), 96% ($N = 183$) of the athletes reported that they have knowledge about at least one mental technique (e.g., imagery, PMR, breathing exercises). Of these athletes, 67% are not using such a technique during training; whereas, 88% use a mental technique before competition. This shows that despite having knowledge of a mental technique, it is not used as a popular recovery strategy. This is further shown by only 7% of these athletes reporting the use of a mental technique for recovery purposes. Reasons for these results are possibly due to insufficient access to sport psychologists, lack of awareness of psychological issues of athletes, uninformed coaching staff, or no referral of athletes to sport psychologists (Keilani et al., 2016).

Communication with significant others include discussions with teammates and coaches or socializing with friends and family. The use of communication as a possible debriefing recovery strategy (Hogg, 2002) has been rated as more important to women than to men (Venter, 2014), possibly because women are in general more willing to seek help from, reach out to and interact with more individuals for social support, including coaches compared to men (Yang et al., 2010). Furthermore, rugby players from all levels of play rated communication as the least important recovery technique (Venter, 2014). It seems that athletes generally differ in their responses to communication as socialising, which is also a form of communication, was rated as an important recovery strategy by all players from all sport codes, regardless of gender, type of sport or level of participation (Venter, 2014).

Yang and colleagues (2010) determined that 93% ($N = 133$) of the athletes in their study reported that they relied on their friends for social support. Effective social support can have a beneficial influence on performance (Rees & Freeman, 2010), protect players from the negative impact of stressors (Rees & Hardy, 2000) and decrease stress (Barefield & McCallister, 1997). Social networks can help the player deal with problems, disappointments, joys, and stresses of life (Quinn & Fallon, 1999). Friends and teammates could provide listening and emotional support; challenge evaluation of attitudes, values, and feelings; express appreciation; and motivate the player to greater excitement and involvement (Barefield & McCallister, 1997).

The use of prayer and other religious-spiritual practises is one of the regularly used psychological techniques before competition (Keilani et al., 2016). Also, Venter and colleagues (2010) reported that prayer was used by 72% ($N = 597$) of the players for recovery purposes. Prayer activity seems to be present throughout various levels of sport participation (Todd & Brown, 2003). The therapeutic potential of spirituality is acknowledged increasingly as it can be seen as a moderator of stress. Ridnour and Hammermeister (2008) indicated that spiritual well-being may be a construct that is useful in developing an enhanced coping-aptitude necessary for excellence in sport. The use of prayer in coping with the uncertainties in sport is prevalent among athletes and more so for athletes playing elite sport (Venter et al., 2010). Jones (2003) mentioned that many people reported using prayer as a stress management technique. This is supported by the study by Plaatjie (2006) where soccer players indicated that they used prayer as a post-match coping strategy.

Players used music for recovery purposes more after matches than after training sessions. The most popular types of music were rock and gospel music; however, other types of music included house music, R&B, hip-hop, kwaito, dance beats, calm music, chants and Gregorian music, love songs, panpipes, soul, and traditional African music (Venter et al., 2010). This wide range of music types suggests that the choice is related to personal preference. Considering that music preferences are diverse, listening to music needs to be a pleasant and meaningful experience to have a positive effect on recovery. The athlete's preferences must therefore be taken into account when music is used for recovery purposes (Venter et al., 2010).

Complementary/alternative medicine strategies

Cohen, Penman, Pirotta, and Da Costa (2005) as well as Johnson and Blanchard (2006) mentioned the substantial increase in the popularity of alternative medicine for a variety of illnesses and symptoms, as well as for preventative health practises and general self-care. MacLennan, Myers, and Taylor (2006) identified an increase in complementary and alternative medicine strategies (CAM) used in Australia, while Johnson and Blanchard (2006) found that 58% of the graduates in their survey used at least one type of CAM during the previous 12 months. White (1998) stated that many athletes use CAM when conventional medicine, according to them, fails to relieve their musculoskeletal symptoms. Ahmedov (2010) mentioned that acupuncture is one of the most popular alternative methods applied in Western medical practise. In the study by Venter and colleagues (2010), athletes indicated that they seldom used complementary and alternative therapies for recovery purposes. Rugby players used acupuncture more than netball and soccer players, possibly to address their contact-related bodily pain and discomfort. As expected, national-level players used acupuncture significantly more than club- and provincial-level players (Venter et al., 2010).

Overall reasons why recovery modalities are/are not used

There might be various reasons why athletes do not apply recovery modalities regularly. Firstly, if athletes did not have more than one training session per day, they might not regard recovery as important (Venter et al., 2010). Secondly, it might be that players did not know what to do if they wanted to use a specific modality. Thirdly, the lack of application of recovery modalities could be money-related, as money has to be paid for specific services (e.g., massage) and players might not want to pay for services related to their recovery. Simjanovic, Hooper, Leveritt, Kellmann, and Rynne (2009) mentioned time and cost as key considerations of factors influencing the use of different recovery modalities.

Regardless of these reasons, athletes that utilise recovery strategies after training are in the belief that it will assist successful performance, despite the lack of scientific evidence for the particular recovery modality (Hohenauer et al., 2016; Sellwood et al., 2007). Athletes often develop their own recovery strategies after training or competition over time (Sellwood et al., 2007). Sellwood and colleagues (2007) suggested that the perceived psychological benefit of a familiar recovery modality may enhance performance even to a greater extent than the actual physiological benefit of the modality itself. Bérdi, Köteles, Hevesi, Bárdos, and Szabo (2014) reported that 92% of their participants who had past placebo experiences in recovery modalities, believed placebos could affect their performance. From this it is thought that athletes' expectancy of the recovery intervention is created from learned information in a social context and not by scientific evidence. The knowledge about specific interventions trigger neurological processes and subjectively utilise neurobiological mechanisms that points the brain and body in the expected direction (Bérdi et al., 2014).

Athletes are often exposed to recovery strategies by their coaching and conditioning staff (Bahnert et al., 2013). It has recently been reported that athletes' experiences of recovery techniques stem from the information and feedback given to them about the particular intervention (Bérdi et al., 2014). Considering that 97% ($N = 77$) of respondents in the study by Bérdi and colleagues (2014) was under the impression that a placebo effect could positively influence their performance (even though 56% of the respondents did not understand the meaning or relevance of the placebo effect), the crucial role of the coaching team in shaping beliefs and expectations about performance are highlighted.

Despite the reasons for athletes not to use recovery techniques, the coaching staff also play an important role in recovery strategies. Van Wyk and Lambert (2009) reported that the recovery modalities most often used by coaches were low-intensity activity, stretching, nutrition, massage, CWT, CWI, sleep, and rest. Van Wyk and Lambert (2009) indicated that medical support staff often give advice to rugby players with regards to recovery modalities. However, according to Kellmann (2010), despite coaches recognising that recovery is crucial, they often have limited knowledge of what recovery modalities are available. Moreover, coaches often use trial-and-error methods or mimic strategies used by other higher level or more successful athletes (Bahnert et al., 2013). Due to the variability in evidence regarding recovery strategies, coaching staff do not have ample evidence-based approaches to manage the recovery of athletes. Therefore, many coaches use a 'something is better than nothing' approach (Van Wyk & Lambert, 2009).

By analysing the relationship between individual recovery behaviours, perception of recovery, and performance, Moreno and colleagues (2015) showed that each player had a distinct recovery strategy from the others. The most probable reason for this is that the athletes are responsible of carrying out their recovery regime themselves, for example with regards to nutrition, hydration, and rest. Contrary to this, other recovery techniques are performed at the training facility under the direction of the coaching staff, for example massage, icing, hot baths, sauna, muscle relaxation, and stretching (Moreno et al., 2015). Many athletes, even in team sports, differ in their preferred combination of recovery strategies after training or competition. These different recovery combinations are determined by personal preference and perceived benefit. Moreover, the coaching team often cannot confidently give specific guidance for optimal recovery (Bahnert et al., 2013). Bérdi and colleagues (2014) reported that most athletes (84%) easily accept a strategy from their coach and are more concerned with the legitimacy or effectiveness of the strategy than its specific (physiological or psychological) mode of action, even though both should be regarded as important. Only 10% of the respondents (who were elite athletes) would perform such a new strategy without questioning its effects or legitimacy (Bérdi et al., 2014). This shows that the remaining 90% were questioning the use of the recovery modality and that coach-athlete communication is important in the process of choosing a recovery strategy. Despite this, 67% of elite athletes questioned by Bérdi and colleagues (2014) would not have a problem in being deceived by their coach regarding the legitimacy of a recovery modality, as long as the strategy exerted a positive effect and it assists in their sporting performance. Despite these ratings, health care professionals should integrate psychological and social factors in the recovery strategy by having effective communication with athletes regarding their behaviour, beliefs, rest schedules, and their experience of stress, fatigue, and pain (Van Wilgen & Verhagen, 2012). Furthermore, sport psychologists could assist coaches with effective debriefing procedures after matches for mental and emotional recovery as well as facilitating team cohesion to address aspects of psychosocial recovery (Venter, 2014).

Conclusion and recommendations for practise

Team players of different levels perceive a variety of recovery modalities as important. Furthermore, when given the choice, it seems that athletes chose three components of the RICE principle (rest, ice, compression, elevation) for recovery. That is rest by not performing active recovery; ice by utilizing CWI; and compression by wearing compression garments (Bahnert et al., 2013). Different situations have different demands, and coaches and players should be educated with regards to protocols for physical, as well as psychosocial recovery modalities, especially as it has been shown that the psychological perception of recovery is strongly associated with performance (Cook & Beaven, 2013).

Many reviews illustrate that recovery strategies vary between different types of sports, position played, age groups, genders, participation levels, and individual preference (Cook & Beaven, 2013). For example, athletes competing at lower levels have different physiological and psychological responses to exercise than elite athletes in terms of coping with aspects of fatigue and bodily discomfort and therefore, apart from the availability of recovery strategies, possibly have different views and usage thereof (Cook & Beaven, 2013). Even within a team setting, the use of recovery modalities should be individualised. It may be unrealistic for athletes to only use a single recovery strategy after exercise. Therefore, athletes should use a combination of recovery modalities (Bieuzen et al., 2013). Strategies that cannot be used while travelling should be avoided as this may induce psychological difficulties to participating individuals when they cannot use a recovery strategy they became accustomed to and reliant on (Van Wyk & Lambert, 2009).

It seems that recovery plans are dependent on individual training schedules, available facilities and equipment, and athlete preferences. Also, the success of a recovery strategy is individualised to the perceived benefits of the modality (Sellwood et al., 2007). On an elite level, the coaching team and team managers play a major role in the decision making process of recovery modalities (Venter, 2014). When recovery interventions are implemented, both scientific evidence as well as the beliefs of the users thereof should be considered. Moreover, behavioural and cognitive aspects of all involved parties, i.e., coaches, athletes, researchers, policy makers, and healthcare professionals, should be considered when designing recovery interventions (Van Wilgen & Verhagen, 2012). The ideal recovery strategy would entail an approach that elicits a desirable perception of recovery while also addressing the appropriate physiological mechanisms necessary to effectively recover from training (Cook & Beaven, 2013).

References

Ahmedov, S. (2010). Ergogenic effect of acupuncture in sport and exercise: A brief review. *Journal of Strength & Conditioning Research, 24*(5), 1421–1427.

Bahnert, A., Norton, K., & Lock, P. (2013). Association between post-game recovery protocols, physical and perceived recovery, and performance in elite Australian Football League players. *Journal of Science and Medicine in Sport, 16*(2), 151–156.

Barefield, S., & McCallister, S. (1997). Social support in the athletic training room: Athletes' expectations of staff and student athletic trainers. *Journal of Athletic Training, 32*(4), 333–338.

Berdejo-del-Fresno, D., Moore, R., & Laupheimer, M.W. (2015). VO$_2$max changes in English futsal players after a 6-week period of specific small-sided games training. *American Journal of Sports Science and Medicine, 3*(2), 28–34.

Bérdi, M., Köteles, F., Hevesi, K., Bárdos, G., & Szabo, A. (2014). Elite athletes' attitudes towards the use of placebo-induced performance enhancement in sports. *European Journal of Sport Science, 15*(4), 315–312.

Bieuzen, F., Bleakley, C., & Costello, J. (2013). Contrast water therapy and exercise induced muscle damage: A systematic review and meta-analysis. *PLoS One, 8*(4), e62356.

Bird, S. (2013). Sleep, recovery, and athletic performance: A brief review and recommendations. *Strength & Conditioning Journal, 35*(5), 43–47.

Bodin, M., & Hartig, T. (2003). Does the outdoor environment matter for psychological restoration gained through running? *Psychology of Sport and Exercise, 4*(2), 141–153.

Bompa, T. O. (2009). *Periodization: Theory and methodology of training* (5th ed.). Champaign, IL: Human Kinetics.

Botterill, C., & Wilson, C. (2002). Overtraining: Emotional and interdisciplinary dimensions. In M. Kellmann (Ed.), *Enhancing recovery: Preventing underperformance in athletes* (pp. 143–159). Champaign, IL: Human Kinetics.

Broatch, J. R., Petersen, A., & Bishop, D. J. (2014). Postexercise cold water immersion benefits are not greater than the placebo effect. *Medicine and Science in Sports and Exercise, 46*(11), 2139–2147.

Calder, A. (2000). *Advanced coaching study pack: Recovery training*. Belconnen, ACT: Australian Sports Commission.

Carney, C. E., & Waters, W. F. (2006). Effects of a structured problem-solving procedure on presleep cognitive arousal in college students with insomnia. *Behavioral Sleep Medicine, 4*(19), 13–28.

Carrasco, L., Sañudo, B., De Hoyo, M., Pradas, M., & Da Silva, M. (2011). Effectiveness of low-frequency vibration recovery method on blood lactate removal, muscle contractile properties and on time to exhaustion during cycling at VO_2max power output. *European Journal of Applied Physiology, 111*(9), 2271–2279.

Cheung, K., Hume, P. A., & Maxwell, L. (2003). Delayed onset muscle soreness: Treatment strategies and performance factors. *Sports Medicine, 33*, 145–164.

Cohen, M. M., Penman, S., Pirotta, M., & Da Costa, C. (2005). The integration of complementary therapies in Australian general practice: Results of a national survey. *Journal of Alternative and Complementary Medicine, 11*(6), 995–1004.

Cook, C. J., & Beaven, C. M. (2013). Individual perception of recovery is related to subsequent sprint performance. *British Journal of Sports Medicine, 47*(11), 705–709.

Eliakim, M., Bodner, E., Meckel, Y., Nemet, D., & Eliakim, A. (2013). Effect of rhythm on the recovery from intense exercise. *Journal of Strength & Conditioning Research, 27*(4), 1019–1024.

Elias, G. P., Wyckelsma, V. L., Varley, M. C., McKenna, M. J., & Aughey, R. J. (2013). Effectiveness of water immersion on post-match recovery in elite professional footballers. *International Journal of Sports Physiology and Performance, 8*, 243–253.

Fullagar, H., Skorski, S., Duffield, R., Hammes, D., Coutts, A., & Meyer, T. (2015). Sleep and athletic performance: The effects of sleep loss on exercise performance, and physiological and cognitive responses to exercise. *Sports Medicine, 45*(2), 161–186.

Fuller, K., & Paccagnella, M. (2004). Revitalising body and soul–physiological and psychological strategies for recovery. *Sports Coach, 27*(3), 14–16.

Halson, S. L. (2008). Nutrition, sleep and recovery. *European Journal of Sport Science, 8*(2), 119–126.

Halson, S. L. (2011). Does the time frame between exercise influence the effectiveness of hydrotherapy for recovery? Less than 60 minutes between bouts of exercise. *International Journal of Sports Physiology and Performance, 6*(2), 147–159.

Hamid, N., Nawawi, M., Abdullah, N., & Latif, R. (2013). Efficacy of cubed-ice and wetted-ice as a cryotherapeutic agent in the Malaysian climate. *Procedia – Social and Behavioral Sciences*, *105*(3), 211–219.

Hanton, S., Fletcher, D., & Coughlan, G. (2005). Stress in elite sport performers: A comparative study of competitive and organizational stressors. *Journal of Sports Sciences*, *23*(10), 1129–1141.

Harris, J., & Elbourn, J. (2002). Cooling down theory. *Sports Coach*, *25*(3), 23–25.

Hogg, J. M. (2002). Debriefing: A means to increasing recovery and subsequent performance. In M. Kellmann (Ed.), *Enhancing recovery: Preventing underperformance in athletes* (pp. 181–198). Champaign, IL: Human Kinetics.

Hohenauer, E., Clarys, P., Baeyens, J.-P., & Clijsen, R. (2016). The effect of local cryotherapy on subjective and objective characteristics following an exhaustive jump protocol. *Open Access Journal of Sports Medicine*, *7*, 89–97.

Hohenauer, E., Taeymans, J., Baeyens, J.-P., Clarys, P., & Clijsen, R. (2015). The effect of post-exercise cryotherapy on recovery characteristics: A systematic review and meta-analysis. *PLoS One*, *10*(9), e0139028.

Holway, F. E., & Spriet, L. L. (2011). Sport-specific nutrition: Practical strategies for team sports. *Journal of Sport Sciences*, *29*(1), S115–S125.

Jeffreys, I. (2005). A multidimensional approach to enhancing recovery. *Strength and Conditioning Journal*, *27*(5), 78–85.

Johnson, S. K., & Blanchard, A. (2006). Alternative medicine and herbal use among university students. *Journal of the American College of Health*, *55*(3), 163–169.

Jones, K. (2003). *Health and human behavior*. Melbourne, VIC: Oxford University Press.

Keilani, M., Hasenöhrl, T., Gartner, I., Krall, C., Fürnhammer, J., Cenik, F., & Crevenna, R. (2016). Use of mental techniques for competition and recovery in professional athletes. *Wiener Klinische Wochenschrift*, *128*(9–10), 315–319.

Kellmann, M. (2002). Underrecovery and overtraining: Different concepts – similar impact? In M. Kellmann (Ed.), *Enhancing recovery: Preventing underperformance in athletes* (pp. 3–24). Champaign, IL: Human Kinetics.

Kellmann, M. (2010). Preventing overtraining in athletes in high-intensity sports and stress/recovery monitoring. *Scandinavian Journal of Medicine and Science in Sports*, *20*(Suppl 2), 95–102.

Kellmann, M., & Kallus, K. W. (2001). *Recovery-Stress Questionnaire for Athletes: User manual*. Champaign, IL: Human Kinetics.

Kenttä, G., & Hassmén, P. (2002). Underrecovery and overtraining: A conceptual model. In M. Kellmann (Ed.), *Enhancing recovery: Preventing underperformance in athletes* (pp. 57–77). Champaign, IL: Human Kinetics.

Lambert, M., & Borresen, J. (2006). A theoretical basis of monitoring fatigue: A practical approach for coaches. *International Journal of Sports Science and Coaching*, *1*(4), 371–388.

Lee, J., Park, B.-J., Tsunetsugu, Y., Ohira, T., Kagawa, T., & Miyazaki, Y. (2011). Effect of forest bathing on physiological and psychological responses in young Japanese male subjects. *Public Health*, *125*, 93–100.

Leeder, J., Gissane, C., Van Someren, K., Gregson, W., & Howatson, G. (2012). Cold water immersion and recovery from strenuous exercise: A meta-analysis. *British Journal of Sports Medicine*, *46*(4), 233–240.

MacLennan, A. H., Myers, S. P., & Taylor, A. W. (2006). The continuing use of complementary and alternative medicine in South Australia: Costs and beliefs in 2004. *Medical Journal of Australia*, *184*(1), 27–32.

Malone, J., Blake, C., & Caulfield, B. (2014). Neuromuscular electrical stimulation during recovery from exercise: A systematic review. *Journal of Strength & Conditioning Research*, *28*(9), 2478–2506.

Mashiko, T., Umeda, T., Nakaji, S., & Sugawara, K. (2004). Position related analysis of the appearance of and relationship between post-match physical and mental fatigue in university rugby football players. *British Journal of Sports Medicine, 38*, 617–621.

McGee, B. (2000). *Magical running*. Boulder, CO: Bobbysez Publishing.

Moreno, J., Ramos-Castro, J., Rodas, G., Tarragó, J., & Capdevila, L. (2015, April). Individual recovery profiles in basketball players. *The Spanish Journal of Psychology, 18*, E24. doi10.1017/sjp.2015.23

Nédélec, M., McCall, A., Carling, C., Legall, F., Berthoin, S., & Dupont, G. (2012). Recovery in soccer: Part I – post-match fatigue and time course of recovery. *Sports Medicine, 42*(12), 997–1015.

Nédélec, M., McCall, A., Carling, C., Legall, F., Berthoin, S., & Dupont, G. (2013). Recovery in soccer: Part II – recovery Strategies. *Sports Medicine, 43*(1), 9–22.

Öhrström, E., & Skånberg, A. (2004). Sleep disturbances from road traffic and ventilation noise laboratory and field experiments. *Journal of Sound and Vibration, 271*(1–2), 279–296.

Pearcey, G., Bradbury-Squires, D., Kawamoto, J.-E., Drinkwater, E., Behm, D., & Button, D. (2015). Foam rolling for Delayed-Onset Muscle Soreness and recovery of dynamic performance measures. *Journal of Athletic Training, 50*(1), 5–13.

Pelka, M., Kölling, S., Ferrauti, A., Meyer, T., Pfeiffer, M., & Kellmann, M. (2017). Acute effects of psychological relaxation techniques between two physical tasks. *Journal of Sports Sciences, 35*(3), 216–223.

Plaatjie, M. R. (2006). *A comparison of coping strategies of ethnically diverse football players*. Unpublished PhD dissertation, Stellenbosch University, Stellenbosch.

Quinn, A. M., & Fallon, B. J. (1999). The changes in psychological characteristics and reactions of elite athletes from injury onset until full recovery. *Journal of Applied Sport Psychology, 11*, 210–229.

Rees, T., & Freeman, P. (2010). The effect of experimentally provided social support on golf-putting performance. *The Sport Psychologist, 18*, 333–348.

Rees, T., & Hardy, L. (2000). An examination of the social support experiences of high-level sports performers. *The Sport Psychologist, 14*, 327–347.

Reilly, T., & Edwards, B. (2007). Altered sleep – wake cycles and physical performance in athletes. *Physiology & Behavior, 90*(2–3), 274–284.

Ridnour, H., & Hammermeister, J. (2008). Spiritual well-being and its influence on athletic coping profiles. *Journal of Sport Behavior, 31*(1), 81–92.

Sands, W., McNeal, J., Murray, S., Ramsey, M., Sato, K., Mizuguchi, S., & Stone, M. (2013). Stretching and its effects on recovery: A review. *Strength & Conditioning Journal, 35*(5), 30–36.

Sargent, C., Halson, S. L., & Roach, G. D. (2014). Sleep or swim? Early-morning training severely restricts the amount of sleep obtained by elite swimmers. *European Journal of Sport Science, 14*(Suppl. 1), S310–S315.

Scopelliti, M., & Giuliani, M. V. (2004). Choosing restorative environments across the lifespan: A matter of place experience. *Psychology, 24*(4), 423–437.

Selfe, J., Alexander, J., Costello, J., May, K., Garratt, N., Atkins, S., . . . Richards, J. (2014). The effect of three different (-135°C) whole body cryotherapy exposure durations on elite Rugby League players. *PLoS One, 9*(1), e86420.

Sellwood, K. L., Brukner, P., Williams, D., Nicol, A., & Hinman, R. (2007). Ice-water immersion and delayed-onset muscle soreness: A randomized controlled trial. *British Journal of Sports Medicine, 41*, 392–397.

Simjanovic, M., Hooper, S., Leveritt, M., Kellmann, M., & Rynne, S. (2009). The use and perceived effectiveness of recovery modalities and monitoring techniques in elite sport [Abstract]. *Journal of Science and Medicine in Sport, 12*(Suppl.), S22.

Solberg, E., Ingjer, F., Holen, A., Sundgot-Borgen, J., Nilsson, S., & Holme, I. (2000). Stress reactivity to and recovery from a standardized exercise bout: A study of 31 runners practicing relaxation techniques. *British Journal of Sports Medicine, 34*(4), 268–272.

Stanley, J., Buchheit, M., & Peake, J. M. (2012). The effect of post-exercise hydrotherapy on subsequent exercise performance and heart rate variability. *European Journal of Applied Physiology, 112*(3), 951–961.

Todd, M., & Brown, C. (2003). Characteristics associated with superstitious behavior in track and field athletes: Are there NCAA Divisional level differences? *Journal of Sport Behavior, 26*(2), 168–188.

Van Wilgen, C. P., & Verhagen, E. (2012). A qualitative study on overuse injuries: The beliefs of athletes and coaches. *Journal of Science and Medicine in Sport, 15*(2), 116–121.

Van Wyk, D., & Lambert, M. (2009). Recovery strategies implemented by sport support staff of elite rugby players in South Africa. *South African Journal of Physiotherapy, 65*(1), 1–15.

Venter, R. E. (2014). Perceptions of team athletes on the importance of recovery modalities. *European Journal of Sport Science, 14*, S69–76.

Venter, R. E., Potgieter, J. R., & Barnard, J. G. (2010). The use of recovery modalities by elite South African team athletes. *South African Journal for Research in Sport, Physical Education & Recreation, 32*(1), 133–145.

White, J. (1998). Alternative sports medicine. *The Physician and Sportsmedicine, 26*(6), 92–98.

Williams, C. (2007). Carbohydrate as an energy source for sport and exercise. In D. MacLaren (Ed.), *Nutrition and sport* (pp. 41–71). Philadelphia, PA: Churchill Livingstone.

Yang, J., Yao, S., Zhu, X., Zhang, C., Ling, Y., Abela, J., . . . McWhinnie, C. (2010). The impact of stress on depressive symptoms is moderated by social support in Chinese adolescents with subthreshold depression: A multi-wave longitudinal study. *Journal of Affective Disorders, 127*(1–3), 113–121.

PART II
Psychophysiological determinants of underrecovery

PART II

Psychophysiological
Assessments of
Intimacy

4

OVERTRAINING – WHAT DO WE KNOW?

Romain Meeusen and Kevin De Pauw

Introduction

This chapter emphasises the (dis)balance between training and recovery, the definitions of the terms 'functional overreaching', 'nonfunctional overreaching', and the 'overtraining syndrome', as well as the diagnosis, prevalence, assessment, and prevention of the overtraining syndrome. This chapter is derived from the joint consensus statement of the European College of Sport Science and the American College of Sports Medicine regarding the prevention, diagnosis, and treatment of the Overtraining Syndrome (Meeusen et al., 2013).

Terminology

'Overtraining' is a word that is used in many different contexts. In many scientific papers *Overtraining* is used as a 'verb', a process of intensified training with possible outcomes of short-term *Overreaching* (functional overreaching [FOR]), extreme or nonfunctional OR [NFOR]), or the overtraining syndrome (OTS). By using the expression 'syndrome', we emphasise the multifactorial aetiology and acknowledge that exercise (training) is not necessarily the sole causative factor of the syndrome. In many cases 'overtraining' is used as a 'noun', where it indicates the state of an athlete that is underperforming without an obvious reason. Therefore, OTS is put forward as the end stage of a process. This is illustrated in Figure 4.1, where we present the different stages that differentiate normal training from OR (FOR and NFOR) and from OTS. Training is an overload process that is used to disturb

PROCESS	TRAINING	INTENSIFIED →		
	(overload)	TRAINING		
OUTCOME	ACUTE FATIGUE	FUNCTIONAL OVERREACHING (short-term OR)	NONFUNCTIONAL OVERREACHING (extreme OR)	OVERTRAINING SYNDROME (OTS)
RECOVERY	Day(s)	Days - weeks	Weeks - months	Months - ...
PERFORMANCE	INCREASE	Temporary performance decrement (e.g., training camp)	STAGNATION DECREASE	DECREASE

FIGURE 4.1 Possible presentation of the different stages of training, OR and OTS (based on Meeusen et al., 2006, p. 3)

homeostasis, which can result in acute fatigue. When this acute fatigue and the subsequent recovery leads to an adaptation, the athlete's performance can improve. When training continues or when athletes deliberately use a short-term overload period (e.g., training camp), they can experience a short-term performance decrement without severe psychological or other lasting negative symptoms. This FOR will eventually lead to an improvement in performance after recovery. However, when athletes do not sufficiently respect the balance between training and recovery, NFOR can occur. At this stage, the first signs and symptoms of prolonged training distress such as performance decrements, psychological disturbance (decreased vigour, increased fatigue), and hormonal disturbances will occur, and the athletes will need weeks or months to recover. Several confounding factors such as inadequate nutrition (insufficient energy and/or carbohydrate intake), illness (most commonly, upper respiratory tract infections [URTI]), psychosocial stressors (work, study, team, coach, and family related), and sleep disorders may be present. At this stage, the distinction between NFOR and OTS is very difficult and will depend on the clinical outcome and exclusion diagnosis.

Diagnosis

OTS is characterised by a 'sport-specific' decrease in performance together with disturbances in mood state. Importantly, because there is no diagnostic tool to identify (e.g., rule in) an athlete as experiencing OTS, the solution to the differential diagnosis can only be made by excluding all other possible influences on changes in performance and mood state. Therefore, if no alternative explanation for the observed changes can be found, OTS is diagnosed. Early and unequivocal recognition of OTS is virtually impossible because the only certain sign is a decrease in performance during competition or training. The definitive diagnosis of OTS always requires the exclusion of an organic disease, e.g., endocrinological disorders (thyroid or adrenal gland and diabetes), iron deficiency with anaemia, or infectious diseases (including myocarditis, hepatitis, and glandular fever). Other major disorders or feeding behaviours such as anorexia nervosa and bulimia should also be excluded. However, it should be emphasised that many endocrinological and clinical findings due to NFOR and OTS can mimic other diseases.

One of the most certain triggers is training errors, the monotony of training, too many competitions, personal and emotional (psychological) problems, and emotional demands of occupation, resulting in an imbalance between load and recovery. Less commonly cited possibilities are sleep disturbance, altitude exposure, and exercise heat stress.

Assessment of overtraining syndrome

OTS represents the sum of multiple life stressors, such as physical training, sleep loss, exposure to environmental stresses (e.g., exposure to heat, high humidity, cold, and high altitude), occupational pressures, change of residence, and interpersonal difficulties. Concomitant to this 'stress disturbance', the endocrine system is called upon to counteract the stress situation. The primary hormone products (adrenaline, noradrenaline, and cortisol) all serve to redistribute metabolic fuels, maintain blood glucose, and enhance the responsiveness of the cardiovascular system. Repeated exposure to stress may lead to altered responsiveness to subsequent stressful experiences depending on the stressor as well as on the stimuli paired with the stressor, either leading to an unchanged, increased, or decreased neurotransmitter and receptor function. Behavioural adaptation (neurotransmitter release, receptor sensitivity, receptor binding, etc.) in higher brain centres will certainly influence hypothalamic output (Lachuer, Delton, Buda, & Tapaz, 1994). Lehmann, Foster, and Keul (1993) introduced the concept that hypothalamic function reflects the state of OR or OTS because the hypothalamus integrates many of the stressors. Acute stress increases not only hypothalamic monoamine release but also consequently corticotropin-releasing hormone and adrenocorticotropic hormone (ACTH) secretion (Shintani et al., 1995). Chronic stress and the subsequent chronically elevated adrenal glucocorticoid secretion could play an important role in the desensitisation of higher brain centres' response to acute stressors, because in acute and chronic stress, the responsiveness of hypothalamic corticotropin-releasing hormone neurons rapidly falls (Lehmann et al., 1993; Urhausen, Gabriel, & Kindermann, 1998).

The lack of definitive diagnostic criteria for OTS is reflected in much of the 'OR' and 'OT' research by a lack of consistent findings. There are several criteria that a reliable marker for the onset of the OTS must fulfil:

- The marker should be sensitive to the training load and ideally be unaffected by other factors (e.g., diet and chronobiological rhythms).
- Changes in the marker should occur before the establishment of the OTS, and changes in response to acute exercise should be distinguishable from chronic changes.

- The marker should be relatively easy to measure with a quick availability of the result, not too invasive (e.g., repeated venous blood samplings are not well accepted) and not too expensive.
- The marker should be derived at rest from submaximal or standardised exercise of relatively short duration in order not to interfere with the training process.

However, none of the currently available or suggested markers meets all these criteria.

Hormones

Hormonal responses during exercise will influence their responses during exercise recovery (Duclos, Corcuff, Rashedi, Faugere, & Manier, 1997), and it is therefore important to study both phases of exercise. For this reason, a multiple exercise test that not only gives the opportunity to measure the recovery capacity of the athlete but also can assess the ability to normally perform the second bout of exercise could be useful to detect signs of OTS and distinguish them from normal training responses or FOR. Meeusen and colleagues (2004) published a test protocol with two consecutive maximal exercise tests separated by 4 hours. The use of a double-exercise bout to volitional exhaustion to study neuroendocrine variations showed an exercise-induced increase of ACTH, prolactin, and GH to a two-exercise bout (Meeusen et al., 2004). The test could be used as an indirect measure of hypothalamic-pituitary reactivity. In normal healthy subjects, the test reveals an increase in the circulating concentrations of the hormones after both the first and the second exercise bout. Depending on the "training" status of the athlete, hormonal output after the second exercise test will be different. This test has the ability to distinguish a state of NFOR from the OTS. In a FOR stage, a less pronounced neuroendocrine response to a second bout of exercise on the same day is found (Meeusen et al., 2004), whereas in a NFOR stage, the hormonal response to a two-bout exercise protocol shows a markedly higher elevation after the second exercise trigger (Meeusen et al., 2004). With the same protocol, athletes experiencing OTS have an extremely large increase in circulating hormone concentration after the first exercise bout, followed by a complete suppression in the second exercise bout (Meeusen et al., 2004, 2010). This could indicate a hypersensitivity of the pituitary followed by an insensitivity or exhaustion afterward. Previous reports that used a single-exercise protocol found similar effects (Meeusen et al., 2004). In a follow-up study, they could clearly distinguish between NFO and OTS athletes (Meeusen et al., 2010). It appears that the use of two-exercise bouts is more useful in detecting OR for preventing OT. Early detection of OR may be very important in the prevention of OTS.

Thus, the endocrine system is one of the major systems involved in the responses to acute stress and adaptation to chronic stress. A great diversity of mechanisms is involved in such adaptation, potentially acting at all levels in the cascade, leading to the biological effects of the hormones. However, the current information regarding the endocrine system and OR/OTS shows that basal (resting) hormone measurements cannot distinguish between athletes who successfully adapt to OR and those who fail to adapt and develop symptoms of OTS. Further studies using multiple exercise tests and/or multiple hormone analyses will be necessary for evaluating the possibility of a hormonal diagnostic test for NOR/OTS.

Performance testing

In athletes being diagnosed with OTS, several signs and symptoms have been associated with this imbalance between training and recovery. However, reliable diagnostic markers for distinguishing between well-trained athletes, OR athletes, and athletes having OTS are lacking. A hallmark feature of OTS is the inability to sustain intense exercise, a decreased sport-specific performance capacity when the training load is maintained or even increased (Meeusen et al., 2004). Athletes experiencing OTS are usually able to start a normal training sequence or a race at their normal training pace but are not able to complete the training load they are given, or race as usual. The key indicator of OTS can be considered an unexplainable decrease in performance. Therefore, an exercise/performance test is considered to be essential for the diagnosis of OTS (Budgett et al., 2000). It appears that both the type of performance test used and the intensity/duration of the test are important in determining the changes in performance associated with OTS. Debate exists as to which performance test is the most appropriate when attempting to diagnose OR and OTS. In general, time-to-fatigue tests will most likely show greater changes in exercise capacity as a result of OR and OTS than incremental exercise tests (Halson & Jeukendrup, 2004). In addition, these tests allow that the assessment of substrate kinetics, hormonal responses, and submaximal measures can be made at a fixed intensity and duration. Time trials reflect more accurately the sport-specific task of most sports but have only rarely been used to objectively quantify the performance loss in OR (Halson, Lancaster, Jeukendruk, & Gleeson, 2003). To detect subtle performance decrements, it might be better to use sport-specific performance tests.

Psychology

The presence of psychological symptoms in cases of OTS has long been acknowledged, but systematic study on this topic did not begin until William Morgan's research in the 1980s on college swimmers and athletes in other sports (Morgan, Brown, Raglin, Conner, & Ellickson, 1987). Using the Profile of Mood States (POMS; McNair, Lorr, & Droppleman, 1992), a questionnaire that measures both general and specific moods, athletes were found to consistently report elevations in negative moods (tension, depression, anger, fatigue, and confusion) and decreases in the positive mood of vigour during periods of rigorous training. More frequent assessments indicated that mood state exhibits a predictable dose-response relationship with training whereby disturbances increase in a stepwise fashion as training loads rise in volume or intensity, with the peak of training and mood disturbance coinciding. Conversely, training tapers usually result in a reduction in negative moods and an increase in vigour such that at the end of a taper the mood scores return to the positive pattern typically observed at the outset of the season, called the iceberg profile (Morgan, Brown, et al., 1987; Morgan, O'Connor, Sparling, & Pate, 1987).

More important for the standpoint of monitoring, athletes with signs of OTS typically exhibit both a greater increase in total mood disturbance and a different pattern of mood disturbance (i.e., more fatigue, less vigour and an increase in depression), compared with athletes undergoing the same training who remain free from symptoms (Raglin & Morgan, 1994).

Several sport-specific OTS scales have been developed using theoretical assumptions about what psychological and behaviour factors should be associated with OTS. Among them, the most extensively studied has been the Recovery-Stress Questionnaire for Athletes (RESTQ-Sport; Kellmann & Kallus, 2001, 2016), a 76-item questionnaire encompassing 19 separate scales that assess both stress and recovery activities in athletes. Monitoring the current levels of both stress and recovery has the possible advantage that problems may be detected before symptoms of OT and staleness (e.g., drowsiness, apathy, fatigue, and irritability) are likely to appear. However, stress and recovery are often different in their time course. Although concerns with its factor structure have been expressed by other researchers (Davis, Orzec, & Keelan, 2007), research indicates the RESTQ-Sport is responsive to changes in training load, particularly in athletes with signs of OTS (Kellmann & Günther, 2000).

Physiology

There have been several proposals as to which physiological measures might be indicative of OR or OTS. Reduced maximal heart rates after increased training may be the result of reduced sympathetic nervous system activity, of a decreased tissue responsiveness to catecholamines, and of changes in adrenergic receptor activity; or it may simply be the result of a reduced power output achieved with maximal effort. Several other reductions in maximal physiological measures (oxygen uptake, heart rate, blood lactate) might be a consequence of a reduction in exercise time and not related to abnormalities per se, and it should be noted that changes of resting heart rate are not consistently found in athletes experiencing OTS (Urhausen & Kindermann, 2002).

Heart rate variability (HRV) analysis has been used as a measure of cardiac autonomic balance, with an increase in HRV indicating an increase in vagal (parasympathetic) tone relative to sympathetic activity (Uusitalo, Uusitalo, & Rusko, 2000). The problems with this physiological measure are as follows: HRV seems to be a promising tool in theory, but does not provide consistent results (Le Meur, Buchheit, Aubry, Coutts, & Hausswirth, 2017). One needs to be careful when using HRV as an outcome measure because there are many different ways to record and calculate the data. Currently, there is no consensus regarding the required standardisation and the method of measurement. The present data do not allow to distinguish between changes in physiological measures resulting from FOR, NFOR, and OTS.

Immune system

There are many reports on URTI due to increased training, and also in OR and OTS athletes. It seems possible that intensified training (leading to OR or OTS) may increase both the duration of the so-called 'open window' (the period directly post-exercise when the athlete is more susceptible to infections), and the degree of the resultant immunodepression. However, the amount of scientific information to substantiate these arguments is limited. More data are available that each bout of prolonged and intensive exercise has transient but significant, wide ranging effects on the immune system (Gleeson, 2007). Heavy exertion leads to alterations in immunity and host pathogen defence and elevations in stress hormones, pro and anti-inflammatory cytokines, and reactive oxygen species.

Prevention

Because OTS is difficult to diagnose, authors agree that it is important to prevent OTS (Foster, Snyder, Thompson, & Kuettel, 1998). Moreover, because OTS is mainly due to an imbalance in the training/recovery ratio (too much training and competitions and too little recovery), it is of utmost importance that athletes record daily their training load, using a daily training diary or training log (Foster, Daines, Hector, Snyder, & Welsh, 1996). The four methods most frequently used to monitor training and prevent OT are as follows: Retrospective questionnaires, training diaries, physiological screening, and the direct observational method (Hopkins, 1991). Also, the psychological screening of athletes and the RPE (Foster et al., 1996) have received more and more attention.

Foster and colleagues (1996) have determined training load as the product of the subjective intensity of a training session using 'session RPE' and the total duration of the training session expressed in minutes. The 'session RPE' has been shown to be related to the average percent heart rate reserve during an exercise session and to the percentage of a training session during which the heart rate is in blood lactate–derived heart rate training zones. With this method of monitoring training, they have demonstrated the utility of evaluating experimental alterations in training and have successfully related training load to the athlete's performance (Foster et al., 1996). Foster, Heimann, Esten, Brice, and Porcari (2000) have demonstrated that athletes often do not perform the same training load prescribed by coaches. In particular, they noted that on days the coaches intended to be 'easy', athletes often performed meaningfully longer and/or more intense training. These data fit well with the concept that OTS is a failure of the work-recovery relationship, often in the direction of athletes failing to take appropriate recovery. However, training load is clearly not the only training-related variable contributing to the genesis of OTS. So additional to the weekly training load, daily mean training load as well as the SD of training load was calculated during each week. The daily mean divided by the SD was defined as the monotony. The product of the weekly training load and monotony was calculated as strain. The incidence of simple illness and injury was noted and plotted together with the indices of training load, monotony, and strain. They noted the correspondence between spikes in the indices of training monotony and strain and subsequent illness or injury, and thresholds that allowed for optimal explanation of illnesses were computed (Foster, 1998).

Rest and sleep

One of the most obvious methods for managing fatigue and enhancing recovery is adequate passive rest and obtaining sufficient sleep. It is generally recommended that athletes should have at least one passive rest day each week, because the absence of a recovery day, especially during intensified training periods, is closely related to the onset of signs of OR and underrecovery (Bruin, Kuipers, Keizer, & Vander Vusse, 1994). A passive rest day can also act as a 'time-out' period for athletes and prevent them from becoming totally preoccupied with their sport and possibly encourage them to pursue a different (passive) interest. Such distractions from the daily routine of training may alleviate boredom and reduce stress perception. Sleep is an essential part of fatigue management, because persistent sleep loss can negatively affect the quality of a training session and general well-being (Hausswirth et al., 2014). The primary need for sleep has been hypothesised as being neurally based rather than a requirement for restitution of other biological tissues (Horne & Pettitt, 1984). Therefore, with inadequate sleep, cognitive functions are likely to be impaired, especially the ability to concentrate. Individuals have different requirements for sleep, and to prescribe the dose of sleep that a highly trained athlete requires would be erroneous. The general advice is to sleep for the amount of time that is required to feel wakeful during the day, which may vary considerably between individuals.

Nutrition

Because OR is brought about by high-intensity training with limited recovery, it is thought that the fatigue and underperformance associated with OR are at least partly attributable to a decrease in muscle glycogen levels. Decreased glycogen levels can result in disturbances of the endocrine milieu. Glycogen depletion results in higher circulating levels of catecholamines, cortisol, and glucagon in response to exercise while insulin levels are very low. Such hormonal responses will result in changes in substrate mobilisation and utilisation (for instance, high adrenaline levels in combination with low insulin will increase lipolysis and stimulate the mobilisation of fatty acids). Because repeated days of hard training and carbohydrate depletion seem to be linked to the development of OR, it is tempting to think that carbohydrate supplementation can reverse the symptoms (Snyder, 1998).

Considerations for coaches and physicians

Until a definitive diagnostic tool for the OTS is present, coaches and physicians need to rely on performance decrements as verification that an OTS exists. However, if sophisticated laboratory techniques are not available, the following considerations may be useful:

- Maintain accurate records of performance during training and competition. Be willing to adjust daily training intensity/volume or allow a day of complete rest, when performance declines, or the athlete complains of excessive fatigue.
- Avoid excessive monotony of training.
- Always individualise the intensity of training.
- Encourage and regularly reinforce optimal nutrition, hydration status, and sleep.
- Be aware that multiple stressors such as sleep loss or sleep disturbance (e.g., jet lag), exposure to environmental stressors, occupational pressures, change of residence, and interpersonal or family difficulties may add to the stress of physical training.
- Treat OTS with rest. Reduced training may be sufficient for recovery in some cases of OR.
- Resumption of training should be individualised on the basis of the signs and symptoms because there is no definitive indicator of recovery.
- Communication with the athletes (maybe through an online training diary) about their physical, mental, and emotional concerns is important.
- Include regular psychological questionnaires to evaluate the emotional and psychological state of the athlete.
- Maintain confidentiality regarding each athlete's condition (physical, clinical, and mental).
- Importance of regular health checks performed by a multidisciplinary team (physician, nutritionist, psychologist, etc.).
- Allow the athlete time to recover after illness/injury.
- Note the occurrence of URTI and other infectious episodes; the athlete should be encouraged to suspend training or reduce the training intensity when experiencing an infection.
- Always rule out an organic disease in cases of performance decrement.
- Unresolved viral infections are not routinely assessed in elite athletes, but it may be worth investigating this in individuals experiencing fatigue and underperformance in training and competition.

Moreover, when OTS is suspected, it is also of utmost importance to standardise the criteria used for diagnosis and/or, at least, as tools for the diagnosis of OTS are lacking, to standardise the criteria of exclusion of OTS.

Conclusion and recommendations for practise

A difficulty with recognizing and conducting research on athletes with OTS is defining the point at which OTS develops. Many studies claim to have induced OTS, but it is more likely that they have induced a state of OR in their subjects. Consequently, the majority of studies aimed at identifying markers of ensuing OTS are actually reporting markers of excessive exercise stress resulting in the acute condition of OR and not the chronic condition of OTS. The mechanism of OTS could be difficult to examine in detail maybe because the stress caused by excessive training load, in combination with other stressors, might trigger different 'defence mechanisms' such as the immunological, neuro-endocrine, and other physiological systems that interact and therefore cannot be pinpointed as the 'sole' cause of OTS. It might be that as in other syndromes (e.g., chronic fatigue syndrome or burnout), the psychoneuroimmunology (study of brain-behaviour-immune interrelationships) might shed a light on the possible mechanisms of OTS, but until there is no definite diagnostic tool, it is of utmost importance to standardise measures that are now thought to provide a good inventory of the training status of the athlete. A primary indicator of OR or OTS is a decrease in sport-specific performance, and it is very important to emphasise the need to distinguish OTS from OR and other potential causes of temporary underperformance such as anaemia, acute infection, muscle damage, and insufficient carbohydrate intake.

The physical demands of intensified training are not the only elements in the development of OTS. It seems that a complex set of psychological factors are important in the development of OTS, including excessive expectations from a coach or family members, competitive stress, personality structure, social environment, relationships with family and friends, monotony in training, personal or emotional problems, and school- or work-related demands. Although no single marker can be taken as an indicator of impending OTS, the regular monitoring of a combination of performance, physiological, biochemical, immunological, and psychological variables would seem to be the best strategy to identify athletes who are failing to cope with the stress of training.

References

Bruin, G., Kuipers, H., Keizer, H. A., & Vander Vusse, G. J. (1994). Adaptation and overtraining in horses subjected to increasing training loads. *Journal of Applied Physiology, 76*, 1908–1913.

Budgett, R., Newsholme, E., Lehmann, M., Sharp, C., Jones, D., Peto, T., . . . & White, P. (2000). Redefining the overtraining syndrome as the unexplained underperformance syndrome. *British Journal of Sport Medicine, 34*, 67–68.

Davis, H., Orzec, T., & Keelan, P. (2007). Psychometric item evaluations of the Recovery-Stress Questionnaire for Athletes. *Psychology of Sport and Exercise, 8*, 917–938.

Duclos, M., Corcuff, J. B., Rashedi, M., Fougere, V., & Manier, G. (1997). Trained versus untrained men: Different immediate post-exercise responses of pituitary – adrenal axis. *European Journal of Applied Physiology, 75*, 343–350.

Foster, C. (1998). Monitoring training in athletes with reference to overtraining syndrome. *Medicine and Science in Sports and Exercise, 30*(7), 164–168.

Foster, C., Daines, E., Hector, L., Snyder, A., & Welsh, R. (1996). Athletic performance in relation to training load. *Wisconsin Medical Journal, 95,* 370–374.

Foster, C., Heimann, K. M., Esten, P. L., Brice, G., & Porcari, J. (2000). Differences in perceptions of training by coaches and athletes. *South African Journal of Sports Medicine, 8,* 3–7.

Foster, C., Snyder, A., Thompson, N., & Kuettel, K. (1998). Normalisation of the blood lactate profile. *International Journal of Sport Medicine, 9,* 198–200.

Gleeson, M. (2007). Immune function in sport and exercise. *Journal of Applied Physiology, 103*(2), 693–699.

Halson, S., & Jeukendrup, A. (2004). Does overtraining exist? An analysis of overreaching and overtraining research. *Sports Medicine, 34,* 967–981.

Halson, S., Lancaster, G., Jeukendrup, A., & Gleeson, M. (2003). Immunological responses to overreaching in cyclists. *Medicine and Science in Sports and Exercise, 35*(5), 854–861.

Hausswirth, C., Louis, J., Aubry, A., Bonnet, G., Duffield, R., & Le Meur, Y. (2014). Evidence of disturbed sleep and increased illness in overreached endurance athletes. *Medicine and Science in Sports and Exercise, 46*(5), 1036–1045.

Hopkins, W. (1991). Quantification of training in competitive sports. Methods and applications. *Sports Medicine, 12,* 161–183.

Horne, J. A., & Pettitt, A. N. (1984). Sleep deprivation and the physiological response to exercise under steady-state conditions in untrained subjects. *Sleep, 7,* 168–179.

Kellmann, M., & Günther, K. (2000). Changes in stress and recovery in elite rowers during preparation for the Olympic Games. *Medicine and Science in Sports and Exercise, 32,* 676–683.

Kellmann, M., & Kallus, K. W. (2001). *Recovery-Stress Questionnaire for Athletes; User manual.* Champaign, IL: Human Kinetics.

Kellmann, M., & Kallus, K. W. (2016). The Recovery-Stress Questionnaire for Athletes. In K. W. Kallus & M. Kellmann (Eds.), *The Recovery-Stress Questionnaires: User manual* (pp. 86–131). Frankfurt am Main: Pearson Assessment.

Lachuer, J., Delton, I., Buda, M., & Tappaz, M. (1994). The habituation of brainstem catecholaminergic groups to chronic daily restraint stress is stress specific like that of the hypothalamo – pituitary – adrenal axis. *Brain Research, 638,* 196–202.

Lehmann, M., Foster, C., & Keul, J. (1993). Overtraining in endurance athletes: A brief review. *Medicine and Science in Sports and Exercise, 25,* 854–861.

Le Meur, Y., Buchheit, M., Aubry, A., Coutts, A., & Hausswirth, C. (2017). Assessing overreaching with HRR: What is the minimal exercise intensity required? *International Journal of Sports Physiology and Performance, 12,* 569–573.

McNair, D. M., Lorr, M., & Droppleman, L. F. (1992). *Revised manual for the Profile of Mood States.* San Diego, CA: Educational and Industrial Testing Service.

Meeusen, R., Duclos, M., Foster, C., Fry, A., Gleeson, M., Nieman, D., . . . Urhausen, A. (2013). Prevention, diagnosis, and treatment of the overtraining syndrome: Joint consensus statement of the European College of Sport Science and the American College of Sports Medicine. *Medicine and Science in Sports and Exercise, 45*(1), 186–205.

Meeusen, R., Duclos, M., Gleeson, M., Rietjens, G., Steinacker, J., & Urhausen, A. (2006). Prevention, diagnosis and treatment of the overtraining syndrome – ECSS position statement 'task force'. *European Journal of Sport Science, 6*(1), 1–14.

Meeusen, R., Nederhof, E., Buyse, L., Roelands, B., De Schutter, G., & Piacentini, M. F. (2010). Diagnosing overtraining in athletes using the two bout exercise protocol. *British Journal of Sport Medicine, 44*(9), 642–648.

Meeusen, R., Piacentini, M. F., Busschaert, B., Buyse, L., De Schutter, G., & Stray-Gundersen, J. (2004). Hormonal responses in athletes: The use of a two bout exercise protocol to detect subtle differences in (over)training status. *European Journal of Applied Physiology, 91*, 140–146.

Morgan, W. P., Brown, D. R., Raglin, J. S., O'Conner, P. J., & Ellickson, K. A. (1987). Psychological monitoring of overtraining and staleness. *British Journal of Sport Medicine, 21*, 107–114.

Morgan, W. P., O'Connor, P. J., Sparling, P., & Pate, R. (1987). Psychological characterization of the elite female distance runner. *International Journal of Sport Medicine, 8*(2), 124–131.

Raglin, J., & Morgan, W. P. (1994). Development of a scale for use in monitoring training-induced distress in athletes. *International Journal of Sport Medicine, 15*, 84–88.

Shintani, F., Nakaki, T., Kanba, S., Sato, K., Yagi, G., Shiozawa, M. Asai, M. (1995). Involvement of interleukin-1 in immobilisation stress-induced increase in plasma adrenocorticotropic hormones and in release of hypothalamic monoamines in rat. *Journal of Neuroscience, 15*, 1961–1670.

Snyder, A. (1998). Overtraining and glycogen depletion hypothesis. *Medicine and Science in Sports and Exercise, 30*(7), 1146–1150.

Urhausen, A., Gabriel, H., & Kindermann, W. (1998). Impaired pituitary hormonal response to exhaustive exercise in overtrained endurance athletes. *Medicine and Science in Sports and Exercise, 30*(3), 407–414.

Urhausen, A., & Kindermann, W. (2002). Diagnosis of overtraining – what tools do we have? *Sports Medicine, 32*, 95–102.

Uusitalo, A. L., Uusitalo, A. J., & Rusko, H. (2000). Heart rate and blood pressure variability during heavy training and overtraining in the female athlete. *International Journal of Sport Medicine, 21*, 45–53.

5
RECOVERY-STRESS BALANCE AND PSYCHOBIOSOCIAL STATES MONITORING OF ROAD CYCLISTS

Claudio Robazza, Fabio Forzini, Selenia di Fronso, and Maurizio Bertollo

Introduction

Cycling stage races are among the most strenuous endurance sports in which performers must cope with huge physical and psychological demands (Lombardi et al., 2013; Taylor & Kress, 2006). Cyclists have to deal with a high variability of course and weather conditions, dehydration, exhaustion, and pain over extensive periods. Monitoring the athletes' progression toward possible health issues and related poor performance is essential for the planning of training load and recovery. Thus, maintaining a healthy recovery-stress balance is fundamental in multi-stage cycling competitions. As in any other challenging tasks, the athlete needs to effectively recruit, use, and recover physical and psychological resources to attain consistent successful performance. The fatigue arising from the high depletion level of energy is usually accompanied by feelings of emotional discomfort indicating that the functional capacities of the individual are decreasing (Hanin, 2002).

Attempts to predict endurance performance exclusively on the basis of physiological variables have been unsuccessful. In a systematic review of measures related to acute and chronic training loads, Saw, Main, and Gastin (2016) reported that objective measures of athletes' well-being generally did not correlate with subjective measures. Objective assessments included, among others, blood markers, heart rate, oxygen consumption, and heart rate response, while subjective measures encompassed mood, anxiety, and perceived stress. Noteworthy, subjective measures were shown to reflect acute and chronic training loads more accurately and consistently than objective measures. This evidence provides strong support for the use

Robazza, C., Forzini, F., di Fronso, S., & Bertollo, M. (2018). Recovery-stress balance and psychobiosocial states monitoring of road cyclists. In M. Kellmann & J. Beckmann (Eds.), *Sport, Recovery, and Performance: Interdisciplinary Insights* (pp. 63–73). Abingdon: Routledge.

of subjective assessments alone, or together with objective measures, to monitor changes in well-being of athletes in response to training and/or races.

Recovery-stress balance and psychological states have been examined in cyclists participating in the 2012 Girobio competition. This was a major multi-stage cycling race held in Italy for Under 23 and Elite categories, and was considered one of the most important races in the world. Participants were approximately 22 years old and had about 11 years of extensive international cycling experience. The race involved nine stages of various lengths and topographies, and covered approximately 1,300 km. In particular, the stages involved flat (stages 1, 2, and 7), low-mountain (stages 3, 4, 5, and 6), and high-mountain (stages 8 and 9) terrains, ranging from 75.6 to 193.3 km in length and from 642 to 5190 m in cumulative elevation. Of the 170 cyclists from four countries (i.e., Italy, Netherlands, Switzerland, and the USA), who entered the competition, about 70 finished the race and agreed to participate in the study. Given the broad focus of this research, findings have been published in the three studies reviewed herein. Additional unpublished results are presented in this chapter as well.

Recovery-stress factors before and after the race

The purposes of the first study (Filho et al., 2013) were to examine the magnitude of pre-post recovery and stress of cyclists involved in the Girobio and to identify those recovery-stress balance factors that remained constant from pre- to post-race testing. The recovery-stress balance has been addressed in previous research on athletic activities requiring long-term and intensive endurance training, such as swimming and rowing (Kellmann, 2010; Kellmann, Altenburg, Lormes, & Steinacker, 2001). Earlier studies in cycling have also focused on detecting changes in recovery and stress variables linked to demanding training regimens or competitions (Halson et al., 2002). In a study reported by Kallus and Kellmann (2000), for example, recovery-stress states of 16 mountain bikers were monitored weekly during the 1997 World Cup. Individual profiles reflected the athletes' recovery and stress condition according to their level of preparation over the season. However, more research was needed to examine those specific stress and recovery-related factors that are likely to vary, as well as those less likely to change as a consequence of highly effortful endurance tasks. Identifying both changeable and stable factors linked to high-level performance in endurance sports may indicate which training loads, behaviours, activities, and mental training procedures are most beneficial in helping athletes enhance their resilience and mental toughness (Gucciardi & Gordon, 2011).

The importance of concurrently assessing various recovery and stress factors is presented in Kellmann's (2002) view of the interrelation between stress states and recovery demands. This interrelation needs to be balanced for optimal performance. During the competitive season, for instance, athletes can balance an increase in social stress derived from pressure that coaches and media exert on them by engaging in various forms of passive (e.g., sleeping), active (e.g., stretching), and pro-active (e.g., purposefully travelling to visit family and friends) recovery activities. When the balance between recovery demands and stress states is compromised (i.e., high stress/low recovery), athletes are more likely to perform poorly. This view of the interrelation between stress states and recovery demands has been psychometrically operationalised through the multidimensional Recovery-Stress Questionnaire for Athletes (RESTQ-Sport; Kellmann & Kallus, 2001, 2016). The RESTQ-Sport includes 76 questions linked to 19 scales. In particular, the instrument assesses the frequency of current stress symptoms together with the frequency of recovery-associated activities and states over the three days and nights prior to the test. The items are included within (a) seven general stress scales (i.e., *General Stress, Emotional Stress, Social Stress, Conflict/Pressure, Fatigue, Lack of Energy*, and *Physical Complaints*), (b) five general recovery scales (i.e., *Success, Social Recovery, Physical Recovery, General Well-being*, and *Sleep Quality*), (c) three sport-specific stress scales (i.e., *Disturbed Breaks, Emotional Exhaustion*, and *Injury*), and (d) four sport-specific recovery scales (i.e., *Being in Shape, Personal Accomplishment, Self-Efficacy*, and *Self-Regulation*). The RESTQ-Sport has one 'warm-up' item, and each scale contains four items measured on a Likert-type frequency scale with anchors 0 (*never*) and 6 (*always*). High scores in the stress-related activity scales denote levels of stress, whereas high scores in the recovery-related scales imply good recovery activities. A conceptual strength of the RESTQ-Sport regards its multidimensional structure in the assessment of recovery-stress balance. Indeed, this instrument taps a multitude of specific indicators of overtraining and dysfunctional overreaching (Kellmann, 2010). The RESTQ-Sport also gauges functional factors and psychological skills (e.g., self-regulation, self-efficacy) that are important in the prevention of under-performance and dysfunctional overreaching. The multifactorial structure and the predictive validity of the RESTQ-Sport has been confirmed in a number of studies across different sport disciplines (e.g., di Fronso, Nakamura, Bortoli, Robazza, & Bertollo, 2013; Kellmann, 2010; Kellmann & Kallus, 2001; Matos, Winsley, & Williams, 2011). A shorter version (RESTQ-Sport-52) with 52 items is also available as well as a reduced version (RESTQ-Sport-36) with 36 items and 12 scales (see Kellmann & Kallus, 2016).

The RESTQ-Sport was administered to the athletes of the Girobio one day before the first stage and the day of the final stage, with a ten-racing-day interval between pre- and post- assessment. In general, post-assessment scores were in the expected direction, with lower values found on both general and sport-specific recovery scales, and higher scores for stress-related scales ($\eta_p^2 = .70$). Within-subjects analysis showed differences in 14 of the 19 scales, with no effect observed for one general stress (i.e., *Conflict/Pressure*), two general recovery (i.e., *Success* and *Social Recovery*), and two sport-specific recovery scales (i.e., *Personal Accomplishment*, and *Self-Efficacy*). Overall results were in the expected direction and in accordance with previous findings (e.g., Kallus & Kellmann, 2000; Kellmann, 2010; Matos et al., 2011) showing higher stress and lower recovery states in the retest scores after a highly demanding competition. From an applied perspective, findings indicate the need to pay attention to changes of large magnitude such as those observed for stress-related scales (i.e., *General Stress, Physical Complaints, Emotional Exhaustion*, and *Injury*), and especially to the high values noticed for *Fatigue* and *Disturbed Breaks*. *Fatigue*, indeed, is a main limiting factor on performance in sports, which is influenced by both physiological and psychological factors (Marcora, Staiano, & Manning, 2009). Thus, athletes may benefit from effective recovering activities, as well as psychological strategies – especially during multi-stage competitions – aimed at improving motivation, control of attentional focus (e.g., through associative and dissociative strategies), and resilience to over-fatigue.

Mood state changes during the race

The objectives of the second study (Murgia et al., 2016) were to investigate how mood states of high and low performers change throughout the race, and the predictive validity of mood states toward performance. Mood states were assessed through the Profile of Mood States (POMS; McNair, Lorr, & Droppleman, 1971). Initially developed to assess mood states in clinical settings, the scale has been extensively used in sport and exercise psychology research thereafter (Prapavessis, 2000; Raglin, 2001). The POMS contains 65 items gauging five negative dimensions (*Anxiety, Anger, Depression, Confusion*, and *Fatigue*) and one positive dimension (*Vigor*). Substantial research evidence indicates that successful athletes score low in negative factors of *Tension, Depression, Anger, Fatigue*, and *Confusion*, and above average in the positive factor of *Vigor*. The POMS factors are often combined by summing the negative dimension scores and subtracting the vigour score to create a higher order factor referred to as total mood disturbance. Research findings suggest that continued training stress leads to mood state disturbance and decreased performance (e.g., Morgan, Costill, Flynn, Raglin, & O'Connor, 1988; Urhausen, Gabriel, & Kindermann, 1995). In endurance athletes, for example, a substantial increase in fatigue and decrease in vigour scores after an overload period resulted in impaired cognitive and physical performance (Dupuy et al., 2014).

In the study of Murgia and colleagues (2016), cyclists were asked to rate the items on a Likert scale ranging from 0 (*not at all*) to 4 (*extremely*) thinking of how they felt over the past week until the current day. Participants were assessed the day prior to the first and last stage. At the end of the race, athletes were classified as high or low performers based on the actual outcome (i.e., the total time spent to complete the race) and perceived performance (i.e., self-evaluation on a 0–10 scale). Time (pre- and post-test) × group (high and low performers) interaction results on mood disturbance level were significant (actual performance ranking, $\eta_p^2 = .20$; perceived performance ranking, $\eta_p^2 = .22$). Compared to high performers, low performers reported higher levels of mood disturbance at the end of the race. The changes in mood disturbance levels observed in low performers suggest that this sample could benefit from mental training and attention control strategies aimed at improving the athletes' resilience and coping skills to better cope with strenuous endurance tasks (Bertollo et al., 2015). Regarding the second purpose of the study, mood states were not found to predict performance.

Recovery-stress balance and cycling performance

Findings of the previous study did not support the predictive validity of mood states toward cycling performance (Murgia et al., 2016). The predictive validity of recovery-stress states on performance was investigated in a third study (Filho et al., 2015) using the RESTQ-Sport (Kellmann & Kallus, 2001, 2016). In particular, the study purposes were to examine the relationship among several perceived recovery-stress states and performance outcomes, and to further explore whether this relationship differed from the initial to the final stage of the Girobio competition. As underlined previously, the ability to balance recovery demands and stress stimuli is critical for the development and maintenance of skilled performance (Kellmann, 2010; Meeusen et al., 2013). Consequently, monitoring recovery-stress balance is fundamental in order to help athletes perform up to their potential, particularly in multi-stage competitions when athletes are exposed to high-stress demands over extensive periods.

The correlation pattern indicated that the relationship among recovery and stress factors was subjected to change over time, with the exception of the strong association between *Self-Regulation* and *Being in Shape* that remained high ($r \leq .70$) on both the initial and final stage. This large association suggests that the ability to self-regulate can enable individuals to stay physically and mentally fit (Robazza, Pellizzari, & Hanin, 2004). Multiple regression analysis was also conducted to estimate the relationship among the RESTQ-Sport recovery factors (nine scales; e.g., *Physical Recovery* and *Sleep Quality*) and stress factors (ten scales; e.g., *Lack of Energy* and *Physical Complaints*) in relation to performance. Results showed that *Physical Recovery*, *Injury*, and *General Well-being* predicted performance in the initial stage. Moreover, *Conflicts/Pressure* and *Lack of Energy* were associated with performance at the final stage. Taken together, these findings suggest that the linkage among recovery scales and stress scales changes greatly over time, and dynamically influences performance in multi-stage competitions.

Recovery-stress balance and psychobiosocial states

In addition to recovery-stress scales and mood states, psychobiosocial states of cyclists were also assessed during the Girobio. Psychobiosocial states related to performance are defined in the individual zones of optimal functioning (IZOF) model as situational, multimodal, and dynamic manifestation of the total human functioning (Hanin, 2007, 2010). Ruiz, Hanin, and Robazza (2016) have proposed an individualised profiling approach to the assessment of functional and dysfunctional psychobiosocial states surrounding successful and unsuccessful performances. This comprehensive assessment encompasses eight basic forms (modalities): *Affective,*

Cognitive, Motivational, Volitional (psychological), *Bodily-somatic, Motor-behavioural* (biological), *Operational*, and *Communicative* (social) modalities. The eight modalities are interconnected and provide a widespread description of a performance state that includes emotional and non-emotional experiences and their displays (expression or suppression). In this view, emotion is a main component of a performance-related psychobiosocial state, which is construed within the framework of four categories derived from hedonic tone and functionality distinctions: Pleasant-functional, unpleasant-functional, pleasant-dysfunctional, and unpleasant-dysfunctional emotions (Hanin, 2007). The cognitive modality involves, for example, attention processing, focusing attention, and the ability to orient attention and respond to relevant stimuli (Moran, 2011). The motivational and volitional components include purposes, desires, drives, and commitments toward the achievement of goals (Achtziger & Gollwitzer, 2008). The bodily-somatic modality refers to biological or psychophysiological concomitants of emotions, such as feelings of tension/relaxation (Robazza & Bortoli, 2003), while the motor-behavioural component is related to an individual's perception of motor coordination and movement characteristics. The operational modality refers to one's perception of the effectiveness of action, while the communicative modality regards to verbal and nonverbal messages among interacting persons. Functional and dysfunctional items for each modality contain three or four adjectives. Examples of adjectives included in functional and dysfunctional items are: Enthusiastic and complacent (affective modality), focused and distracted (cognitive), committed and unmotivated (motivational), persistent and undetermined (volitional), energetic and exhausted (bodily-somatic), powerful- and clumsy-movement (motor-behavioural), effective- and ineffective-task execution (operational), and connected and withdrawn (communicative).

Robazza, Bertollo, Ruiz, and Bortoli (2016) have subsequently examined the characteristics and the factor structure of the items comprised in the individualised profiling of psychobiosocial states (Ruiz et al., 2016). The psychobiosocial states scale was administered in a first study to a sample of athletes in a trait-like manner (i.e., asking them to think of how they usually feel within the hour before an important competition). Exploratory Structural Equation Modelling and Confirmatory Factor Analysis of the data showed satisfactory fit indices for a two-factor, 15-item solution comprised of eight functional items and seven dysfunctional items. Results of a second study in a different sample provided evidence of substantial measurement and structural invariance of all dimensions across samples. Concurrent validity of the scale was also examined. Concurrent measures were the five scales (i.e., *Anger, Anxiety, Dejection, Excitement*, and *Happiness*) of the Sport Emotion Questionnaire (SEQ; Jones, Lane, Bray, Uphill, & Catlin, 2005), the two scales (i.e., *Positive* and *Negative Affect*) of the Positive and Negative Affect Schedule (PANAS; Watson, Clark, & Tellegen, 1988), and the four scales (i.e., *Self-Confidence, Emotional Arousal Control, Worry*, and *Concentration Disruption*) of the Sport Performance Psychological Inventory (IPPS-48; Robazza, Bortoli, & Gramaccioni, 2009).

Interestingly, findings revealed a low association between the psychobiosocial scale and the other measures, suggesting that the scale taps unique constructs.

Psychobiosocial states in sport have been assessed in a number of studies. Results showed high individual variability in item content and intensity, and a wide range of interrelated experiences associated with performance. Findings also support the practical utility of assessing psychobiosocial states to help athletes become aware and control their performance-related experiences (for a review, see Ruiz, Raglin, & Hanin, 2017). According to Hanin (2002), underperformance due to a lack of recovery is reflected in the athletes' psychobiosocial states prior to, during, and after performance. Psychobiosocial states are considered sensitive markers of an athlete's level of readiness for performance. These markers are proposed as descriptors of functional or dysfunctional pre- and mid-performance states, and also serve as idiosyncratic indicators of adequate or inadequate recovery. Specifically, psychobiosocial dynamics reflect how athletes recruit, use, and recover their resources in a single or repeated work-recovery cycle. Thus, individual-oriented monitoring of pre-, mid-, and post-performance states and recovery states is useful in preventing underperformance.

As previously stated, cyclists' psychobiosocial states were monitored during the Girobio. On the day before the initial stage, participants rated the perceived intensity of their states on the items of the psychobiosocial states scale (Robazza et al., 2016). As expected, positive correlations (from .28 to .38) were found between functional psychobiosocial states and *Physical Recovery, General Well-being, Being in Shape, Self-Efficacy*, and *Self-Regulation* scales of the RESTQ-Sport (Kellmann & Kallus, 2001, 2016), and between dysfunctional psychobiosocial states and *General Stress, Emotional Stress, Social Stress, Physical Complaints*, and *Emotional Exhaustion*. Furthermore, negative correlations (from -.18 to -.34) were shown between functional psychobiosocial states and Emotional Exhaustion, and between dysfunctional psychobiosocial states and *Social Recovery, Physical Recovery, General Well-being, Being in Shape, Self-Efficacy*, and *Self-Regulation*. These results suggest that functional and dysfunctional psychobiosocial states share some variance with the scales of the RESTQ-Sport, but also that the two measures address unique constructs.

After having administered the psychobiosocial states scale, each cyclist was asked to choose one adjective from the scale deemed most representative of his current state, and to rate it in intensity on a 11-point Borg scale (Borg, 2001). Negative scores were assigned to adjectives representative of dysfunctional states. The same assessment procedure was repeated within the hour preceding each of the nine stages of the race. At the end of the competition, cyclists were classified based on their mean scores of self-assessed performance across the nine stages. Repeated measures analysis of variance indicated differences between Group 1 and the two other groups, $F(2, 54) = 3.218, p = .048, \eta_p^2 = .106$. The trend of differences across the nine stages is represented in Figure 5.1. As can be observed, psychobiosocial states fluctuated over time and enabled discrimination of groups across the races based on the participants' subjective performance level.

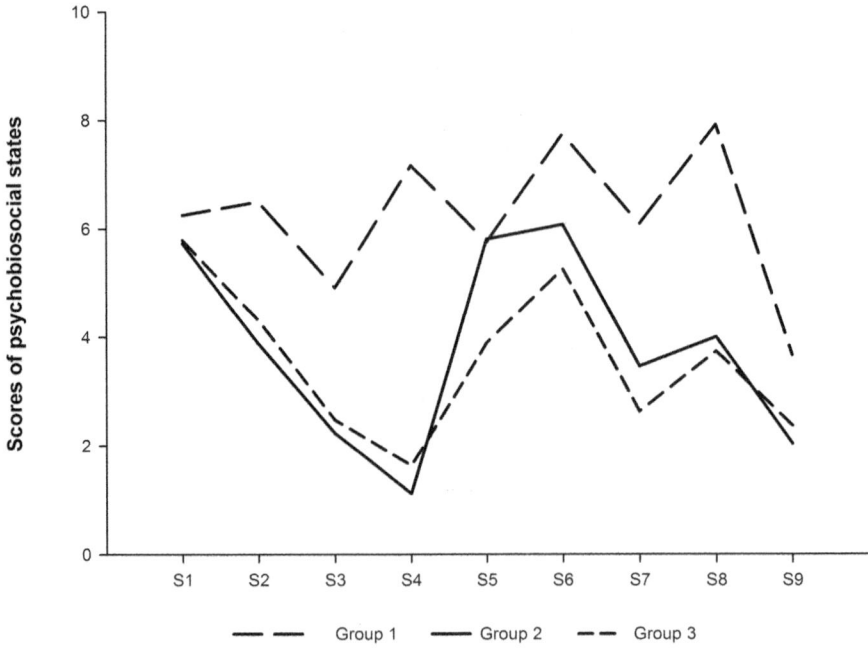

FIGURE 5.1 Mean scores of cyclists' psychobiosocial states across the nine stages (from S1 to S9) of the Girobio. Cyclists were categorised based on their mean scores of self-assessed performance: Group 1 (12 cyclists), good performance scores from 7 to 10; Group 2 (26 cyclists), intermediate performance scores from 6 to 7; Group 3 (19 cyclists), poor performance scores from 0 to 6.

Conclusion and recommendations for practise

The research presented above supports the feasibility and utility of monitoring recovery-stress balance and psychobiosocial states of road cyclists. Cycling presents particular challenges in the athletes' recovery-stress process, which is especially relevant for this type of sport (Taylor & Kress, 2006). There is a general consensus among researchers that the best way to deal with overtraining and underperformance is to prevent it from happening (e.g., Kellmann, 2010; Meeusen et al., 2013). Monitoring the current levels of recovery and stress has the advantage that problems may be detected before symptoms of underperformance occur. From an applied perspective, information derived from psychological measures, such the RESTQ-Sport, the POMS, and an individualised assessment of psychobiosocial states, can be used to implement behavioural, physical, and psychological strategies to facilitate the athletes' recovery and prevent dysfunctional stress, injuries, and illness. Individual optimal performance states are closely tied to individual optimal recovery behaviours such as rest, sleep, nutrition, regenerating activities (e.g., sport massage), distracting activities (e.g., reading a book), and interaction with others. According to Hanin (2002), psychobiosocial markers reflecting an athlete's idiosyncratic experiences are suggested to be sensitive and reliable indicators of optimal performance and optimal recovery. The performance-recovery process in sport needs to be viewed as a unit typified by a balanced and cyclical relationship between the recruitment, utilisation, and recovery of athletes' resources for successful and consistent performance.

Additional strategies to enhance performance and deal with exertion, fatigue, pain, and boredom can be used during the race. In particular, Stevinson and Biddle (1998) expanded Morgan and Pollock's (1977) initial distinction between associative (internal) and dissociative (external) attentional strategies to include task relevance. The four coping strategies deriving from this interaction involve (a) an internal focus of attention and task-relevant thoughts (e.g., physical sensations), (b) an external focus and task-relevant thoughts (e.g., pacing), (c) an internal focus and task irrelevant thoughts (e.g., daydreams), and (d) an external focus and task-irrelevant thoughts (e.g., scenery; for a review, see Brick, MacIntyre, & Campbell, 2014). In a recent study on a cycling task (Bertollo et al., 2015), both external (i.e., focusing attention on a metronome) and internal (e.g., focusing on pacing) strategies were effective, depending on an individual's preference. In conclusion, overall findings of the research carried out throughout the Girobio and other results of recent research add further support to the importance of identifying effective idiosyncratic strategies for both recovery and performance.

References

Achtziger, A., & Gollwitzer, P. M. (2008). Motivation and volition in the course of action. In J. Heckhausen & H. Heckhausen (Eds.), *Motivation and action* (pp. 275–299). New York, NY: Cambridge University Press.

Bertollo, M., di Fronso, S., Filho, E., Lamberti, V., Ripari, P., Reis, M. V., . . . Robazza, C. (2015). To focus or not to focus: Is attention on the core components of action beneficial for cycling performance? *The Sport Psychologist, 29,* 110–119.

Borg, G. (2001). Borg's range model and scales. *International Journal of Sport Psychology, 32,* 110–126.

Brick, N., MacIntyre, T., & Campbell, M. (2014). Attentional focus in endurance activity: New paradigms and future directions. *International Review of Sport and Exercise Psychology, 7,* 106–134.

di Fronso, S., Nakamura, F.Y., Bortoli, L., Robazza, C., & Bertollo, M. (2013). Stress and recovery balance in amateur basketball players: Differences by gender and preparation phase. *International Journal of Sports Physiology and Performance, 8,* 618–622.

Dupuy, O., Lussier, M., Fraser, S., Bherer, L., Audiffren, M., & Bosquet, L. (2014). Effect of overreaching on cognitive performance and related cardiac autonomic control. *Scandinavian Journal of Medicine and Science in Sports, 24,* 234–242.

Filho, E., di Fronso, S., Forzini, F., Agostini, T., Bortoli, L., Robazza, C., & Bertollo, M. (2013). Stress/recovery balance during the Girobio: Profile of highly trained road cyclists. *Sport Sciences for Health, 9,* 107–112.

Filho, E., di Fronso, S., Forzini, F., Murgia, M., Agostini, T., Bortoli, L., . . . & Bertollo, M. (2015). Athletic performance and recovery – stress factors in cycling: An ever changing balance. *European Journal of Sport Science, 15*, 671–680.

Gucciardi, D., & Gordon, S. (Eds.). (2011). *Mental toughness in sport: Developments in theory and research*. Oxon, UK: Routledge.

Halson, S. L., Bridge, M. W., Meeusen, R., Busschaert, B., Gleeson, M., Jones, D. A., & Jeukendrup, A. E. (2002). Time course of performance changes and fatigue markers during intensified training in trained cyclists. *Journal of Applied Physiology, 93*, 947–956.

Hanin, Y. L. (2002). Individually optimal recovery in sports: An application of the IZOF model. In M. Kellmann (Ed.), *Enhancing recovery: Preventing underperformance in athletes* (pp. 199–217). Champaign, IL: Human Kinetics.

Hanin, Y. L. (2007). Emotions in sport: Current issues and perspectives. In G. Tenenbaum & R. Eklund (Eds.), *Handbook of sport psychology* (3rd ed., pp. 31–58). Hoboken, NJ: Wiley.

Hanin, Y. L. (2010). Coping with anxiety in sport. In A. Nicholls (Ed.), *Coping in sport: Theory, methods, and related constructs* (pp. 159–175). New York, NY: Nova Science Publishers.

Jones, M. V., Lane, A. M., Bray, S. R., Uphill, M., & Catlin, J. (2005). Development and validation of the Sport Emotion Questionnaire. *Journal of Sport and Exercise Psychology, 27*, 407–431.

Kallus, K. W., & Kellmann, M. (2000). Burnout in athletes and coaches. In Y. L. Hanin (Ed.), *Emotions in sport* (pp. 209–230). Champaign, IL: Human Kinetics.

Kellmann, M. (2002). Underrecovery and overtraining: Different concepts – similar impact? In M. Kellmann (Ed.), *Enhancing recovery: Preventing underperformance in athletes* (pp. 3–24). Champaign, IL: Human Kinetics.

Kellmann, M. (2010). Preventing overtraining in athletes in high-intensity sports and stress/recovery monitoring. *Scandinavian Journal of Medicine and Science in Sports, 20*, 95–102.

Kellmann, M., Altenburg, D., Lormes, W., & Steinacker, J. M. (2001). Assessing stress and recovery during preparation for the World Championships in rowing. *The Sport Psychologist, 15*, 151–167.

Kellmann, M., & Kallus, K. W. (2001). *Recovery-Stress Questionnaire for Athletes: User manual*. Champaign, IL: Human Kinetics.

Kellmann, M., & Kallus, K. W. (2016). The Recovery-Stress Questionnaire for Athletes. In K. W. Kallus & M. Kellmann (Eds.), *The Recovery-Stress Questionnaires: User manual* (pp. 86–131). Frankfurt am Main: Pearson Assessment.

Lombardi, G., Lanteri, P., Fiorella, P. L., Simonetto, L., Impellizzeri, F. M., Bonifazi, M., . . . Locatelli, M. (2013). Comparison of the hematological profile of elite road cyclists during the 2010 and 2012 GiroBio ten-day stage races and relationships with final ranking. *PLoS One, 8*(4), e63092.

Marcora, S. M., Staiano, W., & Manning, V. (2009). Mental fatigue impairs physical performance in humans. *Journal of Applied Physiology, 106*, 857–864.

Matos, N. F., Winsley, R. J., & Williams, C. A. (2011). Prevalence of nonfunctional overreaching/overtraining in young English athletes. *Medicine and Science in Sports and Exercise, 43*, 1287–1294.

McNair, D. M., Lorr, M., & Droppleman, L. F. (1971). *Manual for the Profile of Mood States*. San Diego, CA: Educational and Industrial Testing Services.

Meeusen, R., Duclos, M., Foster, C., Fry, A., Gleeson, M., Nieman, D., . . . Urhausen, A. (2013). Prevention, diagnosis and treatment of the overtraining syndrome: Joint consensus statement of the European College of Sport Science (ECSS) and the American College of Sports Medicine (ACSM). *European Journal of Sport Science, 13*, 1–24.

Moran, A. (2011). Attention. In D. Collins, A. Button, & H. Richards (Eds.), *Performance psychology: A practitioner's guide* (pp. 319–335). Edinburgh, UK: Churchill Livingstone Elsevier.

Morgan, W. P., Costill, D. L., Flynn, M. G., Raglin, J. S., & O'Connor, P. J. (1988). Mood disturbance following increased training in swimmers. *Medicine and Science in Sports and Exercise, 20*, 408–414.

Morgan, W. P., & Pollock, M. L. (1977). Psychological characteristics of elite cyclers. *Annals of the New York Academy of Sciences, 301*, 382–403.

Murgia, M., Forzini, F., Filho, E., Di Fronso, S., Sors, F., Bertollo, M., & Agostini, T. (2016). How do mood states change in a multi-stage cycling competition? Comparing high and low performers. *Journal of Sports Medicine and Physical Fitness, 56*, 336–342.

Prapavessis, H. (2000). The POMS and sports performance: A review. *Journal of Applied Sport Psychology, 12*, 34–48.

Raglin, J. S. (2001). Psychological factors in sport performance: The Mental Health Model revisited. *Sports Medicine, 31*, 875–890.

Robazza, C., Bertollo, M., Ruiz, M. C., & Bortoli, L. (2016). Measuring psychobiosocial states in sport: Initial validation of a trait measure. *PLoS One, 11*(12), e0167448.

Robazza, C., & Bortoli, L. (2003). Intensity, idiosyncratic content and functional impact of performance-related emotions in athletes. *Journal of Sports Sciences, 21*, 171–189.

Robazza, C., Bortoli, L., & Gramaccioni, G. (2009). L'Inventario Psicologico della Prestazione Sportiva (IPPS-48) [The Sport Performance Psychological Inventory]. *Giornale Italiano di Psicologia dello Sport, 4*, 14–20.

Robazza, C., Pellizzari, M., & Hanin, Y. (2004). Emotion self-regulation and athletic performance: An application of the IZOF model. *Psychology of Sport and Exercise, 5*, 379–404.

Ruiz, M. C., Hanin, Y., & Robazza, C. (2016). Assessment of performance-related experiences: An individualized approach. *The Sport Psychologist, 30*, 201–218.

Ruiz, M. C., Raglin, J. S., & Hanin, Y. L. (2017). The individual zones of optimal functioning (IZOF) model (1978–2014): Historical overview of its development and use. *International Journal of Sport and Exercise Psychology, 15*, 41–63.

Saw, A. E., Main, L. C., & Gastin, P. B. (2016). Monitoring the athlete training response: Subjective self-reported measures trump commonly used objective measures: A systematic review. *British Journal of Sports Medicine, 50*, 281–291.

Stevinson, C. D., & Biddle, S. J. (1998). Cognitive orientations in marathon running and "hitting the wall". *British Journal of Sports Medicine, 32*, 229–234.

Taylor, J., & Kress, J. (2006). Psychology of cycling. In J. Dosil (Ed.), *The sport psychologist's handbook: A guide for sport-specific performance enhancement* (pp. 325–350). Chichester, UK: John Wiley & Sons.

Urhausen, A., Gabriel, H., & Kindermann, W. (1995). Blood hormones as markers of training stress and overtraining. *Sports Medicine, 20*, 251–276.

Watson, D., Clark, L. A., & Tellegen, A. (1988). Development and validation of brief measures of positive and negative affect: The PANAS scales. *Journal of Personality and Social Psychology, 54*, 1063–1070.

6
PSYCHOPHYSIOLOGICAL FEATURES OF SOCCER PLAYERS' RECOVERY-STRESS BALANCE DURING THE IN-SEASON COMPETITIVE PHASE

Maurizio Bertollo, Fabio Yuzo Nakamura, Laura Bortoli, and Claudio Robazza

Introduction

The relationship between training load, fatigue, and recovery-stress balance has received great attention in sports performance literature with special reference to preventing nonfunctional overreaching and overtraining (Meuseen et al., 2013), and reducing the risk of injuries (Soligard et al., 2016) and illness (Schwellnus et al., 2016). Recently, a consensus statement of the International Olympic Committee has defined training load as "the cumulative amount of stress placed on an individual from a single or multiple training sessions (structured or unstructured) over a period of time" (Soligard et al., 2016, Appendix A, p. 1). The combination of external loads and the relative internal responses can lead to fatigue and need of recovery (Halson, 2014). Therefore, monitoring both external load and internal response is important. Fatigue in athletes also derives from stressors in life outside of sports (Schwellnus et al., 2016). Therefore, both general and sport-related sources of stress can determine adaptive or maladaptive changes in the biological system leading to acute and/or chronic fatigue.

According to Soligard and colleagues (2016), "Fatigue is a tiredness resulting from mental or physical exertion or illness in sport, often manifested as failure to maintain the required or expected force (or power output)" (Appendix A, p. 3). A state of fatigue will essentially define the load an individual can tolerate before injury/illness risk increases (Jones, Griffiths, & Mellalieu, 2017). Findings in the current literature reinforce the notion that fatigue (mental and physical) is a natural psychobiological process reflected in physical, cognitive, and perceptual dimensions

(Enoka & Duchateau, 2016; Van Cutsem et al., 2017) and its acute phase is a fundamental stage of training (Morton, Fitz-Clarke, & Banister, 1990). The full return of the biological system to physical and psychological adaptive homeostasis is necessary for performance enhancement and effective training. Indeed, "Recovery is an inter-individual and intra-individual multi-level (e.g., psychological, physiological, social) process in time for the re-establishment of performance abilities. Recovery includes an action-oriented component, and self-initiated activities (proactive recovery), and can be systematically used to optimise situational conditions and to build up and refill personal resources and buffers" (Kellmann & Kallus, 2001, p. 22).

From this perspective, recovery-stress balance is a multidimensional phenomenon which requires a holistic psychophysiological approach to better understand and manage human behaviour. The understanding of psychological, physiological, biochemical, and behavioural components of human performance is expected to advance our knowledge of the recovery-stress balance. "The level of analysis in psychophysiology is not on isolated components of the body, but rather on organismic environmental transactions, with reference to both physical and sociocultural environments" (Cacioppo, Tassinary, & Berntson, 2007, p. 14).

Psychophysiology in sports has a long tradition of applications and investigations of the psychophysiological and behavioural features associated with optimal performance (Bertollo et al., 2013, 2016; Blumenstein & Tsung-Min Hung, 2016; Hatfield & Kerick, 2007; Hatfield & Landers, 1987; Wilson & Somers, 2011). For instance, a well-known application of performance optimisation in soccer players is the 'Milan Lab Mindroom' at AC Milan, which was later also applied at Chelsea FC, and expanded to include neuroscience applications with Real Madrid CF (Wilson, Peper, & Moss, 2006; Zaichkowsky, 2012). The common denominators of these applications with soccer players are the assessment of stress level through a protocol developed by Wilson (2006) and the teaching of self-regulation skills to athletes. Athletes were taught to relax and recover from fatigue as well as control physiological reactions to pressure situations. However, one limitation of this approach is poor ecological validity, given that the protocol is conducted in laboratory settings using non-sport-specific cognitive stimuli. A more ecological and informative psychophysiological approach to assess and monitor the multidimensional nature of recovery-stress balance should be rooted in the analysis of the full scope of human behaviour and its interaction with the environment. Therefore, measuring recovery-stress balance should include observations of kinematic data (e.g., GPS), muscular activity (e.g., EMG), cortical activity (e.g., EEG), and eye movements (e.g., eye tracker), as well as integrative physiological markers (e.g., hormones, ECG) and psychological data (e.g., rating of perceived exertion, psychobiosocial states).

To the best of our knowledge, this psychophysiological holistic approach has never been applied to the investigation of the recovery-stress balance. In daily practise, coaches mainly use cardiac-related indices (e.g., HR, HRR, HRV; Bellenger et al., 2016), biochemical indices (e.g., cortisol and testosterone; Kraemer et al., 2004) and psychological scales (e.g., Recovery-Stress Questionnaire for Athletes, i.e., RESTQ-Sport; Kellmann & Kallus, 2016). However, research on the interactions among different sources of information and their interpretation according to the *principle of converging evidence* (Stanovich, 2013) is missing.

Aligned with this view, we will briefly review the literature on the behavioural, physiological, psychological, and biochemical markers of recovery-stress balance of soccer players; and we will discuss the interactions among internal training load, recovery-stress balance, psychobiosocial states, hormones (cortisol and testosterone), autonomic nervous system indices, and central nervous system activity. We monitored these variables in a sample of professional soccer players during two months of the in-season competitive phase. A preliminary idiographic profile of a professional soccer player is discussed as an example. A better understanding of the ratio between one's resources (e.g., physical, mental, contextual) and demands (e.g., training load, social pressure) can inform intervention strategies intended to prevent dysfunctional overtraining and facilitate recovery.

Psychophysiological assessment of recovery-stress balance and training load

Training load can be assessed by means of external and internal parameters. The total distance, the distance covered at standardised speed zones, and the accelerometer-derived 'body load' are indicators of external load, which can be quantified using global positioning system technologies (Cummins, Orr, O'Connor, & West, 2013). Although the number of teams and athletes using GPS technologies has increased, a high level of technical expertise is required to operate and interpret the information. In addition, the financial cost of purchasing this technology precludes most teams from implementing it in training and competition.

The internal training load is reflected in the physiological and perceptual responses elicited by a given external load (Impellizzeri, Rampinini, & Marcora, 2005). Some individual characteristics (e.g., cardiorespiratory fitness) are regarded given the large inter-subject variation of internal training loads during group activities in team sports. Two principal methods to quantify the internal training load are based on heart rate (HR) and rating of perceived exertion (RPE) responses, namely, the training impulse (TRIMP) and session-rating of perceived exertion (sRPE). The TRIMP can be calculated based on the HR measured continuously during training or competition. However, it is important to note that HR-based methods have limitations in the quantification of very high-intensity activities (e.g., sprints) and exercise intensity during resistance training. The product of RPE (intensity) × duration (volume) has been named sRPE, and represents an alternative to HR-based methods to quantify internal training loads (Foster et al., 2001). This is considered the simplest method, and is probably the most widely used among individual athletes and teams. In team sports, sRPE has been found to be highly correlated with different TRIMP scores, and thus can be used in practical settings in place of HR-derived methods (Alexiou & Coutts, 2008).

One of the most relevant study paradigms to investigate the effects of excessive training loads on different markers of nonfunctional overreaching involves a deliberate increase of the external training load for a known time frame to quantify the resulting internal training load and its impact on biochemical, physiological, and psychological markers in the athletes. In a classic study by Coutts and Reaburn (2008), one group of male semi-professional rugby league players completed significantly greater training loads (21.6%), as measured by sRPE, compared to a 'normal' training group. As a result, the experimental group of players showed a progressive performance loss in a multistage fitness test throughout the six weeks of training intensification, and reduced maximal oxygen consumption (VO_2max). The performance recovery after tapering suggested the occurrence of overreaching during the intensification period. Among the multiple biochemical blood-borne markers, only glutamine to glutamate ratio was different between groups during the overloading period. Several other markers (e.g., testosterone and creatine kinase) increased in both groups, without being able to discriminate the occurrence of fatigue and overreaching. Of note, some scales of the RESTQ-Sport (Kellmann & Kallus, 2001, 2016; for a brief description see also this volume, Chapter 1 and Chapter 5) were sensitive to the training load intensification in these athletes. These findings suggest that psychological questionnaires are more sensitive than biochemical markers in the assessment of athletes' state resulting from training intensification. This conclusion has also been confirmed in other individual and team sports, including soccer (Faude, Steffen, Kellmann, & Meyer, 2014).

In one study of professional soccer players, blood samples were extensively monitored over six months (Heisterberg et al., 2013). Excessive physical strain phases were inferred from increased leucocytes and decreased lymphocytes, suggesting that immune system changes can reveal critical overloading periods in the team as a whole. Nevertheless, conclusions are limited by the absence of internal training load measures and by the lack of subjective assessments of fatigue. The authors suggest that their results do not indicate a severe danger of overreaching in the team. However, conducting analyses of individual players in this study may be warranted given the high inter-individual variability in blood-borne markers (Julian et al., 2017) and the fact that some athletes can suffer from symptoms of excessive match and training loads while their teammates are responding well (Flatt, Esco, Nakamura, & Plews, 2017).

In some studies, simple and non-invasive measures of HRV are combined with subjective ratings of well-being to detect players at risk for overreaching. Recently, several researchers have been using the ultra-short-term measurement of the log-transformed root mean square of successive R-R interval differences (lnRMSSD) to quantify, during several days per week, the activity of the autonomic nervous system on the sinus node (Pereira, Flatt, Ramirez-Campillo, Loturco, & Nakamura, 2016). This simple, 2-minute assessment recorded three to five days per week enabled the calculation of the weekly mean lnRMSSD ($lnRMSSD_{Weekly}$), together with the coefficient of variation ($lnRMSSD_{CV}$). Interestingly, those female soccer players who displayed a reduction in the $lnRMSSD_{Weekly}$ in the early phases of preparation showed reduced VO_2max (after 11 weeks of training), while players who augmented their $lnRMSSD_{Weekly}$ in the first three weeks of training had improvements in their VO$_2$max (Esco, Flatt, & Nakamura, 2016). In addition, higher lnRMSSD$_{CV}$ in female soccer players was associated with greater perceived fatigue and lower cardiorespiratory fitness – evidence that perturbations of the cardiac autonomic homeostasis can be linked to subjective measures and physical capacity (Flatt et al., 2017). Finally, it was shown that high lnRMSSD$_{Weekly}$ was associated with lower lnRMSSD$_{CV}$, suggesting that high vagal activity can protect athletes from the effects of overloading and fatigue (Nakamura et al., 2016). Importantly, HRV is influenced by anxiety and negative emotional states (Laborde, Raab, & Dosseville, 2013; Mateo, Blasco-Lafarga, Martínez-Navarro, Guzmán, & Zabala, 2012).

In-season recovery-stress monitoring of soccer players

We conducted a longitudinal cohort design to assess and monitor psychophysiological states and recovery-stress balance in elite professional soccer players. An idiosyncratic profile of a player is herein presented as an example to highlight the importance of a holistic psychophysiological approach, aligned with the *principle of converging evidence*, in the diagnosis and prevention of overreaching, overtraining, and injuries in athletes, as well as in modulating the weekly individual training load. Twenty-nine male professional players of an Italian soccer team in the second division were monitored during their training sessions (age 24.9 ± 5.3 years; height 178.6 ± 4.84 cm; weight 76 ± 5.07 kg). Data collection was included as part of the professional team's routine and players were frequently assessed across the season. These observations were used to individualise the training load within the weekly training program. The player presented here was 25 years old at the time of assessment (height 180, and weight 76).

The athletes were monitored for two months from November to January during the last competitive period of the first round. The RESTQ-Sport (Kellmann & Kallus, 2001) was administered to the athletes weekly on the day before the match. In the last metabolic session of the week, EEG (ANT system, 32 channels, Enschede, Netherlands) data were also collected immediately before and after the last training session. Moreover, four times per week – before and after training sessions – we collected: (a) HRV measures, obtained using a portable heart rate monitor (team Polar2®, Kempele, Finland) at a sampling of 1000 Hz, for 5 minutes; (b) saliva samples (Salivette©, Sarstedt, Verona, Italy) to assess cortisol and testosterone values; and (c) psychobiosocial state scores through a questionnaire (PBS; Robazza, Bertollo, Ruiz, & Bortoli, 2016). Furthermore, session RPE (Foster et al., 2001) was collected within 15–30 minutes after training sessions. Recovery-stress states were assessed using the RESTQ-Sport, a psychometric tool containing 76 items pertaining to 19 scales (for more details on its use, see this volume, Chapter 1).

EEG data were recorded for five minutes at rest, with eye closed, before and after the last training of the week (sampling frequency: 1024 Hz) from 32 scalp electrodes (waveguard™touch) positioned over the scalp according to the 10–20 system, using an eegosport TM amplifier (ANT, Enschede, Netherlands). EEG signals were recorded with common average reference. The ground electrode was positioned between Fpz and Fz, and the electrode impedance was kept below 10 kΩ. EEG data were off-line band-pass filtered between 0.3 and 40 Hz. Data were visually inspected, and those showing instrumental, ocular, and muscular artefacts were corrected using the artefact reject tool available in the ASA software (Eemagine, Berlin, Germany). Data epochs showing residual artefacts were excluded from further analysis. The Individual Alpha Peak Frequency (IAPF) was calculated based on the Klimesch's (1999) formula for specific gravity frequency between the frequency range of 7.5 to 12.5 over occipital and parietal areas. In our study, the IAPF was used to assess the level of fatigue according to the suggestion by Ng and Raveendran (2007) who showed that IAPF is reduced after physical exertion. However, more recently Gutmann and colleagues (2015) found an increase in IAPF after a bout of exhaustive exercise. The modulation of the IAPF following acute exercise is probably linked to exercise-induced activation of the brain's arousal mechanisms and is due to enhanced alertness during performance. For instance, in pain research it has been found that in healthy patients' noxious stimuli will acutely result in an increased IAPF (Nir, Sinai, Raz, Sprecher, & Yarnitsky, 2010), possibly reflecting a 'fight-or-flight' response. It can be speculated that this increase in IAPF serves to increase alertness in order to respond faster in threatening situations. However, when a threat becomes chronic in nature a slower IAPF is observed, which has also been demonstrated in burnout syndrome (Van Luijtelaar, Verbraak, Van den Bunt, Keijsers, & Arns, 2010). This modulation of IAFP may act as a 'gating function' to reduce the amount of information projected to the cortex in order to better cope with pain or with the information processing demands in burnout syndrome. Similarly, despite the feeling of tiredness, when the athlete is in a situation of overreaching he or she is still cognitively prepared to perform (increase in IAPF), whereas when his or her state shifts toward overtraining the IAPF should decrease.

Resting HRV was recorded half an hour prior to the daily training session (at approximately 14:30) and 15 minutes after the training session (at approximately 17:30). Athletes were assessed collectively to facilitate and shorten data acquisition. The players participated in approximately six training sessions per week consisting of two metabolic sessions, technical and tactical training (i.e., game-based training), exercises aimed at injury prevention (i.e., core training, exercises on unstable surfaces), plyometric and sprinting exercises during warm-up, and two strength-power training sessions (i.e., jump squat, leg press, and deadlift exercises). The total duration of technical and tactical training was 450 ± 90 minutes per week, while the strength/power training sessions lasted ≈120 minutes per week – 1. The athletes were familiar with the monitoring and testing procedures due to routine assessments adopted by the technical and conditioning staff.

The internal training load was recorded using the sRPE method (Foster et al., 2001). Approximately 15 minutes following the completion of every training session, the players were required to report the intensity of the whole session by means of a 100-point rating Borg's scale of perceived exertion following the indication by Fanchini and colleagues (2016). This value was multiplied by the respective total duration of each training session. The psychobiosocial state questionnaire was also administered immediately before RPE. The scale consists of 20 rows of 80 adjectives (from three to six per row) to assess eight functional and dysfunctional state modalities (i.e., affective, cognitive, motivational, volitional, bodily-somatic, motor-behavioural, operational, and communicative; for more details, see this volume, Chapter 5). All assessments were performed by the team's fitness coach with the support of a trained student who was obtaining a Master's Degree in sport science.

Findings showed high levels of inter-individual variability in the rating of perceived exertion for each training session ($M = 45 \pm 20$), given the same external training load (e.g., vigorous physical activity; >VT2) and the same GPS values (e.g., percentage at different threshold of TDC). As a consequence, high variability was also found in sRPE. However, the intra-individual variability can be ascribed to the different training load administered by the coaches during different days, and the individual differences in perception of load based on events in the athletes' personal daily life. These results confirm the importance of an idiographic approach to monitoring temporal trends in stress and recovery indices before and after training sessions. Table 6.1 contains the measures of the player during the eight weeks of monitoring. A comparison among the pre-post training data across the eight weeks provides useful information about the player's recovery level. Findings suggest that functional and/or dysfunctional profiles are not associated with a specific

TABLE 6.1 Idiosyncratic measures of a player. The values are the weekly means of each measure.

	week 1	week 2	week 3	week 4	week 5	week 6	week 7	week 8
sRPE (CR100)	5850	5500	6000	5350	6100	5800	5100	3500
Functional PBSS pre	3.1	3.3	2.5	2.0	2.5	3.0	3.3	3.0
Functional PBSS post	2.9	2.1	3.3	2.5	1.8	2.9	3.5	3.1
Dysfunctional PBSS pre	0.4	0.6	0.9	0.9	0.5	0.8	0.8	0.7
Dysfunctional PBSS post	0.4	0.1	0.3	1.3	0.9	0.4	0.7	0.9
(Ln)SDNN pre	4.0	4.1	4.5	3.9	4.2	4.5	4.2	3.6
(Ln)SDNN post	3.8	3.5	3.0	3.0	3.2	3.4	3.8	3.3
(Ln)RMSSD pre	3.8	3.4	3.7	3.6	3.9	3.4	3.9	4.0
(Ln)RMSSD post	2.7	2.2	2.0	2.0	2.6	2.2	2.2	2.9
(Ln)Cortisol pre	7.4	7.9	7.7	8.2	7.6	8.0	7.6	7.1
(Ln)Cortisol post	8.1	8.6	7.4	7.5	7.3	8.8	7.5	7.0
(Ln)Testosterone pre	4.2	4.3	4.0	4.3	4.3	4.2	3.9	4.4
(Ln)Testosterone post	4.5	4.7	4.3	4.5	4.3	4.7	4.0	4.3
IAFP pre	10.4	10.4	10.3	10.5	10.7	10.3	10.4	10.4
IAFP post	10.7	10.9	11.1	11.1	11.0	11.1	11.0	10.6

Note. sRPE = session-rating of perceived exertion; (Ln) = natural logarithmic; PBSS = psychobiosocial states; SDNN = standard deviation of consecutive RR intervals; RMSSD = root mean square of successive R-R interval differences; IAFP = individual alpha frequency peak

Soccer players' recovery-stress balance **81**

physiological, psychological, or biochemical index, rather the interpretation of the recovery-stress balance requires a more integrated psychophysiological assessment.

Moreover, the comparison of the pre-post training measures provides information about the acute stress profile and the athlete's response to the training load. Figure 6.1 shows the difference between pre- and post-training sessions and the player's day-by-day responses to the workload during one week. The pre-post comparison is strictly related to sport-burden issues. Finally, comparisons between the measures before and after the training session (in particular, in response to the same external training load) can provide an estimate of the non-sport burden. For instance, during the fifth week the IAFP was higher before training, likely indicating the readiness of the Central Nervous System to keep engagement despite physical tiredness (see Guttmann et al., 2015). The other physiological measures were comparable with the values from other weeks. The comparison and/or convergence of these measures with the RESTQ-Sport profile can provide more holistic

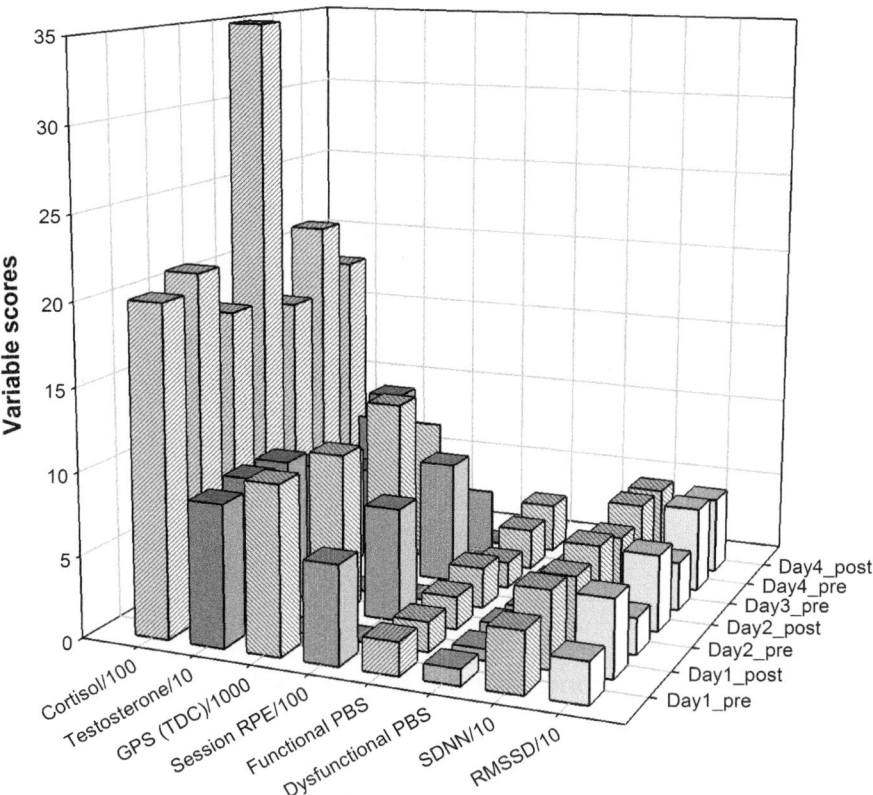

FIGURE 6.1 Acute stress profile. Day-by-day psychological, biochemical, and physiological measures of stress during one week.

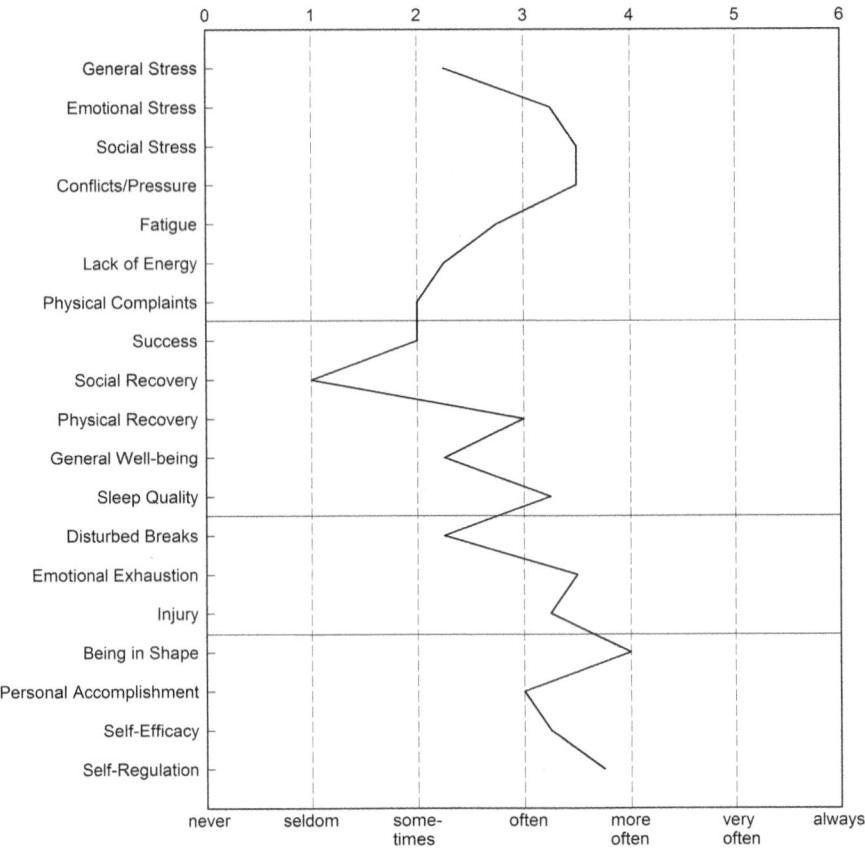

FIGURE 6.2 RESTQ-Sport profile of the fifth week for the player under investigation.

information on the recovery–stress balance. The RESTQ-Sport profile of the player at the end of the week portrayed in Figure 6.2 clearly shows that some degrees of non-sport burden contributed to the recovery-stress balance during the week in this athlete (i.e., high emotional and social stress, and low social recovery).

Conclusion and recommendations for practise

Recovery–stress balance is a multidimensional phenomenon that needs to be monitored in a multimodal way before and after each training session. Each player shows specific and individual responses to training loads that are unique to that player. Comparing the pre-post responses to training sessions using biochemical, physiological, psychological, and behavioural assessments enables the identification of the athlete's idiosyncratic acute stress profile as well as his or her recovery profile.

When evidence from a wide range of tests, information, and indices – which may be vulnerable to measurement error or technical limitations when viewed alone – points in a similar direction, then the evidence has converged and a diagnosis or interpretation is possible. Only recently some authors have suggested combining multiple measures in applied settings (Thorpe et al., 2015) based on the empirical evidence that there is low correlation between subjective and objective measures (Saw, Main, & Gastin, 2016).

In clinical settings, as well as in practical settings, it is important to apply the *principle of converging evidence* (Stanovich, 2013) because of the high 'fuzzy factor' resulting from the complexity of human behaviour. The evaluation of recovery-stress balance is not an exception. Furthermore, in the case of recovery-stress balance there is a need not only to use converging evidence from many methodologies and experimental techniques but also to quantify the different contributions of sport and non-sport stressors. In this case, instruments like the RESTQ-Sport can add specific information.

Future research should further explore individual differences in athletes' responses to training, recovery, and stress, and possibly focus on the development of a simple, integrated, and cost-effective 'recovery index' combining behavioural, psychological, physiological, and biochemical measures. This index is intended to offer a comprehensive picture of the recovery-stress balance for a given individual, and provide practitioners with applied indications to enhance the recovery process.

Acknowledgement

We thank the technical staff and the players of Pescara soccer team, and Lorenzo Paravani and Selenia di Fronso for data collection, screening, and organisation.

References

Alexiou, H., & Coutts, A. J. (2008). A comparison of methods used for quantifying internal training load in women soccer players. *International Journal of Sports Physiology and Performance, 3*, 320–330.

Bellenger, C. R., Fuller, J. T., Thomson, R. L., Davison, K., Robertson, E. Y., & Buckley, J. D. (2016). Monitoring athletic training status through autonomic heart rate regulation: A systematic review and meta-analysis. *Sports Medicine, 46*, 1461–1486.

Bertollo, M., Bortoli, L., Gramaccioni, G., Hanin, Y., Comani, S., & Robazza, C. (2013). Behavioural and psychophysiological correlates of athletic performance: A test of the multi-action plan model. *Applied Psychophysiology Biofeedback, 38*, 91–99.

Bertollo, M., Di Fronso, S., Filho, E., Conforto, S., Schmid, M., Bortoli, L., . . . Robazza, C. (2016). Proficient brain for optimal performance: The MAP model perspective. *PeerJ, 4*, e2082.

Blumenstein, B., & Tsung-Min Hung, E. (2016). Biofeedback in sport. In R. J. Schinke, K. R. McGannon, & B. Smith (Eds.), *Routledge international handbook of sport psychology* (pp. 429–438). New York, NY: Routledge.

Cacioppo, J. T., Tassinary, L. G., & Berntson, G. G. (2007). Psychophysiological science: Interdisciplinary approaches to classic questions about the mind. In J. T. Cacioppo, L. G.

Tassinary, & G. G. Berntson (Eds.), *Handbook of psychophysiology* (pp. 13–16). New York, NJ: Cambridge University Press.

Coutts, A. J., & Reaburn, P. (2008). Monitoring changes in rugby league players perceived stress and recovery during intensified training. *Perceptual and Motor Skills, 106*, 904–916.

Cummins, C., Orr, R., O'Connor, H., & West, C. (2013). Global positioning systems (GPS) and microtechnology sensors in team sports: A systematic review. *Sports Medicine, 43*, 1025–1042.

Enoka, R. M., & Duchateau, J. (2016). Translating fatigue to human performance. *Medicine and Science in Sports and Exercise, 48*, 2228–2238.

Esco, M. R., Flatt, A. A., & Nakamura, F. Y. (2016). Initial weekly HRV response is related to the prospective change in VO_2max in female soccer players. *International Journal of Sports Medicine, 37*, 436–441.

Fanchini, M., Ferraresi, I., Modena, R., Schena, F., Coutts, A. J., & Impellizzeri, F. M. (2016). Use of CR100 scale for session-RPE in soccer and interchangeability with CR10. *International Journal of Sports Physiology and Performance, 11*, 388–392.

Faude, O., Steffen, A., Kellmann, M., & Meyer, T. (2014). The effect of short-term interval training during the competitive season on physical fitness and signs of fatigue: A crossover trial in high-level youth football players. *International Journal of Sports Physiology and Performance, 9*, 936–944.

Flatt, A. A., Esco, M. R., Nakamura, F. Y., & Plews, D. J. (2017). Interpreting daily heart rate variability changes in collegiate female soccer players. *Journal of Sports Medicine and Physical Fitness, 57*, 907–915.

Foster, C., Florhaug, J. A., Franklin, J., Gottschall, L., Hrovatin, L. A., Parker, S., . . . Dodge, C. (2001). A new approach to monitoring exercise training. *Journal of Strength and Conditioning Research, 15*, 109–115.

Gutmann, B., Mierau, A., Hülsdünker, T., Hildebrand, C., Przyklenk, A., Hollmann, W., & Strüder, H. K. (2015). Effects of physical exercise on individual resting state EEG alpha peak frequency. *Neural Plasticity*. Article ID 717312. doi:10.1155/2015/717312

Halson, S. L. (2014). Monitoring training load to understand fatigue in athletes. *Sports Medicine, 44*(Suppl. 2), S139–S147.

Hatfield, B. D., & Kerick, S. E. (2007). The psychology of superior sport performance: A cognitive and affective neuroscience perspective. In G. Tenenbaum & R. C. Eklund (Eds.), *Handbook of sport psychology* (pp. 84–109). Hoboken, NJ: Wiley.

Hatfield, B. D., & Landers, D. M. (1987). Psychophysiology in exercise and sport research: An overview. *Exercise and Sport Science Reviews, 15*, 351–388.

Heisterberg, M. F., Fahrenkrug, J., Krustrup, P., Storskov, A., Kjær, M., & Andersen, J. L. (2013). Extensive monitoring through multiple blood samples in professional soccer players. *Journal of Strength and Conditioning Research, 27*, 1260–1271.

Impellizzeri, F. M., Rampinini, E., & Marcora, S. M. (2005). Physiological assessment of aerobic training in soccer. *Journal of Sports Sciences, 23*, 583–592.

Jones, C. M., Griffiths, P. C., & Mellalieu, S. D. (2017). Training load and fatigue marker associations with injury and illness: A systematic review of longitudinal studies. *Sports Medicine, 47*, 943–974.

Julian, R., Meyer, T., Fullagar, H., Skorski, S., Pfeiffer, M., Kellmann, M., . . . Hecksteden, A. (2017). Individual patterns in blood-borne indicators of fatigue – trait or chance. *Journal of Strength and Conditioning Research, 31*, 608–619.

Kellmann, M., & Kallus, K. W. (2001). *Recovery-Stress Questionnaire for Athletes: User manual.* Champaign, IL: Human Kinetics.

Kellmann, M., & Kallus, K. W. (2016). The Recovery-Stress Questionnaire for Athletes. In K. W. Kallus & M. Kellmann (Eds.), *The Recovery-Stress Questionnaires: User manual* (pp. 86–131). Frankfurt am Main: Pearson Assessment.

Klimesch, W. (1999). EEG alpha and theta oscillations reflect cognitive and memory performance: A review and analysis. *Brain Research Reviews, 29*, 169–195.

Kraemer, W. J., French, D. N., Paxton, N. J., Häkkinen, K., Volek, J. S., Sebastianelli, W. J., . . . Knuttgen, H. G. (2004). Changes in exercise performance and hormonal concentrations over a big ten soccer season in starters and nonstarters. *Journal of Strength and Conditioning Research, 18*, 121–128.

Laborde, S., Raab, M., & Dosseville, F. (2013). Emotions and performance: Valuable insights from the sports domain. In C. Mohiyeddini, M. Eysenck, & S. Bauer (Eds.), *Handbook of psychology of emotions: Recent theoretical perspectives and novel empirical findings* (Vol. 1, pp. 325–358). New York, NY: Nova Publisher.

Mateo, M., Blasco-Lafarga, C., Martínez-Navarro, I., Guzmán, J. F., & Zabala, M. (2012). Heart rate variability and pre-competitive anxiety in BMX discipline. *European Journal of Applied Physiology, 112*, 113–123.

Meeusen, R., Duclos, M., Foster, C., Fry, A., Gleeson, M., Nieman, D., . . . Urhausen, A. (2013). Prevention, diagnosis and treatment of the overtraining syndrome: Joint consensus statement of the European College of Sport Science (ECSS) and the American College of Sports Medicine (ACSM). *European Journal of Sport Science, 13*, 1–24.

Morton, R. H., Fitz-Clarke, J. R., & Banister, E. W. (1990). Modeling human performance in running. *Journal of Applied Physiology, 69*, 1171–1177.

Nakamura, F. Y., Pereira, L. A., Rabelo, F. N., Flatt, A. A., Esco, M. R., Bertollo, M., & Loturco, I. (2016). Monitoring weekly heart rate variability in futsal players during the preseason: The importance of maintaining high vagal activity. *Journal of Sports Sciences, 34*, 2262–2268.

Ng, S. C., & Raveendran, P. (2007). EEG peak alpha frequency as an indicator for physical fatigue. In T. Jarm, P. Kramar, & A. Zupanic (Eds.), *11th Mediterranean conference on medical and biomedical engineering and computing 2007: MEDICON 2007, 26–30 June 2007, Ljubljana, Slovenia* (pp. 517–520). Berlin: Springer.

Nir, R., Sinai, A., Raz, E., Sprecher, E., & Yarnitsky, D. (2010). Pain assessment by continuous EEG: Association between subjective perception of tonic pain and peak frequency of alpha oscillations during stimulation and at rest. *Brain Research, 1344*, 77–86.

Pereira, L. A., Flatt, A. A., Ramirez-Campillo, R., Loturco, I., & Nakamura, F. Y. (2016). Assessing shortened field-based heart-rate-variability-data acquisition in team-sport athletes. *International Journal of Sports Physiology and Performance, 11*, 154–158.

Robazza, C., Bertollo, M., Ruiz, M. C., & Bortoli, L. (2016). Measuring psychobiosocial states in sport: Initial validation of a trait measure. *PLoS One, 11*(12), e0167448.

Saw, A. E., Main, L. C., & Gastin, P. B. (2016). Monitoring the athlete training response: Subjective self-reported measures trump commonly used objective measures: A systematic review. *British Journal of Sports Medicine, 50*, 281–291.

Schwellnus, M., Soligard, T., Alonso, J.-M., Bahr, R., Clarsen, B., Dijkstra, H. P., . . . Engebretsen, L. (2016). How much is too much? (Part 2) International Olympic Committee consensus statement on load in sport and risk of illness. *British Journal of Sports Medicine, 50*, 1043–1052.

Soligard, T., Schwellnus, M., Alonso, J.-M., Bahr, R., Clarsen, B., Dijkstra, H. P., . . . Engebretsen, L. (2016). How much is too much? (Part 1) International Olympic Committee consensus statement on load in sport and risk of injury. *British Journal of Sports Medicine, 50*, 1030–1041.

Stanovich, K. E. (2013). *How to think straight about psychology* (10th ed.). New York, NY: Pearson.

Thorpe, R. T., Strudwick, A. J., Buchheit, M., Atkinson, G., Drust, B., & Gregson, W. (2015). Monitoring fatigue during the in-season competitive phase in elite soccer players. *International Journal of Sports Physiology and Performance, 10*, 958–964.

Van Cutsem, J., Marcora, S., De Pauw, K., Bailey, S., Meeusen, R., & Roelands, B. (2017). The effects of mental fatigue on physical performance: A systematic review. *Sports Medicine, 47*, 1569–1588.

Van Luijtelaar, G., Verbraak, M., Van Den Bunt, M., Keijsers, G., & Arns, M. (2010). EEG findings in burnout patients. *Journal of Neuropsychiatry and Clinical Neurosciences, 22*, 208–217.

Wilson, V. E., Peper, E., & Moss, D. (2006). "The mind room" in Italian soccer training: The use of biofeedback and neurofeedback for optimum performance. *Biofeedback, 34*, 79–81.

Wilson, V. S. (2006). *Optimizing performance and health suite*. Amersfoort, Netherlands: Biofeedback Foundation of Europe.

Wilson, V. S., & Somers, K. (2011). Psychophysiological assessment and training with athletes. Knowing and managing your mind and body. In B. Strack, M. Linden, & V. S. Wilson (Eds.), *Biofeedback and neurofeedback applications in sport psychology* (pp. 45–88). Wheat Ridge, CO: American Association Psychophysiology & Biofeedback.

Zaichkowsky, L. (2012). Psychophysiology and neuroscience in sport: Introduction to the special issue. *Journal of Clinical Sport Psychology, 6*, 1–5.

7
MANAGING THE TRAINING LOAD OF OVERREACHED ATHLETES

Insights from the detraining and tapering literature

Laurent Bosquet, Nicolas Berryman, and Iñigo Mujika

Introduction

One of the numerous challenges for coaches and sport scientists is the early detection of an abnormal fatigue, in order to adjust the training load and prevent nonfunctional overreaching and/or the overtraining syndrome. In the last three decades, a significant effort has been made by the sport science community to identify valid markers of excessive overreaching and to find ways to best use them in the follow-up of athletes. As a consequence, we have much more information at this moment than we had in the nineties of the last century about the interest and limits of many cardiovascular, cognitive, endocrine, immune, metabolic or psychological markers (Meeusen et al., 2013). Sports scientists have also developed monitoring systems using simple statistics like a Z-score or the magnitude of difference that allow a better decision-making process (Batterham & Hopkins, 2006). However, in spite of this improvement in our knowledge and also in our capacity to translate it into practical tools, there are still a lot of athletes concerned by excessive overreaching, which affects approximately 10% of endurance athletes during a competitive season (Raglin & Wilson, 2000) and 30% during a career, whatever the sport (Kenttä, Hassmén, & Raglin, 2001; Meeusen et al., 2013; Raglin, Sawamura, Alexiou, Hassmén, & Kenttä, 2000).

Unfortunately, we must recognise that little is known about the way to manage the situation once overreaching has been diagnosed. The coach could of course continue with the same approach and maintain a training overload. This decision relies on the probability that the athlete will finally manage to cope with this fatigue and adapt to reach a higher level of fitness and performance. Such an approach is probably very efficient when it works, but the probability is very low.

Bosquet, L., Berryman, N., & Mujika, I. (2018). Managing the training load of overreached athletes: Insights from the detraining and tapering literature. In M. Kellmann & J. Beckmann (Eds.), *Sport, Recovery, and Performance: Interdisciplinary Insights* (pp. 87–107). Abingdon: Routledge.

The completely opposite approach would be training cessation. It is obvious that this strategy will be efficient to decrease the level of fatigue. Unfortunately, it will also decrease the level of physical fitness, thus leading to detraining (Mujika & Padilla, 2000a, 2000b). There are many other strategies between these two ends of the training load continuum, most of them consisting in adjusting the training load to the level of fatigue displayed by the athlete.

What are the consequences of total training cessation on the parameters of physical fitness? Should we decrease training intensity or keep it constant but decrease training volume? If so, according to which pattern and for what duration? The present chapter addresses these important questions for the coach when he or she has to design the recovery process of an overreached athlete. In the first part we present the effects of training cessation on the physiological parameters involved in performance, and in the second part we present the general principles that should be followed to decrease the level of fatigue while maintaining physical fitness. The general idea is to provide coaches and sport scientists with theoretical data that will help them in their decision-making process.

Effects of training cessation on metabolism and the cardiovascular system

Since the classic work of Di Prampero, Atchou, Bruckner, and Moia (1986), it is generally considered that endurance performance represents a complex interplay between several physiological factors, including maximal oxygen uptake ($\dot{V}O_2$max), aerobic endurance (AE) and the energy cost of locomotion (Cr).

Maximal oxygen uptake

Maximal oxygen uptake represents the maximal amount of oxygen that can be used at the cellular level for the entire body. It represents the upper limit of the cardiorespiratory system and has long been considered an important determinant of endurance performance (Saltin & Astrand, 1967). According to the Fick principle, any alteration in $\dot{V}O_2$max is the consequence of a modification of maximal cardiac output ($\dot{Q}$max) and/or maximal arteriovenous difference in oxygen (a $- \bar{v}DO_2$max) (Astrand, Rodahl, Dahl, & Straamme, 2003). It is generally accepted that the largest part of the training-induced increase in $\dot{V}O_2$max results from an increase in blood volume, stroke volume, and ultimately $\dot{Q}$max. Nevertheless, the increase in a $- \bar{v}DO_2$max, which results from a more effective distribution of arterial blood from inactive to active muscles, together with a greater oxygen extraction and utilisation capacity by these muscles, also plays an important role in cardiorespiratory adaptations to endurance training. Coyle et al. (1984) studied the effects of 12, 21, 56, and 84 days of training cessation on $\dot{V}O_2$max and its determinants in seven well-trained cyclists. The main results are summarised in Figure 7.1. They observed a ~15% decrease in $\dot{V}O_2$max that followed roughly an exponential kinetics (i.e., a fast decrease at the beginning, followed by a slower rate of decline afterwards).

Very interestingly, there seems to be a time sequence in the physiological mechanisms underlying this loss of adaptation. During a first phase lasting 21 to 28 days, a $- \overline{v}DO_2$max was maintained, suggesting that the decrease in $\dot{V}O_2$max was mainly a consequence of a decrease in oxygen delivery to the muscles. In fact, Coyle, Martin, Bloomfield, Lowry, and Holloszy (1985) reported a rapid decrease in $\dot{Q}$max (~8%) that reached a plateau after 21 to 28 days of training cessation. This loss of adaptation resulted from an important drop in maximal stroke volume (~11%), which was partly compensated for by a ~5% increase in maximal heart rate. The rapid decrease in blood volume after the first few days of training cessation observed in several studies is expected to play a key role in the cascade of events leading to the decrease in $\dot{Q}$max (Coyle, Hemmert, & Coggan, 1986; Cullinane, Sady, Vadeboncoeur, Burke, & Thompson, 1986; Houmard et al., 1992). Once this first 'circulatory detraining' phase is completed, the ongoing decrease in $\dot{V}O_2$max is now the consequence of a continuous decrease in a $- \overline{v}DO_2$max (~9%; Figure 7.1).

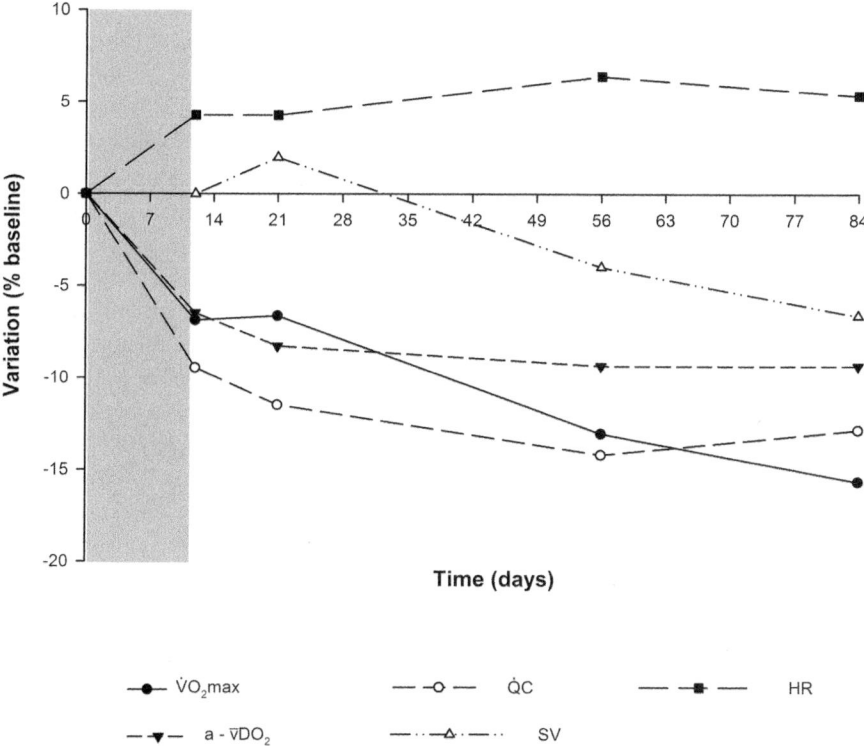

FIGURE 7.1 Effect of training cessation on the physiological determinants of maximal oxygen uptake ($\dot{V}O_2$max). $\dot{Q}$c: Cardiac output; a $- \overline{v}DO_2$: Arteriovenous difference in oxygen; SV: Stroke volume; HR: Heart rate. The shaded part indicates that the exact kinetics of disadaptation is not known in this time frame.

Adapted from Bosquet and Mujika (2012).

Considering that capillary density did not decline during the 84 days of training cessation, this alteration is likely to be the consequence of a decrease in muscle mitochondrial density or other factors such as a reduction in muscle blood flow or capillary transit time (Coyle et al., 1984). In summary, these results suggest the existence of two distinct phases in the physiological mechanisms underlying the continuous decrease in $\dot{V}O_2$max that is observed in well-trained endurance athletes once they stop training. During a first phase lasting 21 to 28 days, the decrease in $\dot{V}O_2$max is mainly the consequence of a loss of central adaptation (i.e., cardiovascular), as shown by a drop in $\dot{Q}$max, while it is peripheral (i.e., specific to the trained muscles) afterwards.

Aerobic endurance

Aerobic endurance represents the capacity to sustain a high fraction of $\dot{V}O_2$max throughout the entire effort duration (Bosquet, Léger, & Legros, 2002). Aerobic endurance is independent from $\dot{V}O_2$max, since two individuals with the same $\dot{V}O_2$max are not necessarily able to sustain the same fraction of $\dot{V}O_2$max for a given effort duration (Peronnet & Thibault, 1989). Both factors contribute to set exercise $\dot{V}O_2$, which is considered an important determinant of endurance performance. In fact, the higher the exercise $\dot{V}O_2$, the higher the energy provision in the form of ATP resynthesis rate. Although physiological mechanisms involved in AE are not fully understood, the capacity to sustain a high fraction of $\dot{V}O_2$max for a given duration has been associated with a combination of several factors, including a high percentage of type I muscle fibres, the capacity to store large amounts of muscle and/or liver glycogen, a high activity of mitochondrial enzymes, and the capacity to spare carbohydrate by using more fatty acids as energy substrate (Bosquet et al., 2002). It is well established that endurance training results in an increased percentage of type I muscle fibres (Pette, 1984). It is worth noting, however, that this progressive shift requires a significant period of time to take place and the magnitude of change is often small (Carter, Rennie, Hamilton, & Tarnopolsky, 2001; Pette, 1984). As expected, the effect of training cessation on muscle fibre distribution depends on the duration of the period of inactivity (Mujika & Padilla, 2001). While short-term training cessation (i.e., three weeks or less) is not enough to induce any changes (Hortobagyi et al., 1993; Houston, Bentzen, & Larsen, 1979), long term inactivity periods (up to several years) have been associated with a progressive return to initial muscle fibre distribution (Coyle et al., 1984; Larsson & Ansved, 1985).

Non-protein respiratory exchange ratio (RER) is commonly used to estimate the respective contribution of fatty acids and glucose to energy provision (Peronnet & Massicotte, 1991). Endurance training has long been associated with a reduced RER at both maximal and submaximal exercise intensities, thus suggesting a reduced reliance on glucose for energy production. Training cessation results in a rapid increase in RER that appears to reach a plateau within 14 days (Coyle et al., 1985; Drinkwater & Horvath, 1972; Houmard et al., 1992; Madsen, Pedersen,

Djurhuus, & Klitgaard, 1993; Mikines, Sonne, Tronier, & Galbo, 1989; Moore et al., 1987), as well as a rapid decrease in muscle glycogen stores (up to 20% within one week of bed rest or training cessation) (Costill et al., 1985; Mikines et al., 1989). The rapid decrease in the glucose transporter protein GLUT-4 concentration reported after six to ten days of training cessation (Vukovich et al., 1996), together with the important drop of glycogen synthase activity after just five days without training (Mikines et al., 1989) is thought to play a major role in this process (Mujika & Padilla, 2000a, 2000b).

Endurance training increases the number and size of the muscle fibre mitochondria, as well as the activity of oxidative enzymes (Abernethy, Thayer, & Taylor, 1990). One of the main characteristics of muscular detraining is an important decrease of this activity (Mujika & Padilla, 2001). Coyle et al. (1984, 1985) reported that citrate synthase activity declined by 23% during the first three weeks of training cessation in endurance trained athletes, by 23% again from the fourth to the eighth week and stabilised thereafter. Succinate dehydrogenase and malate dehydrogenase followed the same pattern of disadaptation. Similar results have been observed in runners (Houmard et al., 1992; Houston et al., 1979), triathletes (McCoy, Proietto, & Hargreaves, 1994) or soccer players (Amigo, Cadefau, Ferrer, Tarrados, & Cusso, 1998). Simsolo, Ong, and Kern (1993) also observed a large reduction of muscle lipoprotein lipase activity after two weeks of training cessation in 16 endurance athletes, which undoubtedly hampered the capacity to spare carbohydrate by using more fatty acids as energy substrate.

The lactate concentration for a given submaximal exercise intensity is one of the numerous methods used to determine AE (Bosquet et al., 2002). The lower its concentration, the better the AE. Considering the short- and long-term loss of adaptation that affect some of the physiological factors underlying AE, it is expected that this important determinant of endurance performance is altered by training cessation. In fact, blood lactate concentration increases exponentially with the duration of training cessation suggesting that aerobic endurance decreases rapidly when the training process is interrupted (Coyle et al., 1985; Mikines et al., 1989; Neufer, Costill, Fielding, Flynn, & Kirwann, 1987). Although a steady state value is reached around 21 to 28 days, one can expect a further decrease in AE that results from the progressive decrease of type I muscle fibres (Coyle et al., 1984; Larsson & Ansved, 1985). In summary, AE decreases very rapidly once training ceases, most probably due to metabolic reasons. An additional and delayed decrease is also possible when the duration of training cessation is long enough to alter muscle fibre distribution.

Energy cost of locomotion

The energy cost of locomotion represents the energy demand to move at a given submaximal power output or speed. The lower the Cr, especially when body mass is accounted for such as in running, the lower the energy expenditure to move at a given velocity. Factors affecting Cr are numerous and have been thoroughly reviewed by Saunders, Pyne, Telford, and Hawley (2004). Some of them are not changeable (e.g., height), while others can be manipulated (e.g., stride biomechanics, strength, elastic store-recoil capacity). Numerous interventions such as plyometric (Berryman, Maurel, & Bosquet, 2010) or high-intensity interval training (Saunders et al., 2004) are effective to decrease Cr and improve performance. In addition to $\dot{V}O_2$max and its determinants, Coyle et al. (1985) also examined the response to submaximal intensity exercise after 12, 21, 56, and 84 days of training cessation. Interestingly, the $\dot{V}O_2$ response to the same absolute intensity remained stable during this period, suggesting that the energy required to develop this power output was not affected by the lack of training. This is in agreement with the finding by Houmard et al. (1992) that Cr was not altered by a 14-day training cessation period in 12 distance runners. However, it is important to keep in mind that although the oxygen demand remains stable, the predominant metabolic pathways used by the subjects to match this energy demand changed significantly over time, since the RER increased linearly with the duration of training cessation (from 0.93 ± 0.01 at baseline to 1.00 ± 0.01 at day 84, corresponding to a ~8% difference). Considering the decrease in $\dot{V}O_2$max we already discussed, the relative intensity of this power output increased with the duration of training cessation from 74 ± 2% at baseline to 90 ± 3% at day 84 (~22% difference). As a consequence, perceived exertion logically increased from 12.3 ± 0.4 at baseline to 17.1 ± 0.4 at day 84 (~39% difference). In view of the increase in RER and the likely concomitant decrease in glycogen stores (see the preceding section), one can easily hypothesise that although Cr is not affected, time to exhaustion at a given intensity is significantly altered. In summary, the oxygen uptake required to run at a given speed does not appear to be altered by training cessation of up to 84 days. However, the concomitant increase in RER and decrease in $\dot{V}O_2$max result in a decreased exercise tolerance at a given speed, since it corresponds to a higher relative intensity and more glucose is needed for ATP resynthesis while the glycogen stores are markedly decreased.

Effects of training cessation on the neuromuscular system

Muscular strength is a major determinant of sport performance, both in explosive (Delecluse, 1997) and long-duration events (Saunders et al., 2004). The capacity of the skeletal muscle to generate a high level of force is a complex interplay between several factors, including muscle fibre type (Gollnick & Matoba, 1984), muscle cross-sectional area (Jones, Bishop, Woods, & Green, 2008), muscle architecture (Aagaard et al., 2001), and neural drive to the muscle (Gandevia, 2001). The relative weight of these factors is mainly determined by the expression of force, whether we are talking about maximal force, maximal power, or submaximal force. Like cardiovascular and metabolic training-induced adaptations, neuromuscular adaptations are transitory and may disappear when training ceases. The question is to determine whether this loss of adaptation is rapid and uniform, or whether it depends on the type of force and/or the duration of training cessation.

Maximal force

Maximal force represents the peak force or peak torque reached during a maximal voluntary contraction. A meta-analysis performed by the authors of this chapter revealed a small decrease in maximal force once training ceases [standardised mean difference (SMD; 95% interval of confidence): -0.46 (-0.54 to -0.37)] (Bosquet et al., 2013), but this decrement grew bigger with the duration of training cessation. As shown in Figure 7.2, the decrease in maximal force became significant from the third week of inactivity, and its magnitude increased thereafter as a function of time. Many physiological factors are involved in this process. They are typically classified as central (or neural) and peripheral (or morphological) factors. Central factors refer to motor unit recruitment and synchronisation, firing frequency, and intermuscular coordination (Cormie, McGuigan, & Newton, 2011a). Central adaptations occur rapidly with training and are thought to explain the greatest part of short-term strength gains in previously untrained individuals (Folland & Williams, 2007; Hakkinen, 1989; Moritani & deVries, 1979). Peripheral factors refer to muscle fibre

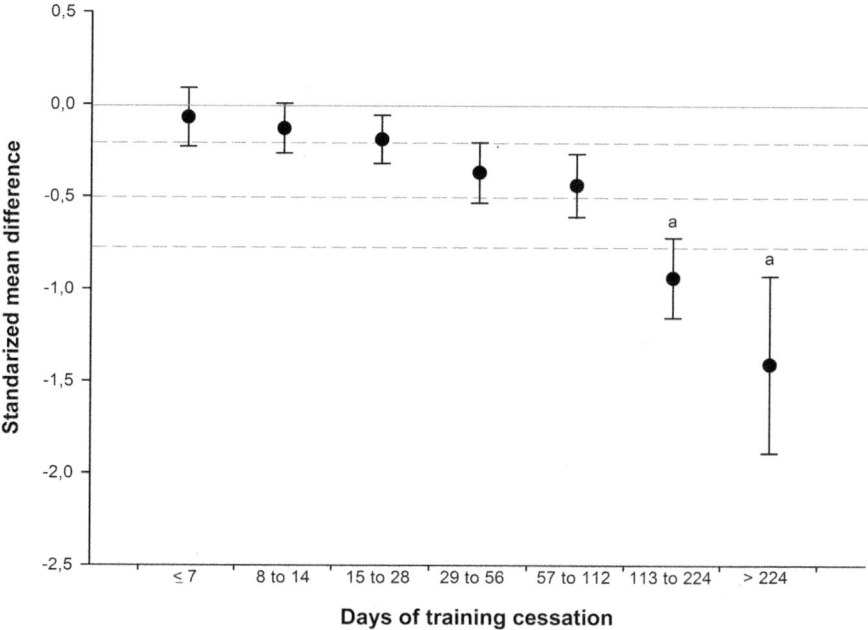

FIGURE 7.2 Dose-response curve for the effect of the duration of training cessation on maximal force. Standardised mean difference interpretation: < 0.2: Trivial; 0.2 to 0.5: Small; 0.5 to 0.8: Moderate; and > 0.8: Large. a: Different from standardised mean differences computed for ≤ 112 days of training cessation.

Adapted from Bosquet et al. (2013).

type and architecture, as well as tendon properties (Cormie et al., 2011a). Although the cellular adaptations that subtend muscle hypertrophy are observed early in a training program (DeFreitas, Beck, Stock, Dillon, & Kasishke, 2011), it is generally considered that the relative contribution of morphological adaptations increases gradually as training proceeds (Folland & Williams, 2007; Narici et al., 1996), with an increasing role of the endocrine system (Crewther, Cronin, & Keogh, 2006; Crewther, Cook, Cardinale, Weatherby, & Lowe, 2011). Although it was beyond the scope of our meta-analysis to study specifically these underlying factors, one may hypothesise that this sequence of events also exists in the disadaptation process, the factors underpinning the continuous decrease in maximal force being mainly central during the first weeks of training cessation, and mainly peripheral afterwards. This hypothesis is in accordance with the data published by the group of Häkkinen (Häkkinen, Alen, Kallinen, Newton, & Kraemer, 2000; Häkkinen & Komi, 1983), who reported a rapid decrease (of small amplitude) in the neural activation once training ceases, followed by a muscular atrophy when the period of inactivity exceeds 24 weeks.

Maximal power

Maximal power represents the ability to produce high amounts of force over a short period of time, and plays a crucial role in many athletic events (Duthie, Pyne, & Hooper, 2003; Mero, Komi, & Gregor, 1992; Stolen, Chamari, Castagna, & Wisloff, 2005). Considering that training cessation results in a significant reduction of maximal force, it would be expected to reduce maximal power as well. However, maximal power is also determined by factors related to velocity that are independent from maximal force (Cormie, McGuigan, & Newton, 2011b; Kraemer et al., 2002). Therefore, depending on the effect of training cessation on these factors, the rates of decline of maximal power and maximal force are not necessarily the same. Indeed, we observed that the magnitude of the effect of training cessation on maximal power was smaller than that observed for maximal force [standardised mean difference (95% interval of confidence): -0.20 (-0.28 to -0.13)] (Bosquet et al., 2013). This difference between both muscular properties concerned overall SMD, but also the kinetics of the disadaptation process. As shown in Figures 7.2 and 7.3, the effect of training cessation on maximal force and maximal power was quite similar during the first weeks, although a small improvement may be expected in maximal power after short-term training cessation (i.e., two weeks or less), while this was less probable in maximal force. Noteworthy, there appears to be dissociation after 16 weeks of inactivity, since we found a large decrease in maximal force while maximal power was not different from the previous weeks (Bosquet et al., 2013). Andersen and Aagaard (2000) provided some experimental data in healthy young males that could explain this discrepancy. Of all muscle fibres, type IIx represented $10.2 \pm 2.5\%$ at pretraining measurement time. After 38 resistance training sessions within a 90-day period, this proportion decreased to $4.1 \pm 1.2\%$. Surprisingly,

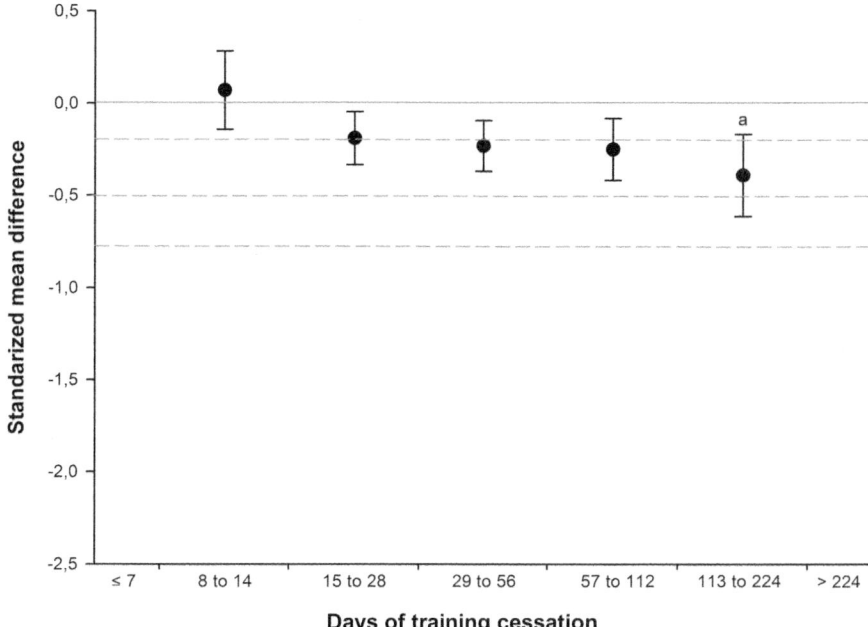

FIGURE 7.3 Dose-response curve for the effect of the duration of training cessation on maximal power. Standardised mean difference interpretation: < 0.2: Trivial; 0.2 to 0.5: Small; 0.5 to 0.8: Moderate; and > 0.8: Large. a: Different from the standardised mean difference computed for ≤ 14 days of training cessation.

Adapted from Bosquet et al. (2013).

this proportion increased to 18.8 ± 3.5% after three months of training cessation. Andersen, Andersen, Magnusson, and Aagaard (2005) later showed that this training cessation-induced overshoot in IIx muscle fibre proportion was accompanied by an increase in the electrically evoked twitch rate of force development, and in the maximal unloaded knee extension velocity and power, while cross-sectional area and peak torque decreased to baseline level. Although other factors may contribute to explaining the difference in the effect of training cessation on maximal force and maximal power, this overshoot of IIx muscle fibres is probably central since the resulting increase in maximal velocity may compensate for the loss in maximal force to maintain maximal power.

Submaximal strength

Submaximal strength represents the ability of the neuromuscular system to sustain a high fraction of maximal force for a long period of time or a high number of repetitions. This specific ability is particularly important in many long-duration events such as cycling or triathlon (Marcora, Bosio, & de Morree, 2008). We found a moderate decrease in submaximal strength once training ceases [standardised mean difference (95% interval of confidence): -0.62 (-0.80 to -0.45)] (Bosquet et al., 2013). As shown in Figure 7.4, the negative impact of training cessation duration on submaximal strength was more important than on maximal force and maximal power. Physiological factors related to oxygen transport and energy production should be added to the neural and morphological factors to explain the detrimental effect of training cessation on muscular force and power. As previously discussed, the rapid decrease in blood volume that is observed very shortly once training ceases (Houmard et al., 1992) is the starting point of a cascade of events leading to a decrease in cardiac output (Coyle et al., 1984, 1985). Training cessation is also associated with a greater reliance on glucose for energy provision that is concomitant with a rapid decrease in muscle glycogen stores (Costill et al., 1985; Mikines et al., 1989) and a rapid decrease in the activity of oxidative enzymes

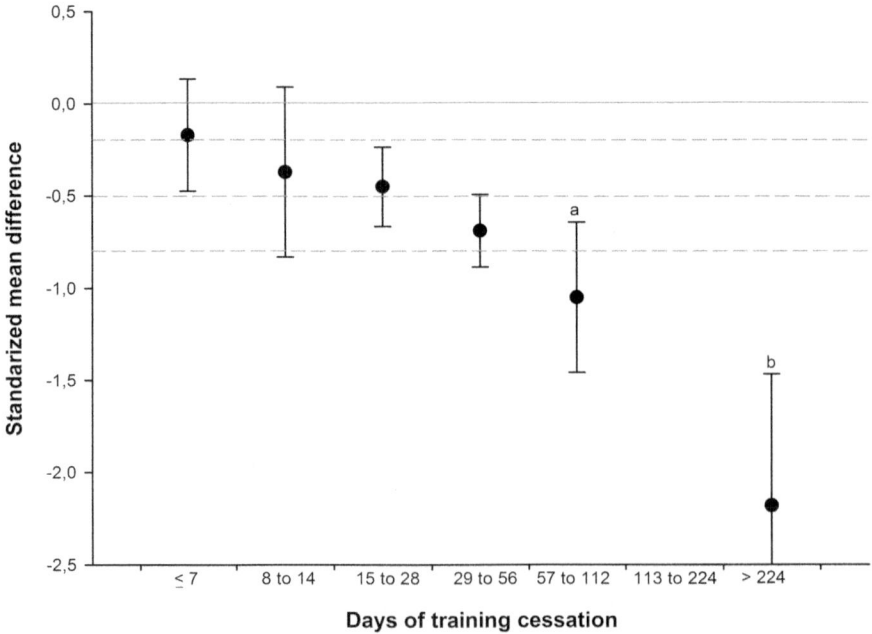

FIGURE 7.4 Dose-response curve for the effect of the duration of training cessation on submaximal strength. Standardised mean difference interpretation: < 0.2: Trivial; 0.2 to 0.5: Small; 0.5 to 0.8: Moderate; and > 0.8: Large. a: Different from the standardised mean difference computed for ≤ 7 days of training cessation. b: Different from standardised mean differences computed for ≤ 112 days of training cessation.

Adapted from Bosquet et al. (2013).

such as citrate synthase, succinate dehydrogenase and malate dehydrogenase (Coyle et al., 1984, 1985). All together, these disadaptations clearly compromise oxygen transport, aerobic energy production, and submaximal strength. Through an additive effect to neural and morphological disadaptations, they probably contribute to the larger decrease we found in submaximal strength in comparison with maximal force and maximal power.

In summary, training cessation is associated with a more or less rapid loss of cardiovascular, metabolic and neuromuscular adaptations that will negatively impact physical performance (Mujika & Padilla, 2000a, 2000b). From a practical point of view, two weeks of training cessation appear to represent a good compromise between the decrease in overall fatigue and the decrease in physical fitness. In fact, with the exception of muscle glycogen stores, most of the muscular adaptations remain almost unaltered and detraining is limited to some cardiorespiratory factors like blood volume, stroke volume, and, ultimately, cardiac output.

Effects of training load reduction on performance capacity

As already mentioned, the difficulty for the coach or the sport scientist consists in determining the training load that will maximise the decrease in accumulated fatigue while retaining physical fitness. Interestingly, this is the specific purpose of the tapering strategy, which represents a reduction in the training load of athletes in the final days before important competitions, with the specific aim of optimizing performance capacity (Bosquet, Montpetit, Arvisais, & Mujika, 2007). The main difference with the excessively overreached athlete lies in the fact that the latter is mainly interested in recovering his initial performance level, and not necessarily in reaching a peak performance. However, we will see in this section that these goals are not as different as it could be thought. During a taper, the reduction of the training load can be achieved through the alteration of one or several of its components, including the training volume, intensity, and frequency (Wenger & Bell, 1986), as well as the pattern of the taper (i.e., progressive or step taper) and its duration (Houmard, 1991; Houmard & Johns, 1994; Mujika, 1998; Mujika & Padilla, 2003). Many strategies to decrease the training load have been reported in the tapering literature, most of them leading to an improvement in performance and/or its physiological correlates (Houmard, 1991; Houmard & Johns, 1994; Mujika, 1998; Mujika, Padilla, Pyne, & Busso, 2004; Neufer, 1989). Considering the important heterogeneity between studies in the way they decrease the training load, the question arises to determine whether an optimal strategy exists. To answer this question, we carried out a systematic review of the tapering literature with a meta-analysis (Bosquet et al., 2007). The specific goal of this investigation was to assess the effects of the alteration of training load components on performance in competitive athletes.

Parameters of the training load

In agreement with previous suggestions (Houmard & Johns, 1994; Mujika & Padilla, 2003), our meta-analysis confirmed that performance improvement was more likely to occur as a result of a reduction in training volume. As shown in Figure 7.5, maximal performance gains are obtained with a total reduction in training volume of 41–60% of pretaper value. Training volume can be altered through the decrease of the duration of each training session and/or the decrease of training frequency. It seems that the first strategy should be preferred, since decreasing training frequency does not result in a significant performance improvement (Table 7.1). It should be kept in mind, however, that there is a large variability between studies, as evidenced by the wide 95% confidence interval. In fact, the decrease in training frequency often interacts with other moderator variables like the form and duration of the taper, which makes it difficult to isolate precisely its effect on performance. A more conservative approach would be to recommend maintaining training frequency at 80% or more of the pretaper value (Mujika et al., 2002; Mujika & Padilla, 2003). As already pointed out by other researchers (Houmard & Johns, 1994; Kubukeli, Noakes, & Dennis, 2002; Mujika, 1998; Mujika & Padilla, 2003; Neufer, 1989), it

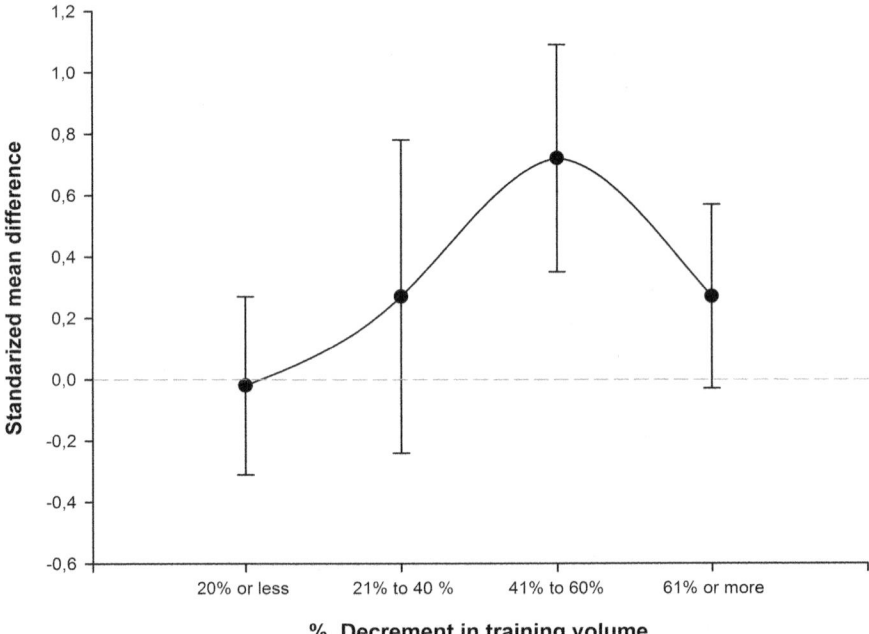

FIGURE 7.5 Dose-response curve for the effect of % decrement in training volume on performance. Standardised mean difference interpretation: < 0.2: Trivial; 0.2 to 0.5: Small; 0.5 to 0.8: Moderate; and > 0.8: Large.

Adapted from Bosquet et al. (2007).

TABLE 7.1 Effects of moderator variables on standardised mean difference (SMD) for tapering-induced changes in performance. Adapted from Bosquet et al. (2007).

Categories	SMD Mean [95% C.I.]
Decrease in training intensity	
Yes	-0.02 [-0.37, 0.33]
No	0.33 [0.19, 0.47]
Decrease in training frequency	
Yes	0.24 [-0.03, 0.52]
No	0.35 [0.18, 0.51]
Pattern of the taper	
Step taper	0.42 [-0.11, 0.95]
Progressive taper	0.30 [0.16, 0.45]

seems clear that the training load should not be reduced at the expense of training intensity (Table 7.1), probably because it is a key parameter in the maintenance of training-induced adaptation during the taper (Mujika et al., 2004).

Duration of the taper

We found a dose-response relationship between the duration of the taper and the performance improvement. A taper duration of eight to 14 days is associated to the larger improvement in performance capacity. It is worth noting that performance improvements can also be expected after one-, three-, or four-week tapers (Figure 7.6). However, as suggested by 95% confidence intervals, some athletes may experience negative results, while the gains are systematic with a two-week taper. This interindividual variability in the optimal taper duration has already been highlighted by some mathematical modelling studies (Mujika et al., 1996; Thomas & Busso, 2005). Differences in the physiological and/or psychological adaptation response to reduced training (Mujika et al., 1996; Mujika, Padilla, & Pyne, 2002) probably account for this variability.

Pattern of the taper

Mujika and Padilla (2003) identified four taper patterns: Linear taper, exponential taper with slow or fast time constant of decay of the training load, and step taper. Because the pattern was not always precisely detailed in the studies included in our meta-analysis, we compiled linear and exponential tapers together into one single pattern named progressive taper. Noteworthy, the majority of studies used a progressive decrease in training load. Our results agree with the study by Banister, Carter, and Zarkadas (1999), who reported larger performance improvements after a progressive taper when compared with a step taper. We were not able to address the effect of the kind of progressive taper (i.e., linear or exponential with fast or slow decay of the training load) on performance. Therefore, actual recommendations

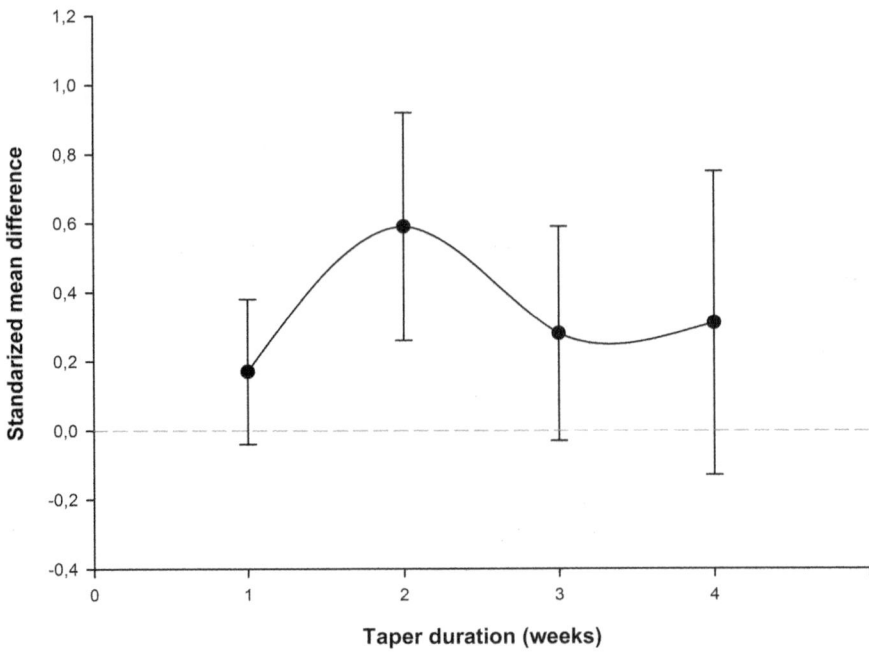

FIGURE 7.6 Dose-response curve for the effect of taper duration on performance. Standardised mean difference interpretation: < 0.2: Trivial; 0.2 to 0.5: Small; 0.5 to 0.8: Moderate; and > 0.8: Large.

Adapted from Bosquet et al. (2007).

rely on the work of Banister et al. (1999), who suggest that a fast decay was more beneficial to performance than a slow decay of the training load.

Performance gains

As we have seen in previous sections, maximal gains are obtained with a tapering intervention of two-week duration, where the training volume is exponentially decreased by 41–60%, without any modification of either training intensity or frequency. What is the magnitude of the gains we are talking about? When using the scale of Cohen (1988) for the interpretation of standardised mean differences, expected performance improvements are most often small, and occasionally moderate. When expressed as a percent difference, the weighted mean improvement is 1.96%, which is of the same order of magnitude as the mathematical prediction by Thomas and Busso (2005). This difference could be considered as meaningless if the population of interest was not competitive athletes. As highlighted by Hopkins, Hawley, and Burke (1999), the smallest enhancement of performance that has a substantial effect on a top athlete's chance of a medal is about one third of the typical variation of performance in competition. This has been shown to be approximately 0.5–1% in both swimming and running (Hopkins & Hewson, 2001; Stewart & Hopkins, 2000). In this context, the gains that can be expected after a taper intervention, as little as they are, may have a major impact on an athlete's success in major competitions. An illustration was provided by Mujika et al. (2002), who reported that the magnitude of taper-induced improvements in performance in the Olympic swimming events (2.2%) were of similar order to the differences between the gold medallist and the fourth place (1.62%) or between third and eighth place (2.02%) at the 2000 Sydney Olympics.

Implications for the overreached athlete

An important feature of the tapering literature is the large interindividual variability in the response to the taper, thus suggesting that individualisation is probably one of the most important keys for success (Bosquet et al., 2007). The main practical implication of this observation, which also applies to overreached athletes, is that the simplest of most efficient way to adapt the taper strategy to each individual consists in accounting for the level of fatigue. A recreational runner with four sessions per week, has probably a low level of cumulated fatigue. Then the decrease in training volume does not need to be so important. Conversely, an elite athlete training 12 sessions per week and aiming at peaking for an important event will probably need a larger and/or longer decrease in training volume to fully recover from the physiological and psychological cumulated fatigue, particularly if he or she is severely overreached. This approach was well illustrated by Thomas and Busso (2005). These authors used a nonlinear modelling approach to determine whether the optimal taper depended on the severity of fatigue an athlete carries into the taper process. They clearly showed that using an overload procedure before the taper (which could result in functional overreaching) resulted in higher performance gains, but also that taper duration and percentage decrease in training load should be adapted (i.e., increased) to dissipate this extra accumulated fatigue (Figure 7.7). Despite this sound theoretical background, very few experimental studies addressed this topic. This situation probably arises from the difficulty to quantify fatigue. The overreaching/overtraining literature of the past two decades clearly indicates that there exists no pathognomonic clinical sign of severe fatigue (Mujika et al., 2002). However, an affordable and very interesting tool to estimate overall fatigue is probably the use of questionnaires like the Profile of Mood States (McNair, Lorr, & Droppleman, 1992) or the Recovery-Stress Questionnaire for Athletes (Kellmann & Kallus, 2001, 2016).

Conclusion and recommendations for applied practise

The purpose of this chapter was to provide coaches and sport scientists with theoretical data obtained from the detraining and tapering literature in order

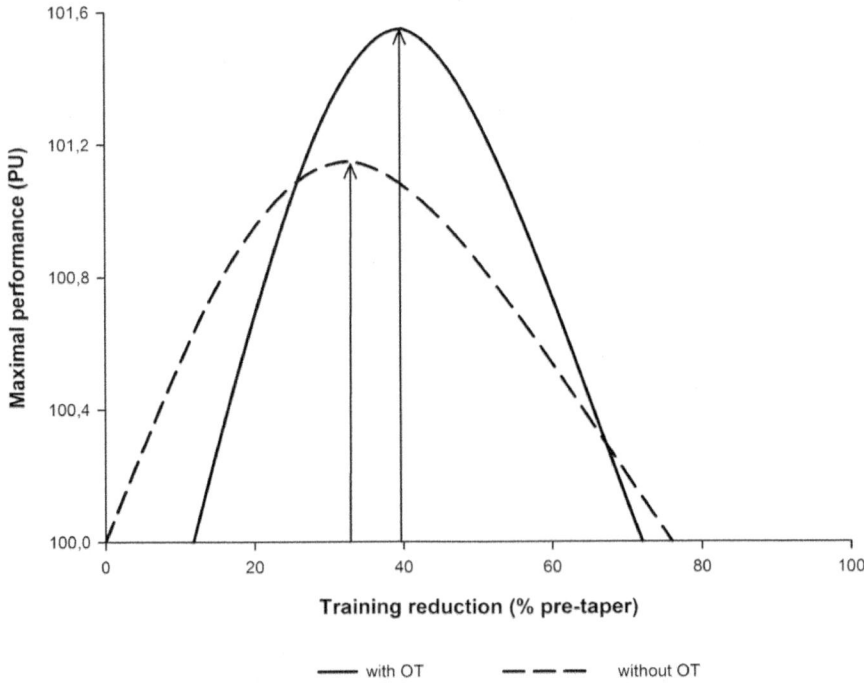

FIGURE 7.7 Dose-response curve for the effect of training load reduction on performance. Adapted from Thomas and Busso (2005).

to help them in the decision-making process when they have to deal with an overreached athlete. Being aware of these data is a prerequisite in the management of overreaching. However, it does not warrant efficiency. The diversity of causes involved in the development of overreaching and the complexity of its aetiology is not compatible with a unique strategy suitable for all athletes and all sports. In the simplest case, overreaching originates from overload training. Then a well-designed taper should be relevant. Most often, overreaching is a consequence of a negative interaction between training load and other sources of stress including family, work, school, and so on. The situation is then more complex, and it is likely that a complete training cessation of one to two weeks would be more beneficial than a taper. In fact, it would probably allow a better psychological recovery, and from a physiological point of view we can consider that most determinants of performance would not be significantly altered, with the exception of blood volume and glycogen stores, thus warranting a quick return to baseline when the athlete is ready to resume training. In conclusion, it is not possible to give a general recipe to cope with this issue. There are almost as many strategies as there are individual athletes, and the key for individualisation is a global multimodal approach incorporating all the dimensions of fatigue and performance.

References

Aagaard, P., Andersen, J. L., Dyhre-Poulsen, P., Leffers, A. M., Wagner, A., Magnusson, S. P., & Simonsen, E. B. (2001). A mechanism for increased contractile strength of human pennate muscle in response to strength training: Changes in muscle architecture. *Journal of Physiology, 534*(Pt. 2), 613–623.

Abernethy, P. J., Thayer, R., & Taylor, A. W. (1990). Acute and chronic responses of skeletal muscle to endurance and sprint exercise. A review. *Sports Medicine, 10*(6), 365–389.

Amigo, N., Cadefau, J. A., Ferrer, I., Tarrados, N., & Cusso, R. (1998). Effect of summer intermission on skeletal muscle of adolescent soccer players. *Journal of Sports Medicine and Physical Fitness, 38*(4), 298–304.

Andersen, J. L., & Aagaard, P. (2000). Myosin heavy chain IIX overshoot in human skeletal muscle. *Muscle Nerve, 23*(7), 1095–1104.

Andersen, L. L., Andersen, J. L., Magnusson, S. P., & Aagaard, P. (2005). Neuromuscular adaptations to detraining following resistance training in previously untrained subjects. *European Journal of Applied Physiology, 93*(5–6), 511–518.

Astrand, P., Rodahl, K., Dahl, H., & Straamme, S. (2003). *Textbook of work physiology – physiological bases of exercise*. Champaign, IL: Human Kinetics.

Banister, E. W., Carter, J. B., & Zarkadas, P. C. (1999). Training theory and taper: Validation in triathlon athletes. *European Journal of Applied Physiology, 79*(2), 182–191.

Batterham, A. M., & Hopkins, W. G. (2006). Making meaningful inferences about magnitudes. *International Journal of Sports Physiology and Performance, 1*(1), 50–57.

Berryman, N., Maurel, D., & Bosquet, L. (2010). Effect of plyometric vs. dynamic weight training on the energy cost of running. *Journal of Strength and Conditioning Research, 24*(7), 1818–1825.

Bosquet, L., Berryman, N., Dupuy, O., Mekary, S., Arvisais, D., Bherer, L., & Mujika, I. (2013). Effect of training cessation on muscular performance: A meta-analysis. *Scandinavian Journal of Medicine & Science in Sport, 23*(3), e140–149.

Bosquet, L., Léger, L., & Legros, P. (2002). Methods to determine aerobic endurance. *Sports Medicine, 32*(11), 675–700.

Bosquet, L., Montpetit, J., Arvisais, D., & Mujika, I. (2007). Effects of tapering on performance: A meta-analysis. *Medicine and Science in Sports and Exercise, 39*(8), 1358–1365.

Bosquet, L., & Mujika, I. (2012). Detraining. In I. Mujika (Ed.), *Endurance training – science and practice* (pp. 99–106). Vitoria-Gasteiz, Basque Country: Iñigo Mujika S.L.U.

Carter, S. L., Rennie, C. D., Hamilton, S. J., & Tarnopolsky. (2001). Changes in skeletal muscle in males and females following endurance training. *Canadian Journal of Physiology and Pharmacology, 79*(5), 386–392.

Cohen, J. (1988). *Statistical power analysis for the behavioral sciences*. Hillsdale, NJ: Lawrence Erlbaum Associates.

Cormie, P., McGuigan, M. R., & Newton, R. U. (2011a). Developing maximal neuromuscular power: Part 1 – biological basis of maximal power production. *Sports Medicine, 41*(1), 17–38.

Cormie, P., McGuigan, M. R., & Newton, R. U. (2011b). Developing maximal neuromuscular power: Part 2 – training considerations for improving maximal power production. *Sports Medicine, 41*(2), 125–146.

Costill, D. L., Fink, W. J., Hargreaves, M., King, D. S., Thomas, R., & Fielding, R. (1985). Metabolic characteristics of skeletal muscle during detraining from competitive swimming. *Medicine and Science in Sports and Exercise, 17*(3), 339–343.

Coyle, E. F., Hemmert, M. K., & Coggan, A. R. (1986). Effects of detraining on cardiovascular responses to exercise: Role of blood volume. *Journal of Applied Physiology, 60*(1), 95–99.

Coyle, E. F., Martin, W. H., Bloomfield, S. A., Lowry, O. H., & Holloszy, J. O. (1985). Effects of detraining on responses to submaximal exercise. *Journal of Applied Physiology, 59*(3), 853–859.

Coyle, E. F., Martin, W. H., Sinacore, D. R., Joyner, M. J., Hagberg, J. M., & Holloszy, J. O. (1984). Time course of loss of adaptations after stopping prolonged intense endurance training. *Journal of Applied Physiology, 57*(6), 1857–1864.

Crewther, B. T., Cook, C., Cardinale, M., Weatherby, R. P., & Lowe, T. (2011). Two emerging concepts for elite athletes: The short-term effects of testosterone and cortisol on the neuromuscular system and the dose-response training role of these endogenous hormones. *Sports Medicine, 41*(2), 103–123.

Crewther, B. T., Cronin, J., & Keogh, J. (2006). Possible stimuli for strength and power adaptations: Acute metabolic responses. *Sports Medicine, 36*(1), 65–78.

Cullinane, E. M., Sady, S. P., Vadeboncoeur, L., Burke, M., & Thompson, P. D. (1986). Cardiac size and VO_2max do not decrease after short-term exercise cessation. *Medicine and Science in Sports and Exercise, 18*(4), 420–424.

DeFreitas, J. M., Beck, T. W., Stock, M. S., Dillon, M. A., & Kasishke, P. R., 2nd. (2011). An examination of the time course of training-induced skeletal muscle hypertrophy. *European Journal of Applied Physiology, 111*(11), 2785–2790.

Delecluse, C. (1997). Influence of strength training on sprint running performance. *Sports Medicine, 24*(3), 147–156.

Di Prampero, P. E., Atchou, G., Bruckner, J. C., & Moia, C. (1986). The energetics of endurance running. *European Journal of Applied Physiology, 55*, 259–266.

Drinkwater, B. L., & Horvath, S. M. (1972). Detraining effects on young women. *Medicine and Science in Sports, 4*(2), 91–95.

Duthie, G., Pyne, D., & Hooper, S. (2003). Applied physiology and game analysis of rugby union. *Sports Medicine, 33*(13), 973–991.

Folland, J. P., & Williams, A. G. (2007). The adaptations to strength training: Morphological and neurological contributions to increased strength. *Sports Medicine, 37*(2), 145–168.

Gandevia, S. C. (2001). Spinal and supraspinal factors in human muscle fatigue. *Physiological Reviews, 81*(4), 1725–1789.

Gollnick, P. D., & Matoba, H. (1984). The muscle fiber composition of skeletal muscle as a predictor of athletic success. An overview. *American Journal of Sports Medicine, 12*(3), 212–217.

Häkkinen, K. (1989). Neuromuscular and hormonal adaptations during strength and power training. A review. *Journal of Sports Medicine and Physical Fitness, 29*(1), 9–26.

Häkkinen, K., Alen, M., Kallinen, M., Newton, R. U., & Kraemer, W. J. (2000). Neuromuscular adaptation during prolonged strength training, detraining and re-strength-training in middle-aged and elderly people. *European Journal of Applied Physiology, 83*(1), 51–62.

Häkkinen, K., & Komi, P. V. (1983). Electromyographic changes during strength training and detraining. *Medicine and Science in Sports and Exercise, 15*(6), 455–460.

Hopkins, W. G., Hawley, J. A., & Burke, L. M. (1999). Design and analysis of research on sport performance enhancement. *Medicine and Science in Sports and Exercise, 31*(3), 472–485.

Hopkins, W. G., & Hewson, D. J. (2001). Variability of competitive performance of distance runners. *Medicine and Science in Sports and Exercise, 33*(9), 1588–1592.

Hortobagyi, T., Houmard, J. A., Stevenson, J. R., Fraser, D. D., Johns, R. A., & Israel, R. G. (1993). The effects of detraining on power athletes. *Medicine and Science in Sports and Exercise, 25*(8), 929–935.

Houmard, J. A. (1991). Impact of reduced training on performance in endurance athletes. *Sports Medicine, 12*(6), 380–393.

Houmard, J. A., Hortobagyi, T., Johns, R. A., Bruno, N. J., Nutte, C. C., Shinebarger, M. H., & Welborn, J. W. (1992). Effect of short term training cessation on performance measures in distance runners. *International Journal of Sports Medicine, 13*, 572–576.

Houmard, J. A., & Johns, R. A. (1994). Effects of taper on swim performance: Practical implications. *Sports Medicine, 17*(4), 224–232.

Houston, M. E., Bentzen, H., & Larsen, H. (1979). Interrelationships between skeletal muscle adaptations and performance as studied by detraining and retraining. *Acta Physiologica Scandinavica, 105*(2), 163–170.

Jones, E. J., Bishop, P. A., Woods, A. K., & Green, J. M. (2008). Cross-sectional area and muscular strength: A brief review. *Sports Medicine, 38*(12), 987–994.

Kellmann, M., & Kallus, K. W. (2001). *Recovery-Stress Questionnaire for Athletes: User manual.* Champaign, IL: Human Kinetics.

Kellmann, M., & Kallus, K. W. (2016). The Recovery-Stress Questionnaire for Athletes. In K. W. Kallus & M. Kellmann (Eds.), *The Recovery-Stress Questionnaires: User manual* (pp. 86–131). Frankfurt am Main: Pearson Assessment.

Kenttä, G., Hassmén, P., & Raglin, J. S. (2001). Training practices and overtraining syndrome in Swedish age-group athletes. *International Journal of Sports Medicine, 22*(6), 460–465.

Kraemer, W. J., Koziris, L. P., Ratamess, N. A., Hakkinen, K., Triplett-McBride, N. T., Fry, A. C., . . . Fleck, S. J. (2002). Detraining produces minimal changes in physical performance and hormonal variables in recreationally strength-trained men. *Journal of Strength and Conditioning Research, 16*(3), 373–382.

Kubukeli, Z. N., Noakes, T. D., & Dennis, S. C. (2002). Training techniques to improve endurance exercise performances. *Sports Medicine, 32*(8), 489–509.

Larsson, L., & Ansved, T. (1985). Effects of long-term physical training and detraining on enzyme histochemical and functional skeletal muscle characteristic in man. *Muscle Nerve, 8*(8), 714–722.

Madsen, K., Pedersen, P. K., Djurhuus, M. S., & Klitgaard, N. A. (1993). Effects of detraining on endurance capacity and metabolic changes during prolonged exhaustive exercise. *Journal of Applied Physiology, 75*(4), 1444–1451.

Marcora, S. M., Bosio, A., & de Morree, H. M. (2008). Locomotor muscle fatigue increases cardiorespiratory responses and reduces performance during intense cycling exercise independently from metabolic stress. *American Journal of Physiology. Regulatory, Integrative and Comparative Physiology, 294*(3), R874–883.

McCoy, M., Proietto, J., & Hargreaves, M. (1994). Effect of detraining on GLUT-4 protein in human skeletal muscle. *Journal of Applied Physiology, 77*, 1532–1536.

McNair, D. M., Lorr, M., & Droppleman, L. F. (1992). *Revised manual for the Profile of Mood States.* San Diego, CA: Educational and Industrial Testing Service.

Meeusen, R., Duclos, M., Foster, C., Fry, A., Gleeson, M., Nieman, D., . . . Urhausen, A. (2013). Prevention, diagnosis, and treatment of the overtraining syndrome: Joint consensus statement of the European College of Sport Science and the American College of Sports Medicine. *Medicine and Science in Sports and Exercise, 45*(1), 186–205.

Mero, A., Komi, P. V., & Gregor, R. J. (1992). Biomechanics of sprint running. *Sports Medicine, 13*(6), 376–392.

Mikines, K. J., Sonne, B., Tronier, B., & Galbo, H. (1989). Effects of acute exercise and detraining on insulin action in trained men. *Journal of Applied Physiology, 66*(2), 704–711.

Moore, R. L., Thacker, E. M., Kelley, G. A., Musch, T. I., Sinoway, L. I., Foster, V. L., & Dickinson, A. L. (1987). Effect of training/detraining on submaximal exercise responses in humans. *Journal of Applied Physiology, 63*(5), 1719–1724.

Moritani, T., & deVries, H. A. (1979). Neural factors versus hypertrophy in the time course of muscle strength gain. *American Journal of Physical Medicine, 58*(3), 115–130.

Mujika, I. (1998). Influence of training characteristics and tapering on the adaptation in highly trained individuals: A review. *International Journal of Sports Medicine, 19,* 439–446.

Mujika, I., Busso, T., Lacoste, L., Barale, F., Geyssant, A., & Chatard, J. (1996). Modeled responses to training and taper in competitive swimmers. *Medicine and Science in Sports and Exercise, 28*(2), 251–258.

Mujika, I., Goya, A., Ruiz, E., Grijalba, A., Santisteban, J., & Padilla, S. (2002). Physiological and performance responses to a 6-day taper in middle-distance runners: Influence of training frequency. *International Journal of Sports Medicine, 23*(5), 367–373.

Mujika, I., & Padilla, S. (2000a). Detraining: Loss of a training induced physiological and performance adaptation. Part I. *Sports Medicine, 30*(2), 79–87.

Mujika, I., & Padilla, S. (2000b). Detraining: Loss of training-induced physiological and performance adaptations: Part II. *Sports Medicine, 30*(3), 145–154.

Mujika, I., & Padilla, S. (2001). Muscular characteristics of detraining in humans. *Medicine and Science in Sports and Exercise, 33*(8), 1297–1303.

Mujika, I., & Padilla, S. (2003). Scientific bases for precompetition tapering strategies. *Medicine and Science in Sports and Exercise, 35*(7), 1182–1187.

Mujika, I., Padilla, S., & Pyne, D. (2002). Swimming performance changes during the final 3 weeks of training leading to the Sydney 2002 Olympic Games. *International Journal of Sports Medicine, 23*(8), 582–587.

Mujika, I., Padilla, S., Pyne, D., & Busso, T. (2004). Physiological changes associated with the pre-event taper in athletes. *Sports Medicine, 34*(13), 891–927.

Narici, M. V., Hoppeler, H., Kayser, B., Landoni, L., Claassen, H., Gavardi, C., . . . Cerretelli, P. (1996). Human quadriceps cross-sectional area, torque and neural activation during 6 months strength training. *Acta Physiologica Scandinavica, 157*(2), 175–186.

Neufer, P. D. (1989). The effect of detraining and reduced training on the physiological adaptations to aerobic exercise training. *Sports Medicine, 8*(5), 302–321.

Neufer, P. D., Costill, D. L., Fielding, R. A., Flynn, M. G., & Kirwann, J. P. (1987). Effect of reduced training on muscular strength and endurance in competitive swimmers. *Medicine and Science in Sports and Exercise, 19*(5), 486–490.

Peronnet, F., & Massicotte, D. (1991). Table of nonprotein respiratory quotient: An update. *Canadian Journal of Applied Physiology, 16*(1), 23–29.

Peronnet, F., & Thibault, G. (1989). Mathematical analysis of running performance and world running records. *Journal of Applied Physiology, 67*(1), 453–465.

Pette, D. (1984). J.B. Wolffe memorial lecture. Activity-induced fast to slow transitions in mammalian muscle. *Medicine and Science in Sports and Exercise, 16*(6), 517–528.

Raglin, J., Sawamura, S., Alexiou, S., Hassmén, P., & Kenttä, G. (2000). Training practices and staleness in 13–18-year-old swimmers: A cross-cultural study. *Pediatric Exercise Science, 12*(1), 61–70.

Raglin, J., & Wilson, G. (2000). Overtraining and staleness in athletes. In Y. Hanin (Ed.), *Emotions in sports* (pp. 191–207). Champaign, IL: Human Kinetics.

Saltin, B., & Astrand, P. O. (1967). Maximal oxygen uptake in athletes. *Journal of Applied Physiology, 23*(3), 353–358.

Saunders, P. U., Pyne, D. B., Telford, R. D., & Hawley, J. A. (2004). Factors affecting running economy in trained distance runners. *Sports Medicine, 34*(7), 465–485.

Simsolo, R. B., Ong, J. M., & Kern, P. A. (1993). The regulation of adipose tissue and muscle lipoprotein lipase in runners by detraining. *Journal of Clinical Investigation, 92*(5), 2124–2130.

Stewart, A. M., & Hopkins, W. G. (2000). Consistency of swimming performance within and between competitions. *Medicine and Science in Sports and Exercise, 32*(5), 997–1001.

Stolen, T., Chamari, K., Castagna, C., & Wisloff, U. (2005). Physiology of soccer: An update. *Sports Medicine, 35*(6), 501–536.

Thomas, L., & Busso, T. (2005). A theoretical study of taper characteristics to optimize performance. *Medicine and Science in Sports and Exercise, 37*(9), 1615–1621.

Vukovich, M. D., Arciero, P. J., Kohrt, W. M., Racette, S. B., Hansen, P. A., & Holloszy, J. O. (1996). Changes in insulin action and GLUT-4 with 6 days of inactivity in endurance runners. *Journal of Applied Physiology, 80*(1), 240–244.

Wenger, H. A., & Bell, G. J. (1986). The interactions of intensity, frequency and duration of exercise training in altering cardiorespiratory fitness. *Sports Medicine, 3*(5), 346–356.

8
RECOVERY-STRESS BALANCE AND INJURY RISK IN TEAM SPORTS

Michel Brink and Koen Lemmink

Introduction

Sport participation involves a considerable risk of injury for both recreational and elite athletes (Fuller, Junge, & Dvorak, 2012). Even in a small country like the Netherlands with approximately 17 million inhabitants, every year 1.4 million people receive medical attention because of an athletic injury (Schmikli, Backx, Kemler, & Van Mechelen, 2009). Of these injuries, 59% occur in organised sport settings. Especially team sports have a relatively high injury risk. Soccer, field hockey, and volleyball together are responsible for 41% of all injuries (Schmikli et al., 2009). These injuries can be divided into traumatic and overuse injuries. Traumatic injuries are characterised by a sudden event, where overuse injuries develop over time and result from repeated micro trauma.

The consequences of these injuries are not only physical (e.g., tissue damage) (Dvorak & Junge, 2000), but also psychosocial (e.g., anxiety for re-injury) (Larson, Starkey, & Zaichkowsky, 1996). In professional football, it has been found that due to these consequences, players are on average unable to compete for about 12% of the time per season (Ekstrand, Hägglund, & Waldén, 2011). As a result, coaches cannot play in optimal team formation. This unavailability of players hinders performance and can lead to serious financial losses, which are caused by reduced commercial income and medical care (Woods, Hawkins, Hulse, & Hodson, 2002). Therefore, there is a need for injury prevention that targets evidence-based risk factors. This is especially relevant in team sports, because of the high injury incidence.

Brink, M., & Lemmink, K. (2018). Recovery-stress balance and injury risk in team sports. In M. Kellmann & J. Beckmann (Eds.), *Sport, Recovery, and Performance: Interdisciplinary Insights* (pp. 108–118). Abingdon: Routledge.

Risk factors

Risk factors are commonly divided into extrinsic and intrinsic risk factors. Extrinsic risk factors include factors as weather, field conditions, rules, and equipment (Meeuwisse, Tyreman, Hagel, & Emery, 2007). Intrinsic risk factors on the other side are internal to the athlete and include factors like age, coordination of movements, flexibility, and risk-taking behaviour (Van der Sluis et al., in press). Together, extrinsic and intrinsic risk factors may predispose an athlete to injury. However, risk factors alone are usually not sufficient to cause an injury. It depends on the inciting event during which the injury occurs (Meeuwisse et al., 2007). Screening of these factors before the start of the season could indicate the individual risk profile (Dallinga, Benjaminse, & Lemmink, 2012). However, some risk factors are unstable and vary from day-to-day or week-to-week. For example, training load and the following recovery are highly variable. In addition, psychological and social factors add weight to this delicate balance. Pressure from parents or coaches, conflicts with fellow players or stress due to relationship problems at home, at school or in the workplace can place an additional load on the players. These psychosocial factors also show high variability (Brink, Visscher, Arends, Zwerver, & Lemmink, 2010). In order to identify some starting points for the development of prevention strategies, this chapter provides an overview of theoretical models and future research while taking recovery into consideration.

Theoretical models on training load, stress, recovery, and injuries

In order to understand the role of stress and recovery in relation to injuries, several theoretical models have been developed. These models focus on training load or psychosocial stress and recovery, or the combination. Depending on the underlying mechanism these models try to explain traumatic injuries or overuse injuries.

The model of Cook and Purdam (2009) focuses on the role of training load (type, frequency, volume, intensity) and the association with tendon structure. This continuum model of tendon pathology assumes that the amount of load is critical and determines if the structure of the tendon improves or worsens. An adequate amount of load results in an increased net collagen synthesis, causing positive adaptations of structural and mechanical properties of the tendon tissue (Cook & Purdam, 2009; Kjaer et al., 2006; Magnusson, Langberg, & Kjaer, 2010). Overload on the other hand can be defined as a mismatch between tendon load and the tendon's load-bearing capacity. This mismatch can lead to changes in the tendon structure resulting in reactive tendinopathy, tendon disrepair and finally degenerative tendon abnormalities (Kjaer et al., 2006; Magnusson et al., 2010). Long-lasting overload can thus result in overuse injuries.

Andersen and Williams (1988) explained the underlying mechanism between psychosocial stress and the occurrence of traumatic injuries. They stated that when athletes experience stressful situations, psychosocial stress contributes to their stress

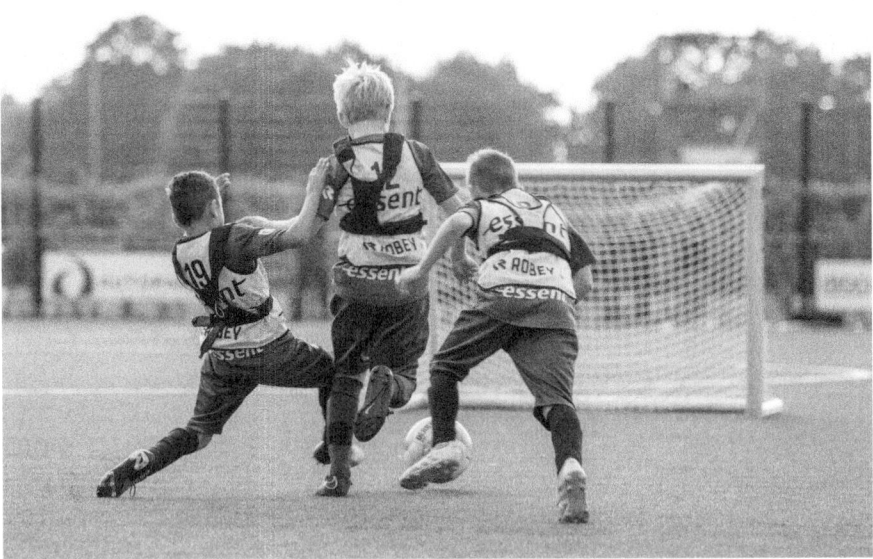

FIGURE 8.1 Young elite soccer players wearing tracking technology to quantify individual training load during a small-sided game.

response. Players may have greater or lesser capacity to deal with these stress factors. For example, having plenty of social support results in a bigger buffer to channel these stress factors. If players are unable to cope with stress it leads to increases in muscle tension, reduced coordination, narrowing of the visual field and an increase in distractibility. These changes make team sport players more susceptible to traumatic injury since they may not see tackles in time or are unable to restore balance due to coordination deficits.

Finally, the model of Kenttä and Hassmén (1998) describes the athletic balance, which consists of both physical and psychosocial stress and recovery components. A disturbed balance between these factors contributes to the development of a general or local overload (overuse injuries). It is assumed that individuals have different capacities and thus respond in various ways to stress and recovery. This balance is especially delicate in younger players that deal with sudden increases in training load as part of youth academies (Figure 8.1). This takes place in a phase of physical and psychosocial maturation (Van der Sluis et al., 2014). Combining sport with school or work causes additional psychological stress. Finally, pressure from teammates, friends, and parents provides social stress. These physical and psychosocial stressors require adequate recovery.

The load-injury relationship

The load-injury relationship has become a popular topic in sport science (Drew & Finch, 2016; Jaspers, Brink, Probst, Frencken, & Helsen, 2017; Windt & Gabbett, 2017). When quantifying training load, a distinction between external load and internal load is made (Impellizzeri, Rampinini, & Marcora, 2005). The external load is then defined as the load that is prescribed by the coach, such as the distance covered or the time spent in certain speed zones or number of accelerations. The internal load on the other hand takes individual characteristics such as fitness into account and is the actual physiological stress placed on the human body. Heartrate and Session-Rating of Perceived Exertion (RPE) are the most commonly used tools in sports practise. As a result of recent technological developments in tracking sensors, advanced monitoring systems are now accessible for sport practise and allow for quantification of training load on a daily basis. Combined with valid injury registration, the association between training load and injury occurrence can be assessed. Over the years, a number of studies assessed whether different load indicators (volume in minutes, distance covered, time spent in high-intensity speed zones, session RPE, and heart rate) increase the injury risk (Figure 8.2)

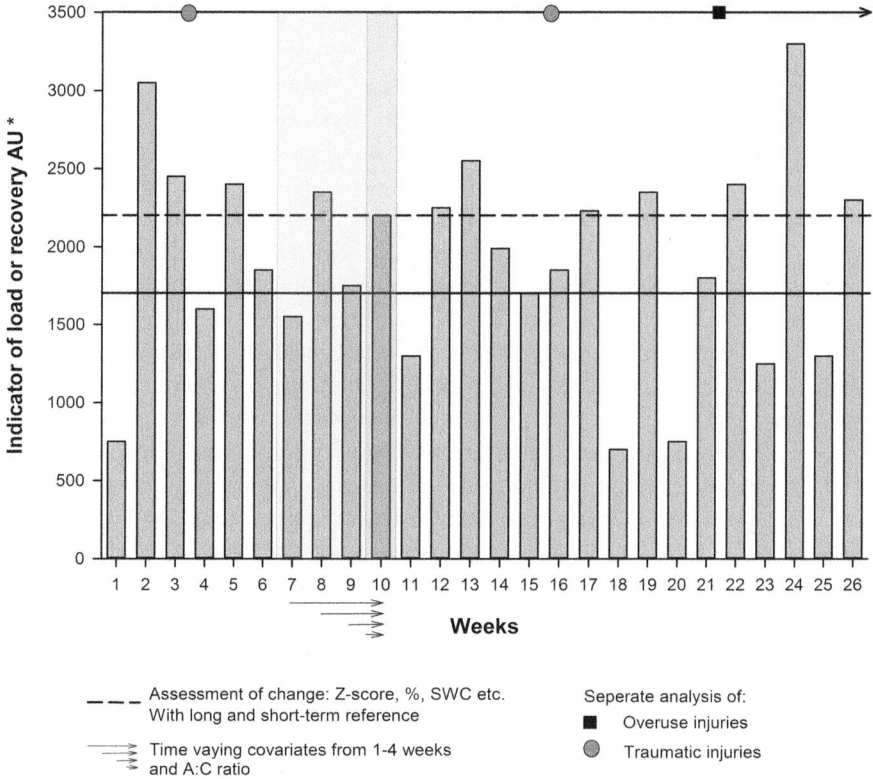

FIGURE 8.2 Visualisation of changes in training load, psychosocial stress or recovery using different time varying co-variates. A distinction between traumatic and overuse injuries is highlighted and individual threshold determined based on a meaningful deviation (Z-score, dotted line) from an individuals' mean (continuous line). AU: Arbitrary Units, A:C ratio: Acute:Chronic ratio, SWC: Smallest Worthwhile Change.

(Drew & Finch, 2016). Since more and more data is collected and stored, several time-varying covariates are introduced. In addition to using the cumulative load of one week, research suggests that cumulative load up to four weeks should be calculated in relation to injury prevention (Drew & Finch, 2016). On top of that, authors introduced outcome measures that compare short-term load (one week) relative to long-term load (four weeks). This so-called acute:chronic ratio assumes that a relative high acute training load compared to the previous four weeks results in increased injury risk (Windt & Gabbett, 2017). Finally, studies included both traumatic and overuse injuries and apply a separate analysis (Brink et al., 2010) or analysis with all injuries combined (Rogalski, Dawson, Heasman, & Gabbett, 2013). It is important to realise that based on the injury mechanism (traumatic or overuse) different load indicators and time varying covariates can be relevant.

Recovery-injury relationship

In contrast to the load-injury relationship, less is known on recovery and its link with injury occurrence. In general, recovery occurs after training or matches and can be indicated by concentrations of biochemical markers (e.g., creatine kinase, cortisol, and testosterone), field performance tests or self-report measures (Nédélec et al., 2012). If the outcome of these tests are restored to normal values at baseline, then it is assumed that for example muscle tissue damage is repaired or mental fatigue is resolved (Kucera et al., 2005; Price, Hawkins, Hulse, & Hodson, 2004; Schwebel, Banaszek, & McDaniel, 2007). After full recovery, the player will be able to reach or exceed benchmark levels (Kucera, Marshall, Kirkendall, Marchak, & Garrett, 2005; Price et al., 2004; Van Mechelen et al., 1996). If this is not the case, the player is not fully recovered. To prevent injuries, it is very important for players to recover properly between the different bouts of exercise. Furthermore, in order to plan subsequent training sessions or prepare for upcoming matches, knowledge is needed about the exact time courses of recovery (Bishop, Jones, & Woods, 2008; Nédélec et al., 2012). This appears particularly relevant during dense in-season weeks with a high number of matches. Indeed, injury risk increases with two matches per week compared to one match (Dupont et al., 2010). Consequently, if the number of rest days between matches is reduced the injury risk increases. Time courses of recovery after matches in team sports indeed indicate that more than two days are needed for full recovery (Nédélec et al., 2012). This supports the need for empirical studies and monitoring tools that are able to detect subtle changes in both load and recovery that can be linked to injuries.

One could argue that recovery can also be distinguished in external and internal recovery (Figure 8.3). External recovery would then be the number of activities that an individual actively executes to promote recovery. An example of this is the Total Quality of Recovery (TQR) action, as proposed by Kenttä and Hassmén (1998). This tool enables players to count points for recovery-related activities such as nutrition, hydration, sleep, relaxation, emotional support, and active rest. The

Recovery-stress balance and injury risk **113**

Tools to monitor external and internal recovery

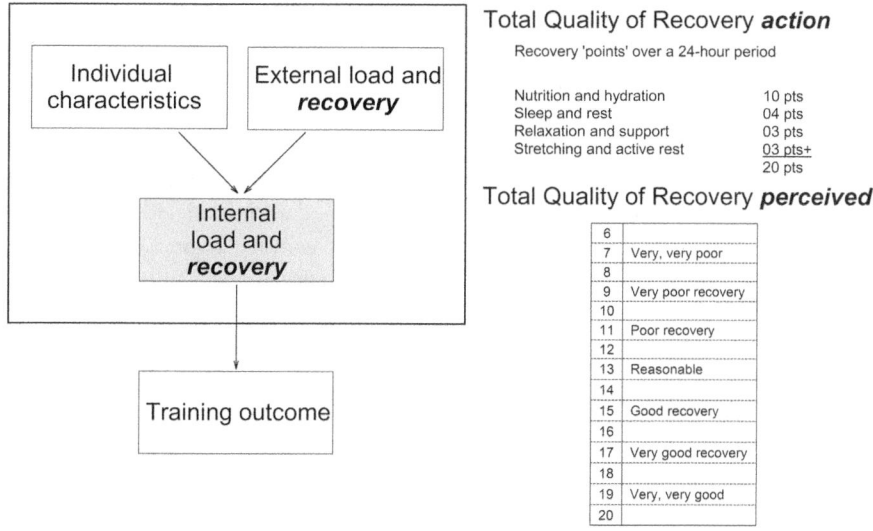

FIGURE 8.3 Adapted version of a theoretical model by Impellizzeri et al. (2005) with a distinction between external and internal recovery.

Examples of tools to monitor external and internal recovery are depicted (Kenttä & Hassmén, 1998).

internal recovery takes individual characteristics into account and indicates the effect of these activities on the human body. For example, the TQR perceived can be seen as a tool to monitor the internal recovery. It should be noted that recovery-related activities often take place outside the organised training setting. As a consequence, it is extremely difficult for coaches to evaluate individual differences in recovery strategies. Indeed, recent studies confirmed a mismatch between the perception of both load (Brink, Frencken, Jordet, & Lemmink, 2014; Brink, Kersten, & Frencken, 2017) and recovery (Doeven, Brink, Frencken, & Lemmink, in press) between coaches and players after matches. Coaches tend to overestimate recovery and the discrepancy is larger two days after matches compared to one day. This indicates that the longer players are out of sight of coaches, the more difficult it is to estimate their recovery. These activities could be very relevant for injury research. Unfortunately, there are no studies available that link different recovery indicators to injury occurrence. Nor are there studies that use time-varying covariates and link these to traumatic injuries, overuse injuries or both.

Psychosocial stress, recovery, and injury risk

Based on the theoretical models it is assumed that not only physical parameters in terms of load and recovery, but also psychosocial stress and recovery increase injury risk. Traditionally, assessment of stress (such as a negative major life events) is solely executed at the start of the season (Junge, 2000). Retrospective stressors over for example the last year are investigated and association with future injuries is then determined via prospective injury registration. In addition, the risk assessment was expanded and also looked into the underlying mechanism, by studying the visual field of players (Williams & Andersen, 1997). Associations between stress levels and narrowing of the visual field appeared to be present. However, just like training load, stress and recovery are known to be unstable factors that vary during the course of a season. Therefore, several authors decided to implement regular assessments of psychosocial stress and recovery across a season, using the Recovery-Stress Questionnaire for Athletes (Kellmann & Kallus, 2001, 2016; Nederhof, Brink, & Lemmink, 2008). High stress levels and poor recovery was present before and at the time of injury occurrence (Brink et al., 2010; Laux, Krumm, Diers, & Flor, 2015). More recently, Van der Does, Brink, Otter, Visscher, and Lemmink (2017) studied individual change in stress and recovery six and three weeks before injuries. Both traumatic and overuse injuries were included and analysed separately. Reduction in general recovery such as social recovery and general well-being was related to a higher risk of traumatic injuries. Relevant changes were seen six weeks before injury occurrence. For overuse, reduced sport-specific recovery were related three weeks before injury occurrence. These findings support the need for using a holistic approach in which physical load and recovery as well as psychosocial stress and recovery should be monitored closely over time to unravel the complex mechanisms that lead to traumatic or overuse injuries.

Future research

Future research should focus at first on the development of theoretical models that include training load, and psychosocial stress and recovery factors, and then describe the underlying mechanism for both traumatic and overuse injuries. Well-designed empirical studies should follow thereafter, particularly in the area of recovery in relation to injury. This requires reliable and valid tools to quantify both external and internal recovery outside the training context, preferably on a 24/7 basis. Once these tools are available, research should link different recovery indicators with time-varying covariates. After identification of sensitive indicators, a holistic approach should be adopted to assess the combination of physical and psychosocial risk factors. It should be considered that physical and psychosocial stress and recovery interact and that these interrelations are relevant in predicting injury risk. The integration of stress and recovery parameters could be an alternative for multifactorial analyses, for example by taking recovery before training into account when interpreting RPE afterwards. The assumption is that if two players perceive training as equally intense, the actual load of a player with perfect recovery before training is higher, compared to a player with poor recovery. Maximal actual load of training is when a player reports perfect recovery before training and maximal perceived exertion after training. Although it is probably a utopia to expect that one single number could capture all relevant elements, this approach may simplify analyses and interpretation. This is especially important with dynamic longitudinal datasets where large amounts of information are stored on a daily basis. This requires analyses of time series at the individual level with advanced modelling techniques such as automated data analysis (Bartlett, O'Connor, Pitchford, Torres-Ronda, & Robertson, 2017; Shyr & Spisic, 2014). Finally, evidence-based feedback needs to be developed and presented in individual player's dashboards. Effectiveness of these feedback interventions needs to be assessed to provide support for use of these monitoring systems in reducing injuries.

Conclusion and recommendations for practise

Careful and systematic monitoring of the recovery-stress balance has the potential to reduce injury risk. Monitoring systems should include physical load of training and recovery afterwards, as well as psychosocial stress and recovery items. At the elite level, recent technological development allows for advanced tracking of players, but the link of these load indicators with injuries has not been established so far. Simple solutions such as session-RPE appear to be relevant at all playing levels and can be used across different time frames from one week up to four weeks. The time frames need to be considered in the context of the training program and taking individual differences into account. Training load monitoring needs to be extended with recovery indicators to evaluate the contribution of recovery to the recovery-stress balance. Finally, to assess changes in psychosocial stress and recovery, regular assessment across a season is needed to be able to warn players at risk and adopt intervention strategies if needed. It should be noted that indicators and time-varying covariates that derive from injury research are not necessary the same as indicators that relate to enhanced performance. Monitoring systems are likely to have separate and shared indicators that link to performance and injuries.

In conclusion, injuries frequently occur in team sports and can have serious physical, psychosocial, and financial consequences. This supports the need for prevention strategies. It is known that the cause of injuries is multifactorial and consist of external and internal risk factors. Stress and recovery are relevant risk factors and can be both physical and psychosocial. Since stress and recovery continuously change over time methodological designs are needed that allow to assess variation across the season. Over the last years, technological developments have led to daily monitoring of training load in professional sports. Research into the load-injury relation provided insight in the sensitivity of these load indicators as well as the application of different time-varying covariates. However, there is a need for new load indicators that take individual variation into account. Besides, the role of recovery in relation to injuries needs to be included in well-designed studies. For a complete understanding, the role of psychosocial stress and recovery needs to be assessed so that relevant indicators can be added to the monitoring system. The interaction of these processes and inter-individual variability in relation to injuries requires more sophisticated models and analysis methods. Whether the use of structured feedback and prevention strategies based on these models will result in a reduction of injuries has yet to be determined.

References

Andersen, M. B., & Williams, J. M. (1988). A model of stress and athletic injury: Prediction and prevention. *Journal of Sport and Exercise Psychology, 10*, 294–306.

Bartlett, J. D., O'Connor, F., Pitchford, N., Torres-Ronda, L., & Robertson, S. J. (2017). Relationships between internal and external training load in team sports athletes: Evidence for an individualised approach. *International Journal of Sports Physiology and Performance, 12*, 230–234.

Bishop, P. A., Jones, E., & Woods, A. K. (2008). Recovery from training: A brief review. *Journal of Strength and Conditioning Research, 22*, 1015–1024.

Brink, M. S., Frencken, W. G. P., Jordet, G., & Lemmink, K. A. M. P. (2014). Coaches' and players' perceptions of training dose: Not a perfect match. *International Journal of Sports Physiology and Performance, 9*, 497–502.

Brink, M. S., Kersten, A. W., & Frencken, W. G. P. (2017). Understanding the mismatch between coaches' and players' perceptions of exertion. *International Journal of Sports Physiology and Performance, 12*, 562–568.

Brink, M. S., Visscher, C., Arends, S., Zwerver, J., & Lemmink, K. A. P. M. (2010). Monitoring stress and recovery: New insights for the prevention of injuries and illnesses in elite youth soccer players. *British Journal of Sports Medicine, 44*, 809–815.

Cook, J. L., & Purdam, C. R. (2009). Is tendon pathology a continuum? A pathology model to explain the clinical presentation of load-induced tendinopathy. *British Journal of Sports Medicine, 43*(6), 409–416.

Dallinga, J. M., Benjaminse, A., & Lemmink, K. A. P. M. (2012). Which screening tools can predict injury to the lower extremities in team sports? A systematic review. *Sports Medicine, 42*, 791–815.

Doeven, S. H., Brink, M. S., Frencken, W. G. P., & Lemmink, K. A. P. M. (in press). Impaired player-coach perceptions of exertion and recovery during match congestion. *International Journal of Sports Physiology and Performance*. doi:10.1123/ijspp.2016-0363

Drew, M. K., & Finch, C. F. (2016). The relationship between training load and injury, illness and soreness: A systematic and literature review. *Sports Medicine, 46*, 861–883.

Dupont, G., Nédélec, M., McCall, A., McCormack, D., Berthoin, S., & Wisløff, U. (2010). Effect of 2 soccer matches in a week on physical performance and injury rate. *American Journal of Sports Medicine, 38*, 1752–1758.

Dvorak, J., & Junge, A. (2000). Football injuries and physical symptoms. A review of the literature. *American Journal of Sports Medicine, 28*, S3–9.

Ekstrand, J., Hägglund, M., & Waldén, M. (2011). Injury incidence and injury patterns in professional football: The UEFA injury study. *British Journal of Sports Medicine, 45*, 553–558.

Fuller, C. W., Junge, A., & Dvorak, J. (2012). Risk management: FIFA's approach for protecting the health of football players. *British Journal of Sports Medicine, 46*, 11–17.

Impellizzeri, F. M., Rampinini, E., & Marcora, S. M. (2005). Physiological assessment of aerobic training in soccer. *Journal of Sports Sciences, 23*, 583–592.

Jaspers, A., Brink, M. S., Probst, S. G. M., Frencken, W. G. P., & Helsen, W. F. (2017). Relationships between training load indicators and training outcomes in professional soccer. *Sports Medicine, 47*, 533–544.

Junge, A. (2000). The influence of psychological factors on sports injuries. Review of the literature. *American Journal of Sports Medicine, 28*, S10–15.

Kellmann, M., & Kallus, K. W. (2001). *Recovery-Stress Questionnaire for Athletes: User manual.* Champaign, IL: Human Kinetics.

Kellmann, M., & Kallus, K. W. (2016). The Recovery-Stress Questionnaire for Athletes. In K. W. Kallus & M. Kellmann (Eds.), *The Recovery-Stress Questionnaires: User manual* (pp. 86–131). Frankfurt am Main: Pearson Assessment.

Kenttä, G., & Hassmén, P. (1998). Overtraining and recovery. A conceptual model. *Sports Medicine, 26,* 1–16.

Kjaer, M., Magnusson, P., Krogsgaard, M., Boysen Moller, J., Olesen, J., Heinemeier, K., ... Langberg, H. (2006). Extracellular matrix adaptation of tendon and skeletal muscle to exercise. *Journal of Anatomy, 208*(4), 445–450.

Kucera, K. L., Marshall, S. W., Kirkendall, D. T., Marchak, P. M., & Garrett, W. E. (2005). Injury history as a risk factor for incident injury in youth soccer. *British Journal of Sports Medicine, 39,* 462–466.

Larson, G. A., Starkey, C., & Zaichkowsky, L. D. (1996). Psychological aspects of athletic injuries as perceived by athletic trainers. *The Sport Psychologist, 10*(1), 37–47.

Laux, P., Krumm, B., Diers, M., & Flor, H. (2015). Recovery – stress balance and injury risk in professional football players: A prospective study. *Journal of Sports Sciences, 33,* 2140–2148.

Magnusson, S. P., Langberg, H., & Kjaer, M. (2010). The pathogenesis of tendinopathy: Balancing the response to loading. *Nature Reviews Rheumatology, 6*(5), 262–268.

Meeuwisse, W. H., Tyreman, H., Hagel, B., & Emery, C. (2007). A dynamic model of etiology in sport injury: The recursive nature of risk and causation. *Clinical Journal of Sport Medicine, 17,* 215–219.

Nédélec, M., McCall, A., Carling, C., Legall, F., Berthoin, S., & Dupont, G. (2012). Recovery in soccer part I – post-match fatigue and time course of recovery. *Sports Medicine, 42,* 997–1015.

Nederhof, E., Brink, M. S., & Lemmink, K. A. P. M. (2008). Reliability and validity of the Dutch Recovery-Stress Questionnaire for Athletes. *International Journal of Sport Psychology, 39,* 301–311.

Price, R. J., Hawkins, R. D., Hulse, M. A., & Hodson A. (2004). The Football Association medical research programme: An audit of injuries in academy youth football. *British Journal of Sports Medicine, 38,* 466–471.

Rogalski, B., Dawson, B., Heasman, J., & Gabbett T. J. (2013). Training and game loads and injury risk in elite Australian footballers. *Journal of Science and Medicine in Sport, 16,* 499–503.

Schmikli, S. L., Backx, F. J., Kemler, H. J., & Van Mechelen, W. (2009). National survey on sports injuries in the Netherlands: Target populations for sports injury prevention programs. *Clinical Journal of Sport Medicine, 19,* 101–106.

Schwebel, D. C., Banaszek, M. M., & McDaniel, M. (2007). Brief report: Behavioral risk factors for youth soccer (football) injury. *Journal of Pediatric Psychology, 32,* 411–416.

Shyr, J., & Spisic, D. (2014). Automated data analysis. *WIREs Computational Statistics, 6,* 359–366.

Van der Does, H. T. D., Brink, M. S., Otter, R. T. A., Visscher, C., & Lemmink, K. A. P. M. (2017). Injury risk is increased by changes in perceived recovery of team sport players. *Clinical Journal of Sport Medicine, 27,* 46–51.

Van der Sluis, A., Brink, M. S., Pluim, B., Verhagen, E. A., Elferink-Gemser, M. T., & Visscher, C. (in press). Is risk-taking in talented junior tennis players related to overuse injuries? *Scandinavian Journal of Medicine & Science in Sports.* doi:10.1111/sms.12729

Van der Sluis, A., Elferink-Gemser, M. T., Coelho-e-Silva, M. J., Nijboer, J. A., Brink, M. S., & Visscher, C. (2014). Sport injuries aligned to peak height velocity in talented pubertal soccer players. *International Journal of Sports Medicine, 35,* 351–355.

Van Mechelen, W., Twisk, J., Molendijk, A., Blom, B., Snel, J., & Kemper, H. C. (1996). Subject-related risk factors for sports injuries: A 1-yr prospective study in young adults. *Medicine & Science in Sports & Exercise, 28*, 1171–1179.

Williams, J. M., & Andersen, M. B. (1997). Psychosocial influences on central and peripheral vision and reaction time during demanding tasks. *Behavioural Medicine, 22*, 160–167.

Windt, J., & Gabbett, T. J. (2017). How do training and competition workloads relate to injury? The workload–injury aetiology model. *British Journal of Sports Medicine, 51*, 428–435.

Woods, C., Hawkins, R., Hulse, M., & Hodson, A. (2002). The Football Association Medical Research Programme: An audit of injuries in professional football – analysis of preseason injuries. *British Journal of Sports Medicine, 36*, 436–441.

9
STRESS, UNDERRECOVERY, AND HEALTH PROBLEMS IN ATHLETES

Raphael Frank, Insa Nixdorf, and Jürgen Beckmann

Introduction

Periods of high-intensity training are part of every training schedule. Prolonged periods of high intensity and extensiveness of training may lead to training overload and eventually overtraining (Kellmann, 2010). Besides a marked decrease in performance, symptoms associated with overtraining are depressed mood, general apathy, irritability, sleep disturbance, increased vulnerability to injuries, and endocrine changes (Kellmann, 2010). Thus, overtraining can be connected to various negative outcomes. For example, it goes along with an increased susceptibility to infections which is attributed to impaired immune system reactions (Kellmann, 2002). Brenner (2007) coined the term overuse injury which refers to microtraumatic damage to a body part that has been subjected to repetitive stress without sufficient time to heal or recover. In addition to physiological changes in overtrained athletes, psychological disturbances such as depressed mood are also apparent and overlaps with relating psychological problems and disorders are discussed. In this chapter we will primarily focus on impaired performance through somatic and psychological health problems resulting from stress and underrecovery. In addition, aspects to prevent negative outcomes resulting from stress and lack of recovery will be highlighted. We will start with a brief summary of the vulnerabilities to a lack of recovery.

Vulnerabilities to lack of recovery

Several risk factors for a lack of recovery resulting in underrecovery have been identified in research. Among those vulnerabilities to underrecovery are various

Frank, R., Nixdorf, I., & Beckmann, J. (2018). Stress, underrecovery, and health problems in athletes. In M. Kellmann & J. Beckmann (Eds.), *Sport, Recovery, and Performance: Interdisciplinary Insights* (pp. 119–131). Abingdon: Routledge.

factors such as insufficient self-regulation, and insufficient knowledge on recovery and individually adequate recovery strategies.

Insufficient and individually inadequate knowledge on recovery

Researchers argue that recovery appears to be individual and can vary across different athletes on an individual level or between gender and country (Kellmann, 2000; Venter, 2014). In addition, training planning is mostly concerned with the optimal amount of training stress in terms of quality, duration, or intensity. Thus, recovery is often treated as a vague term and specific recovery activities are based on the knowledge and personal engagement of recovering athletes. In a case study with players of a German football youth academy (Beckmann & Beckmann-Waldenmayer, in press) insufficient and inadequate knowledge on individual recovery was found as a major reason for insufficient recovery. Young players perceived stress and recovery were assessed with the Recovery-Stress Questionnaire for Athletes (RESTQ-Sport; Kellmann & Kallus, 2016). With a total of 19 scales the RESTQ-Sport provides a thorough evaluation of athletes perceived stress and recovery over the previous three days: General stress (*General Stress, Emotional Stress, Social Stress, Conflicts/Pressure, Fatigue, Lack of Energy, Physical Complaints*), general recovery (*Success, Social Recovery, Physical Recovery, General Well-being, Sleep Quality*) as well as sport-specific stress (*Disturbed Breaks, Emotional Exhaustion, Injury*) and sport-specific recovery (*Being in Shape, Personal Accomplishment, Self-Efficacy, Self-Regulation*) which can be visualised in a recovery-stress profile. According to the RESTQ-Sport profile the level of stress in the young football players (aged 14 to 18) was comparatively low. However, their recovery was also generally very low. Further qualitative investigation revealed that most of the young players had no knowledge on the importance of recovery. Furthermore, they had no access to what would be the optimal recovery for them on an individual level. When asked 'What do you do for recovery?', exemplary answers were, 'I play FIFA Football Manager' (16-year-old) or 'I do 40 push-ups before going to bed' (16-year-old). Thus, the player's low levels of recovery might be explained with insufficient knowledge on recovery.

Insufficient self-regulation

Another vulnerability to a lack of recovery is due to insufficient self-regulation (for discussion see Beckmann, 2002; Beckmann & Kellmann, 2004). When speaking of self-regulation, Kuhl and Beckmann (1994a) referred to auxiliary (usually meta-) processes that aid individuals in generating or maintaining a state that is optimal for his/her transactions with the environment. Self-regulation involves the control of thinking, emotion, attention, and concentration. Stressors constitute adverse conditions that demand the employment of self-regulatory skills to reduce the stress load and to cope with the adverse conditions. Recovery can suffer from adverse external conditions (e.g., a noisy environment when trying to rest between trials, an uncomfortable bed, etc.) as well as from adverse internal conditions (e.g., worrying about being dismissed from the team after a bad performance, conflicts, etc.).

Most important in the context of recovery is the deactivation problem. When athletes do not manage to deactivate the underlying intentions of activities already performed, which is most likely the case after a slump has occurred, their subsequent performance is negatively affected. If an intention is not deactivated after an outcome has been obtained, its activation will remain at a high level. Thoughts related to that activity are likely to intrude into consciousness, thereby interfering with concentration on a new activity (Beckmann, 1994). The intrusions can disturb proactive as well as passive recovery (for a definition of proactive and passive recovery, see Kellmann, 2002). Sleep is an important form of passive recovery. Thoughts about failing to reach a goal during the day may result in sleep disruption. If a change of activity is planned as a form of proactive recovery, the intrusions may impair this new activity and thus ruin recovery. The failure to deactivate will thus lead to proximal underperformance (in the case of reduced concentration for the next activity) or distal underperformance (in the case of regaining motivation for future competitions). Whereas the first is mainly mediated through a lack of concentration, the second is primarily mediated by disturbed recovery.

State orientation is a personality disposition that is related to insufficient self-regulation. State orientation is characterised by chronic negative affect, blocked access to the (implicit) self, and impaired self-regulation (Kuhl, 2001). State-oriented individuals tend to ruminate about experienced failure (failure-related state orientation) and decision alternatives (decision-related state orientation). State-oriented individuals are unable to disengage from a past activity and remain preoccupied with that activity. Empirical findings support the assumption that state-oriented individuals are especially likely to end up in self-evaluation loops (see Beckmann, 1994). Furthermore, state-oriented individuals have an impaired access to their implicit self which results in alienation from their real needs (Kuhl & Beckmann, 1994b) as for example individual optimal recovery.

Thus, state orientation can generate underrecovery in two ways: First, because of impairing recovery through an inability to let go of stress load (e.g., a failure experience); second, because of blocking access to recovery strategies optimally fitting individual needs. In fact, Beckmann and Kellmann (2004) found recovery to be impaired in state-oriented individuals through rumination and high self-discipline. The latter is related to doing one's duty rather than taking care of oneself and probably related to perfectionism.

Young athletes are particularly vulnerable to health problems

Only recently, research has addressed the above stated problems in junior athletes. In fact, junior athletes appear to be especially vulnerable to health problems (Elbe & Beckmann, 2006), frequently resulting in an untimely end of career (Elbe, Beckmann, & Szymanski, 2003). Recovery-stress imbalance was found to be a major determinant in this regard. Therefore, effects of stress and underrecovery in young athletes will be focused in more detail.

In a study with 13- to 18-year-old swimmers across several countries Raglin, Sawamura, Alexiou, Hassmén, and Kenttä (2000) found that 35% had been overtrained at least once. Statistics presented by the Loyola University Health System (2013) trace serious overuse injuries to intense specialised training in young athletes. According to Schubring and Thiel (2014), sickness- and injury-related absence of junior athletes in practise and competition has meanwhile become accepted as 'normal case'. Furthermore, research shows high levels of depressive syndromes in elite athletes (Nixdorf, Frank, Hautzinger, & Beckmann, 2013). Especially junior athletes were found to have relatively high levels of depressive symptoms. Several risk factors are being discussed, such as injuries or adjusting to new conditions (Wolanin, Gross, & Hong, 2015; Yang et al., 2007). Nixdorf and colleagues (2013) found high sport-related stress and low sport-related recovery to be correlated with depression.

Stress experience of junior athletes has largely increased over the last decades due to raised practise and training demands. According to Fessler and colleagues (2002) the overall amount of time junior athletes (German D cadre) spent for training and practise increased by almost 25% between 1979 and 2000. This study did not even take into account travel time spent by travelling between home, school, and training facilities. Several studies (e.g., Gould, Jackson, & Finch, 1993; Puente-Díaz & Anshel, 2005; Reeves, Nicholls, & McKenna, 2009) furnish evidence that, in addition to the stress related to training, practise, and competitions, the amount of daily stress in an athlete's life is sufficient to cause an essential burden. Concerns about personal achievement potential, a lost match accompanied by fear of failure and dissatisfaction, and conflicts with trainers, partners, and family, as well as the time and effort that goes into training, are identified as the main stressors. Thiel and colleagues (2011) conclude that the interaction of continuously increasing demands in elite sports, the recognised importance of education for life, and developmental tasks that need to be dealt with during adolescence constitutes a high-risk potential for junior athletes.

Effects on performance, career, and somatic health

At this point we will briefly address a problem in youth sport that is associated with stress and lack of recovery before turning to athletes' health in more detail: Sport attrition and drop out. Each year approximately 35% of young athletes quit participation in sport, and whether an athlete returns to participation at a later date is unknown (Purcell, 2005). Sports attrition rates are the highest during the transitional years of adolescence, when outside influences have the most impact (Breunner, 2012). According to the 2008 Report on Trends and Participation in Organized Youth Sports by the US National Council of Youth Sports Health Problems the number one reason for dropping out of sports is 'not having fun' (38.5%) with health problems being in second place among boys (29%) and third place among girls (27%). Nixdorf, Frank, and Beckmann (2015) analysed various stressors in athletes and concluded, that especially sport-related stressors such as training loads are related to intentions of dropout. Therefore, excessive training loads and training stress might provoke even ends of careers.

Cresswell and Eklund (2007) found loss of autonomy and experience of powerlessness along with the perception of reduced opportunities for personality development as crucial factors for impaired development of performance. Perceived lack of control over one's life, a lack of autonomy has frequently been shown to be a strong stressor resulting in health problems (e.g., Steptoe & Appels, 1989), Kellmann (2002) has pointed out the role of overtraining (see also Smith, 2004) in performance decrements. Injury is a very prominent cause for a loss of performance capacity (Walker, Thatcher, & Lavallee, 2007).

As mentioned above, serious overuse injuries are associated with intense specialised training (Loyola University Health System, 2013). In addition to injuries diseases, among which infections are most prominent, can interfere with performance. Even minor infections can impair exercise performance or even prevent the athlete from competing. Periods of intensified training have been shown to depress immune function and there is a reduction of resistance to common minor illnesses. In periods of intensified training immune function might not fully recover from successive training sessions and some functions can become chronically depressed (Gleeson, 2005). However, some athletes are more prone to illness than others why differential factors should be taken into account. A factor shown to have an effect on both perceived stress as well as recovery is action versus state orientation (Beckmann & Kellmann, 2004). As already stated above, state orientation is characterised by a tendency to ruminate about current, past and future states (Kuhl & Beckmann, 1994a).

There are a number of studies linking overtraining to a suppression of the immune system and infections as a consequence (see MacKinnon, 2000; Nieman & Pedersen, 1999 for overviews). However, the evidence is not completely unequivocal. Other factors in addition to overtraining have been taken into account, such as individual differences and motivational factors (e.g., training monotony; Foster, 1998). Generally, the clinical mechanisms mediating the effects of training load on the immune system are not sufficiently explained. One of the few research findings in this area is that training load more or less activates the immune system, which can be both, beneficial as well as detrimental (cf. Wolfarth & Blume, 2011).

A study by Zier (2015) shows that not objective load (assessed through the metabolic equivalent) but perceived stress (assessed with the RESTQ-Sport) determines susceptibility to infections (assessed with the Wisconsin Upper Respiratory Symptoms Scale; Barrett et al., 2002). Furthermore, the effect of training load on perceived stress was found to be mediated by social support. Athletes who indicated to have high social support showed less perceived stress than athletes with low social support. The perceived stress in athletes with high-level social support was almost unaffected by training load whereas athletes with low social support showed a pronounced increase in perceived stress with an increase in training load.

Effects on mental health

Periods of stress and lack of recovery can be expected in athletes. However, besides somatic effects, psychological outcomes are also apparent. Most obvious, there seems to be a connection between tremendous physical stress through exercise and negative mood. Many studies showed clear connections between increased training loads and negative or depressed mood (Morgan, Brown, Raglin, O'Connor, & Ellickson, 1987; Raglin, Morgan, & O'Connor, 1991; Steinacker et al., 2000). This connection becomes even more obvious when considering the overtraining syndrome and its relation to depressive syndromes. A long-lasting imbalance between exhaustion and recovery can develop into overtraining. Especially after long periods of intensified training, performance decreases can occur. If this state persists although the athlete took a resting period of at least several weeks or months it is referred to as overtraining syndrome (Meeusen et al., 2013). Besides the mentioned decrease in performance, which is obviously negative for striving athletes, this chronic state can manifest itself in symptoms such as fatigue, loss of weight and appetite, sleep disturbances, emotional instability, anxiety, depressive mood, heavy transpiration, heavy muscles and frequent, small infections (Budgett et al., 2000). Many of these symptoms can be related to symptoms during a depressive disorder. Armstrong and Van Heest (2002) point out, that there are in fact great overlaps in the symptomatology (e.g., depressed mood, loss of appetite and weight, insomnia, or fatigue). The authors also conclude, that there are comparable changes in the vegetative nervous system and the associated neurotransmitters. Following their argumentation, the overtraining syndrome might have a similar aetiology to depression. Puffer and McShane (1992) also highlight the connection between overtraining and depression. They argue that depression may appear without fatigue, but is far more frequent seen with physiological fatigue in athletes. Besides the found effects between training loads and depressed moods, a recent study showed connections between underrecovery and depressive syndromes (Nixdorf et al., 2013). Results showed depressive symptoms to be prone in athletes with high scores in exhaustion and low scores in recovery.

These results clearly highlight the relationship between training stress, lack of recovery and depression (for review see Frank, Nixdorf, & Beckmann, 2013). For stress to be connected to psychological disorders, especially to depression, is little surprising and well recognised in the general population (Hammen, Kim, Eberhart, & Brennan, 2009; Lee, Jeong, Kwak, & Park, 2010; Monroe & Reid, 2009). For elite athletes this has recently been replicated, by findings showing a connection between chronic stress and depressive symptoms (Nixdorf et al., 2013). Besides depressive symptoms experiences of burnout are also recognised as a result of training stress and a lack of recovery (Lemyre, Roberts, & Stray-Gundersen, 2007). According to Angeli, Minetto, Dovio, and Paccotti (2004) burnout is a stress-related condition that consists of alteration of physiological functions and adaptation to performance, impairment of psychological processing, immunological dysfunction and biochemical abnormalities. Also other researchers consider burnout as a stress-related syndrome (Gustafsson, Kenttä, & Hassmén, 2011; Smith, 1986), in which training stress might play an important role. In their review on athlete burnout Goodger, Gorely, Lavallee, and Harwood (2007) report substantial evidence for the association between burnout and training loads or a lack in recovery.

However, stress appears to be a construct which covers a relatively wide range. Therefore, various stressors (including training stress) can lead to experiences of stress. As already pointed out in regards for youth athletes' stressor can be various and impact athletes' lives in various domains. Research on stressors in the context of elite sports point out that stressors can be found in the competitive surrounding as well as in the organisation an athlete is located in (Hanton, Fletcher, & Coughlan, 2005). These stressors are clearly related to the sport organisation or the competitive nature of elite sports athletes. However, athletes are also exposed to stressors such as job insecurity or difficulties balancing sport, study commitments (Noblet & Gifford, 2002) and the physical demand of training (Gould et al., 1993). As summed up above, injuries (Appaneal, Levine, Perna, & Roh, 2009; Leddy, Lambert, & Ogles, 1994) and failure (Hammond, Gialloreto, Kubas, & Davis, 2013) were shown to be important stressors in regards to depressive symptoms. As already mentioned, Nixdorf and colleagues (2015) explored in a qualitative analysis sources of stress in German elite athletes. Results revealed for some stressors to be connected with chronic stress, lack of recovery, depressive symptoms, and intentions of dropout. More specific, stressors which are clearly sport-related such as training loads, training stress or pressure to perform showed the strongest effects. This shows again the importance of managing stress and recovery. It also highlights the importance of sport-related stressors for negative outcomes such as depression, stress, or dropout.

Conclusion and recommendation for applied practise

As highlighted, stress and underrecovery are connected to various and in some instance severe somatic and psychological problems such as depression, susceptibility to infections or dropout. Prevention of such negative outcomes seem therefore a valuable goal for practitioners in the field and to positively manage stress and recovery among athletes appears as an essential task in this regard. Therefore, Kellmann (2010) proposed possibilities for preventing overtraining in athletes, which are highlighted and expanded in the following with consideration of the above stated effects. The author argues according to a model on recovery (scissor model; Kellmann, 2002), ". . . that increased recovery must co-occur with the increasing stress if the stress-state is to remain stable" (Kellmann, 2010, p. 96). It is further argued that negative cycles can lead into greater experiences of stress or lead into overtraining. Considerable factors are hereby the recovery demands which is defined as the amount (quality and quantity) of recovery in order to balance the stress-state. Furthermore, individual resources are limiting the capacity to meet the recovery demands (Kellmann, 2010). Taking a look at this general model, important aspects in preventing stress-based outcomes can be argued. In the following, possible aspects for prevention are focused, which are the monitoring of athletes' stress and recovery level, adjustment of training stress, promotion of recovery, and strengthening of individual resources.

Taking the *scissor model* into consideration, the need to monitor the balance between stress and recovery becomes apparent (Kellmann, 2010). Therefore, the individual state of stress and recovery can be assessed, which would give practitioners clues when to promote recovery in athletes. Psychological and somatic measurements can help illustrate the current stress and recovery state (Kellmann, 2000, for an overview see Chapter 1). Furthermore, this knowledge on current states of stress and recovery builds a basis for subsequent prevention methods of stress-related problems. Interventions might focus on reduction of training loads or building recovery possibilities (see below) and can be based on measured indicators through monitoring. The importance of monitoring stress and recovery states is based on its connection to negative outcomes such as overtraining (Kellmann, Altenburg, Lormes, & Steinacker, 2001) or depression (Nixdorf et al., 2013). It is further important to especially monitor episodes with high levels of stress. This refers to phases of intensified exercise (Meeusen et al., 2013) but also to stressful phases such as competitions (Hammond et al., 2013). Results showed, that high levels of stress and low levels of recovery in phases of competition are associated with greater levels of depressive symptoms in subsequent phases of recovery (Nixdorf, Frank, & Beckmann, in press).

One clear advantage in monitoring athletes' state of stress and recovery is apparent when focusing the influence of (training) stress. Especially in high-intensity sport disciplines, where performance is largely based of high levels of amount of trainings loads, monitoring can provide coaches and athletes important information (Kellmann et al., 2001). Exercise planning can be more precise by balancing training stress in a way to enhance performance rather than lead into stress-based negative outcomes such as overtraining or burnout.

Clearly, from a training perspective the adjustment of training stress is a main factor in building performance and, as pointed out, is also important in preventing overtraining or other potential negative outcomes. However, to argue only from a training perspective would be too narrow. According to the *scissor model* (Kellmann, 2002) possibilities of recovery are necessary to balance the previously exposed stress and thus appear to be a limiting factor. Hence, building recovery might contribute to a greater capacity for (training) stress. This would bare degrees of freedom for training enhancement and build resilience for stress-related problems. Here, possibilities for recovery should be increased (Kellmann, 2010). In addition, individual preferences of recovery modalities can be assessed and further developed. Venter (2014) pointed out, that there are differences based on gender and that there is potential in athletes for enhancing recovery possibilities and activities.

Monitoring and, as a consequence, intervening in exercise and recovery are important possibilities in order to prevent (training) stress-related negative outcomes. However, monitoring illustrates also a strategy which would lead to interventions based on current imbalances and thus would rather lead to reacting instead of proactive building resilience in athletes. By focusing on individual resources, possibilities for optimizing recovery possibilities and coping with stress can be highlighted. In this regard, factors which can be considered as vulnerabilities or personal strengths with connections to stress, recovery and negative psychological outcomes should be focused.

As pointed out earlier, individual knowledge on recovery process and activities should be considered as valuable. Especially in the somewhat vulnerable population of young but ambitious athletes the consideration of knowledge and competence in this regard might be valuable. Therefore, personal skills in self-regulation and development of self-responsibility might be important (Beckmann & Kellmann, 2004). Furthermore, various personal aspects such as skills, cognition or attitudes are discussed. Perfectionism for example is often highlighted as a potential negative cognition for stress based outcomes as burnout (Appleton, Hall, & Hill, 2009; Hill, 2013). More specific research showed longitudinally that perfectionistic concerns can lead to burnout (Madigan, Stoeber, & Passfield, 2015). Therefore, perfectionism might be valuable in an early prevention of negative outcomes based on stress and underrecovery. Furthermore, skills in coping have variously been connected to psychological problems such as burnout and depression (Goodger et al., 2007; Gustafsson et al., 2011; Nixdorf et al., 2013). In a recent study (Nixdorf et al., in press), negative coping was found to explain increased levels of burnout and depression after one season. In addition, the study revealed dysfunctional attitudes – attitudes with excessively high standards and rigid self-evaluation – as another factor with predictive value. Therefore, prevention by focusing individual resources should take personal competences such as coping with stress and general attitudes (perfectionistic and dysfunctional) into consideration. Building and developing adequate coping strategies and functional attitudes might highlight important aspects in putting athletes in a promising position for balancing stress and recovery in a successful manner.

In summary, there are multiple possibilities for prevention of underrecovery and stress-related mental health problems. Monitoring of athletes' stress and recovery states is therefore an important basis. However, research also indicates the importance regarding the promotion of recovery and building individual resources in order to successfully cope with stress. These factors might bare potential for athletes to minimise the risk of negative outcomes in regards to somatic health, psychological health, or dropout and therefore possibly enhance performance.

References

Angeli, A., Minetto, M., Dovio, A., & Paccotti, P. (2004). The overtraining syndrome in athletes: A stress-related disorder. *Journal of Endocrinological Investigation, 27*(6), 603–612.

Appaneal, R. N., Levine, B. R., Perna, F. M., & Roh, J. L. (2009). Measuring postinjury depression among male and female competitive athletes. *Journal of Sport & Exercise Psychology, 31*(1), 60–76.

Appleton, P. R., Hall, H. K., & Hill, A. P. (2009). Relations between multidimensional perfectionism and burnout in junior-elite male athletes. *Psychology of Sport and Exercise, 10*(4), 457–465.

Armstrong, L. E., & Van Heest, J. L. (2002). The unknown mechanism of the overtraining syndrome: Clues from depression and psychoneuroimmunology. *Sports Medicine, 32*(3), 185–209.

Barrett, B., Locken, K., Maberry, R., Schwamman, J., Bobula, J., Brown, R., & Stauffacher, E. (2002). The Wisconsin Upper Respiratory Symptom Survey: Development of an instrument to measure the common cold. *Journal of Family Practice, 51*(3), 265–273.

Beckmann, J. (1994). Rumination and the deactivation of an intention. *Motivation and Emotion, 18*, 317–334.

Beckmann, J. (2002). Interaction of volition and recovery. In M. Kellmann (Ed.), *Optimal recovery: Preventing underperformance in athletes* (pp. 269–282). Champaign, IL: Human Kinetics.

Beckmann, J., & Beckmann-Waldenmayer, D. (in press). Talent development in youth football. In E. Konter, J. Beckmann, & T. Loughead (Eds.), *Football psychology*. Abingdon: Routledge.

Beckmann, J., & Kellmann, M. (2004). Self-regulation and recovery: Approaching an understanding of the process of recovery from stress. *Psychological Reports, 95*, 1135–1153.

Brenner, J. S. (2007). Overuse injuries, overtraining, and burnout in child and adolescent athletes. *Pediatrics, 119*, 1242–1245.

Breunner, C. C. (2012). Avoidance of burnout in the young athlete. *Pediatric Annals, 4*, 335–339.

Budgett, R., Newsholme, E., Lehmann, M., Sharp, C., Jones, D., Peto, T., . . . White, P. (2000). Redefining the overtraining syndrome as the unexplained underperformance syndrome. *British Journal of Sports Medicine, 34*(1), 67–68.

Cresswell, S. L., & Eklund, R. C. (2007). Athlete burnout: A longitudinal qualitative study. *The Sport Psychologist, 21*, 1–20.

Elbe, A.-M., & Beckmann, J. (2006). Psychological factors of talent development and athletic performance. In G. Tenenbaum & D. Hackfort (Eds.), *Essential processes for attaining peak performance* (pp. 137–157). Oxford, UK: Meyer & Meyer Sport Ltd.

Elbe, A.-M., Beckmann, J., & Szymanski, B. (2003). Das Dropout Phänomen an Eliteschulen des Sports – ein Problem der Selbstregulation? [The drop-out phenomena in elite sports academies – a problem of self-regulation?]. *Leistungssport, 33*, 46–49.

Fessler, N., Frommknecht, R., Kaiser, R., Renna, M., Schorer, J., & Binder, M. (2002). *Förderung des leistungssportlichen Nachwuchses – Ergebnisse der Athletenbefragung in der D-Kader-Studie Baden-Württemberg 1999/2000* [Promotion of competitive youth athletes – results from the athlete evaluation of cadre-d-study in Baden-Württemberg 1999/2000]. Schorndorf: Hofmann.

Foster, C. (1998). Monitoring training in athletes with reference to overtraining syndrome. *Medicine and Science in Sports and Exercise, 30*, 1164–1168.

Frank, R., Nixdorf, I., & Beckmann, J. (2013). Depressionen im Hochleistungssport: Prävalenzen und psychologische Einflüsse [Depression in elite athletes: Prevalence and psychological factors]. *Deutsche Zeitschrift für Sportmedizin, 64*(11), 320–326.

Gleeson, M. (2005). Immune function in sport and exercise. *Journal of Applied Physiology, 103*, 693–699.

Goodger, K., Gorely, T., Lavallee, D., & Harwood, C. (2007). Burnout in sport: A systematic review. *The Sport Psychologist, 21*, 127–151.

Gould, D., Jackson, S., & Finch, L. (1993). Sources of stress in national champion figure skaters. *Journal of Sport & Exercise Psychology, 15*(2), 134–159.

Gustafsson, H., Kenttä, G., & Hassmén, P. (2011). Athlete burnout: An integrated model and future research directions. *International Review of Sport and Exercise Psychology, 4*(1), 3–24.

Hammen, C., Kim, E. Y., Eberhart, N. K., & Brennan, P. A. (2009). Chronic and acute stress and the prediction of major depression in women. *Depression and Anxiety, 26*(8), 718–723.

Hammond, T., Gialloreto, C., Kubas, H., & Davis, H. (2013). The prevalence of failure-based depression among elite athletes. *Clinical Journal of Sport Medicine, 23*(4), 273–277.

Hanton, S., Fletcher, D., & Coughlan, G. (2005). Stress in elite sport performers: A comparative study of competitive and organizational stressors. *Journal of Sports Sciences, 23*(10), 1129–1141.

Hill, A. P. (2013). Perfectionism and burnout in junior soccer players: A test of the 2 x 2 model of dispositional perfectionism. *Journal of Sport & Exercise Psychology, 35*(1), 18–29.

Kellmann, M. (2000). Psychologische Methoden der Erholungs-Beanspruchungs-Diagnostik [Psychological methods of stress/recovery diagnostics]. *Deutsche Zeitschrift für Sportmedizin, 51*(7), 253–258.

Kellmann, M. (2002). Underrecovery and overtraining: Different concepts-similar impact. In M. Kellmann (Ed.), *Enhancing recovery: Preventing underperformance in athletes* (pp. 3–24). Champaign, IL: Human Kinetics.

Kellmann, M. (2010). Preventing overtraining in athletes in high-intensity sports and stress/recovery monitoring. *Scandinavian Journal of Medicine and Science in Sports, 20*(2), 95–102.

Kellmann, M., Altenburg, D., Lormes, W., & Steinacker, J. M. (2001). Assessing stress and recovery during preparation for the World Championships in rowing. *The Sport Psychologist, 15*(2), 151–167.

Kellmann, M., & Kallus, K. W. (2016). The Recovery-Stress Questionnaire for Athletes. In K. W. Kallus & M. Kellmann (Eds.), *The Recovery-Stress Questionnaires: User manual* (pp. 86–131). Frankfurt am Main: Pearson Assessment.

Kuhl, J. (2001). *Motivation und Persönlichkeit* [Motivation and personality]. Göttingen: Hogrefe.

Kuhl, J., & Beckmann, J. (Eds.). (1994a). *Volition and personality: Action and state orientation*. Seattle: Hogrefe & Huber Publishers.

Kuhl, J., & Beckmann, J. (1994b). Alienation. Ignoring one's preferences. In J. Kuhl & J. Beckmann (Eds.), *Volition and personality: Action and state orientation* (pp. 375–390). Seattle: Hogrefe & Huber Publishers.

Leddy, M. H., Lambert, M. J., & Ogles, B. M. (1994). Psychological consequences of athletic injury among high-level competitors. *Research Quarterly for Exercise and Sport, 65*(4), 347–354.

Lee, S., Jeong, J., Kwak, Y., & Park, S. K. (2010). Depression research: Where are we now? *Molecular Brain, 3*, 8.

Lemyre, P.-N., Roberts, G. C., & Stray-Gundersen, J. (2007). Motivation, overtraining, and burnout: Can self-determined motivation predict overtraining and burnout in elite athletes? *European Journal of Sport Science, 7*(2), 115–126.

Loyola University Health System. (2013, April 19). Intense, specialized training in young athletes linked to serious overuse injuries. *Science Daily*. Retrieved February 16, 2014, from www.science-daily.com/releases/2013/04/130419132508.htm

MacKinnon, L. T. (2000). Overtraining effects on immunity and performance in athletes. *Immunology and Cell Biology, 78*, 502–509.

Madigan, D. J., Stoeber, J., & Passfield, L. (2015). Perfectionism and burnout in junior athletes: A three-month longitudinal study. *Journal of Sport & Exercise Psychology, 37*(3), 305–315.

Meeusen, R., Duclos, M., Foster, C., Fry, A., Gleeson, M., Nieman, D., . . . & Urhausen, A. (2013). Prevention, diagnosis, and treatment of the overtraining syndrome: Joint consensus statement of the European College of Sport Science and the American College of Sports Medicine. *Medicine and Science in Sports and Exercise, 45*(1), 186–205.

Monroe, S. M., & Reid, M. W. (2009). Life stress and major depression. *Current Directions in Psychological Science, 18*(2), 68–72.

Morgan, W. P., Brown, D. R., Raglin, J. S., O'Connor, P. J., & Ellickson, K. A. (1987). Psychological monitoring of overtraining and staleness. *British Journal of Sports Medicine, 21*(3), 107–114.

National Council of Youth Sports. (2008). *Report on trends and participation in organized youth sports*. Stuart, FL: National Council of Youth Sports.

Nieman, D. C., & Pedersen, B. K. (1999). Exercise and immune function. Recent developments. *Sports Medicine, 27*, 73–80.

Nixdorf, I., Frank, R., & Beckmann, J. (2015). An explorative study on major stressors and its connection to depression and chronic stress among German elite athletes. *Advances in Physical Education, 5*(4), 255–262.

Nixdorf, I., Frank, R., & Beckmann, J. (in press). Preventing burnout and depression in youth football. In E. Konter, J. Beckmann, & T. Loughead (Eds.), *Football psychology*. Abingdon: Routledge.

Nixdorf, I., Frank, R., Hautzinger, M., & Beckmann, J. (2013). Prevalence of depressive symptoms and correlating variables among German elite athletes. *Journal of Clinical Sport Psychology, 7*, 313–326.

Noblet, A. J., & Gifford, S. M. (2002). The sources of stress experienced by professional Australian footballers. *Journal of Applied Sport Psychology, 14*(1), 1–13.

Puente-Díaz, R., & Anshel, M. H. (2005). Sources of acute stress, cognitive appraisal, and coping strategies among highly skilled Mexican and U.S. competitive tennis players. *Journal of Social Psychology, 145*(4), 429–446.

Puffer, J. C., & McShane, J. M. (1992). Depression and chronic fatigue in athletes. *Clinics in Sports Medicine, 11*(2), 327–338.

Purcell, L. K. (2005). Sport readiness in children and youth. *Paediatric Child Health, 10*, 343–344.

Raglin, J. S., Morgan, W. P., & O'Connor, P. J. (1991). Changes in mood states during training in female and male college swimmers. *International Journal of Sports Medicine, 12*(6), 585–589.

Raglin, J., Sawamura, S., Alexiou, S., Hassmén, P., & Kenttä, G. (2000). Training practices and staleness in 13–18-year-old swimmers. A cross-cultural study. *Pediatric Exercise Science, 12*, 61–70.

Reeves, C. W., Nicholls, A. R., & McKenna, J. (2009). Stressors and coping strategies among early and middle adolescent premier league academy soccer players. Differences according to age. *Journal of Applied Sport Psychology, 21*, 31–48.

Schubring, A., & Thiel, A. (2014). Coping with growth in adolescent elite sports. *Sociology of Sport Journal, 31*, 304–326.

Smith, L. L. (2004). Tissue trauma: The underlying cause of overtraining syndrome? *Journal of Strength and Conditioning Research, 18*, 185–193.

Smith, R. E. (1986). Toward a cognitive-affective model of athletic burnout. *Journal of Sport Psychology, 8*(1), 36–50.

Steinacker, J. M., Lormes, W., Kellmann, M., Liu, Y., Reißnecker, S., Opitz-Gress, A., . . . Altenburg, D. (2000). Training of junior rowers before world championships. Effects on performance, mood state and selected hormonal and metabolic responses. *Journal of Sports Medicine and Physical Fitness, 40*(4), 327–335.

Steptoe, A., & Appels, A. (Eds.). (1989). *Stress, personal control, and health*. New York, NY: Wiley.

Thiel, A., Diehl, K., Giel, K., Schnell, A., Schubring, A., Mayer, J., . . . Schneider, S. (2011). The German young Olympic athletes' lifestyle and health management study (GOAL study): Design of a mixed-method study. *BMC Public Health, 11*(1), 410.

Venter, R. E. (2014). Perceptions of team athletes on the importance of recovery modalities. *European Journal of Sport Science, 14*(1), 69–76.

Walker, N., Thatcher, J., & Lavallee, D. (2007). Psychological responses to injury in competitive sport: A critical review. *The Journal of The Royal Society for the Promotion of Health, 127*, 174–180.

Wolanin, A., Gross, M., & Hong, E. (2015). Depression in athletes: Prevalence and risk factors. *Current Sports Medicine Reports, 14*(1), 56–60.

Wolfarth, B., & Blume, K. (2011). Belastbarkeit und Trainierbarkeit aus internistischer Sicht unter besonderer Berücksichtigung des Immunsystems bei Nachwuchsleistungssportlern [Capacity and trainability from an internist point of view, with particular consideration of the immune system in junior elite athletes.]. In E. Müller (Ed.), *BISp-Symposium: Top Forschung für den Spitzensport. Bonn, 15. April 2010* (pp. 125–137). Köln: Sportverlag Strauß.

Yang, J., Peek-Asa, C., Corlette, J. D., Cheng, G., Foster, D.T., & Albright, J. (2007). Prevalence of and risk factors associated with symptoms of depression in competitive collegiate student athletes. *Clinical Journal of Sport Medicine, 17*(6), 481–487.

Zier, E. (2015). *Belastbarkeit von Nachwuchsleistungssportlern- und Sportlerinnen. Über den Zusammenhang zwischen Trainingsbelastung, wahrgenommener Beanspruchung, individuellen Voraussetzungen und Infektanfälligkeit junger Athleten und Athletinnen* [Capacity of junior elite athletes. On the relation between exercise load, perceived stress, individual resources and infect vulnerability of young athletes]. Unpublished Dissertation, Technical University Munich, Germany.

10
QUANTIFICATION OF TRAINING AND COMPETITION LOADS IN ENDURANCE SPORTS

A key to recovery-stress balance and performance

Avish P. Sharma and Iñigo Mujika

Introduction

Training is the systematic application of stress (predominantly in the form of exercise) and recovery to enhance physiological capacity, refine motor patterns, reduce injury/illness risk, and ultimately improve performance. Coaches and trainers generally consider that the outcome of the training process depends on the type and amount of the stimulus, and understanding this cause-and-effect relationship between training dose and response is crucial to prescribe exercise training accordingly (Lambert & Mujika, 2013a). To analyse and establish causal relationships between the training performed by an athlete and the resultant physiological and performance adaptations, it is necessary to quantify precisely and reliably the training load undertaken by the athlete. Indeed, it is difficult to assess a competitive performance without first considering the prior training of an athlete (Mujika, 2013). For this reason, several sport scientists have underlined the importance of proper training quantification in relation to both individual athlete adaptation and scientific research (Foster, Florhaug, et al., 2001; Hopkins, 1991; Pollock, 1973).

To maximise the effectiveness of training and achieve peak performance at a desired time, quantifying the training load of an athlete and its relationship to performance outcomes should be a priority (Borresen & Lambert, 2009). An incorrect training load may lead to excessive accumulated fatigue or detraining; an appropriate load should facilitate optimal improvements in an individual athlete's performance. Given strong links between training and performance/injury, it is surprising that the methodology for measurement of training has not been a focus of attention

---

Sharma, A. P., & Mujika, I. (2018). Quantification of training and competition loads in endurance sports: A key to recovery-stress balance and performance. In M. Kellmann & J. Beckmann (Eds.), *Sport, Recovery, and Performance: Interdisciplinary Insights* (pp. 132–147). Abingdon: Routledge.

in the sport science literature (Hopkins, 1991). Hopkins considered it to be a blind spot that some articles reporting the effects of training neglect to describe the method by which the measures of training were obtained.

More recently, several reviews have described the methods and applications of quantifying the training load in sports and research (Borresen & Lambert, 2009; Lambert, 2012), monitoring training with respect to minimising nonfunctional overreaching, injury and illness (Halson, 2014), and objective and subjective measures of athlete well-being available to guide training and detect any progression towards negative outcomes (Saw, Main, & Gastin, 2016). Irrespective of the quantification methods used, they can be defined as quantifying either external or internal training load (Halson, 2014; Impellizzeri, Rampinini, & Marcora, 2005; Saw et al., 2016). The external training load is an objective measure of the work that an athlete completes either during training or competition (e.g., distance completed, total elevation gain, or running speed). This measure contrasts with the internal workload, which assesses the biological stress imposed by the training session and is typically defined by the disturbance in homeostasis of physiological and metabolic processes during the exercise training session (Lambert, 2012). In a recent investigation studying the relationship between different training load methods and performance in cyclists (Sanders, Abt, Hesselink, Myers, & Akubat, 2017), measures integrating individual physiological characteristics (i.e., relationship between heart rate and blood lactate, measures of internal load) had the strongest dose-response relationships with performance and submaximal aerobic fitness. It is important to emphasise that the external training load does not strictly measure the biological stress imposed by a given training session, rather it provides the context necessary for interpretation of internal load measures. In fact, two athletes may undertake an identical external training load but experience quite different internal loads, depending on their fitness, training background and genetic characteristics (Halson, 2014; Impellizzeri et al., 2005; Lambert, 2012). In this respect, quantifying external load alone is limited, as it may not be sensitive to detecting individual responses to training. However, it is necessary to provide context for the physiological stress imposed by training.

This chapter discusses the application of training load quantification in both endurance sports and research, summarises the most relevant external and internal workload measures in endurance sports, and provides practical examples of their implementation in the context of altitude training to adjust the training programmes of elite athletes in accordance to their individualised recovery-stress balance.

The basics of training load quantification in endurance sports

Performance in most endurance events is determined largely by the maximal sustained power production for a given competition distance and the energy cost of maintaining a given racing speed. In shorter endurance events and during accelerations, establishing breakaways and sprints, anaerobic capacity and maximal speed may also contribute to endurance performance and competition outcomes (Mujika, Rønnestad, & Martin, 2016). This combination implies that both low-to-moderate and high-intensity training are important for the endurance athlete to optimise adaptation to training (Boullosa, Abreu, Varela-Sanz, & Mujika, 2013; Seiler, 2010; Stöggl & Sperlich, 2014). Training load methods should cover the entire range of training intensities, in addition to other training variables such as volume and frequency, and a range of training modalities used by endurance athletes (Table 10.1). With this in mind, it would appear that multiple (and not a single) monitoring tools are required to adequately quantify the training response.

Data relating to training loads and to athletes' responses and adaptations are of interest to athletes, coaches, and sport scientists. Training data, physiological monitoring and direct observation can have a positive motivational impact on the athlete by heightening awareness of their investment in time and effort, as well as others (e.g., coach and sports scientist), and encouraging a more systematic and goal-oriented approach to training (Hopkins, 1991). A systematic approach to training quantification also facilitates better training prescription, with coaches able to modify training based on data, physiological measures of stress and direct observation. Sport scientists can undertake descriptive and experimental studies on training effects, performance prediction and enhancement, recovery, and injury prevention to identify outcomes relevant and easily implementable by coaches into

TABLE 10.1 Training variables quantified daily and individually for an entire season in a group of national and international level swimmers (Mujika et al., 1995; Mujika, Chatard, Busso, et al., 1996).

Training variable
Frequency (sessions per day)
Total volume (km)
Intensity I (km below ≤ 2 mmol blood lactate)
Intensity II (km 2–4 mmol blood lactate)
Intensity III (km 4–6 mmol blood lactate)
Intensity IV (km ≥ 6 mmol blood lactate)
Intensity V (km sprint swimming)
50 m Pool (km)
25 m Pool (km)
Normal swim (km)
Arm pulling (km)
Kicking (km)
Front crawl (km)
Medley (km)
Own stroke (km)
Strength swim (increased resistance to advance, km or min)
Stroke rate (km to develop stroke frequency)
Distance per stroke (km to develop stroke distance)
Weight lifting (dryland strength training, min)

their training environments. Mujika (2013) considers the information about training (i.e., training quantification) the most important information for a study on one or more forms of training intervention, and lack of a precise description of the training contents, in terms of volume, intensity, and frequency before and during a training intervention a substantial limitation of studies. Therefore, precise information about training quantification is absolutely necessary as manipulating the training program is the basis of many studies in our field, and interpretation of findings from such research is difficult without it.

A useful situation whereby research outcomes, and therefore scientific consensus and coaching practise may have been influenced by training quantification (or lack thereof) is altitude training. The general consensus in the athletic community is that altitude training may improve performance, reflected through its continual use by elite endurance athletes (Friedmann-Bette, 2008; Tønnessen et al., 2014). However, scepticism regarding its efficacy for elite athletes persists (Lundby, Millet, Calbet, Bärtsch, & Subudhi, 2012) based on several studies indicating a decrement in performance following altitude training (Adams, Bernauer, Dill, & Bomar, 1975; Jensen et al., 1993; Levine & Stray-Gundersen, 1997). This assertion is despite a large body of data describing physiological adaptations theoretically beneficial to endurance performance arising from altitude training, including improved red cell mass (Gore et al., 2013) and running economy (Saunders et al., 2004). Although most altitude training studies incorporate well-established principles of training design including periodisation, recovery, overload, and specificity, they only report basic metrics such as overall training volume or duration (Bailey et al., 1998; Gore, Hahn, Burge, & Telford, 1997). This shortcoming makes it difficult to determine all the factors that strongly influence subsequent athletic performance and the timing of a peak performance. It is therefore no surprise that both coaches and scientists are conflicted regarding the best training strategies to employ during altitude camps, and the best time to compete after training at altitude (Chapman, Stickford, Lundby, & Levine, 2014). However, in many cases, the performance outcomes of altitude training research, whether negative (Adams et al., 1975; Gough et al., 2012) or positive (Bonne et al., 2014; Levine & Stray-Gundersen, 1997), could be explained by the training completed prior to these performances when it is adequately quantified. In this respect, training monitoring and quantification enhances the interpretation of research findings, allowing practitioners to make informed decisions on implementation of training interventions with their athletes.

There are three distinct aspects of external training load that typically vary in a training program: The load planned before the season (or study) starts; the load prescribed on a daily basis; and the actual load completed by each individual athlete. The actual load should be quantified and reported for both sports training and research purposes (Mujika, 2013). Given that no gold standard method exists that defines the training load that is applicable to all endurance sports under all circumstances, factors like accessibility, feasibility, degree of labour intensity, cost-efficiency, validity, and reliability need to be considered when a decision is made about which method should be used to quantify training and competition load. Above all, any decision regarding the implementation of training monitoring practises needs to be made in concert with the coach, with an understanding of their knowledge, priorities, and overall goals. Practitioners need to understand and accept that all methods present advantages and limitations, and variable levels of accuracy and suitability for sports-specific training and competition (Lambert, 2012). Hopkins (1991) classified quantification methods into four major groups: Retrospective questionnaires, diaries, physiological monitoring, and direct observation. Retrospective questionnaires and diaries obtain data recalled from the athlete's memory after training, and can yield information on any aspect related to training. On the positive side, they are cheap and easy to administer, and do not interfere with the training program. On the negative side, questionnaires and diaries rely on an athlete's self-reported memory and subjectivity, so the information gathered may be intentionally or unintentionally distorted or forgotten. In addition, diaries may present problems of compliance and also management and interpretation of the large volume of data they can generate, though these issues are being overcome to an extent with the development of technology and database systems. Despite these limitations, endurance coaches appear to overwhelmingly prioritise the importance of subjective feedback from their athletes (Roos, Taube, Brandt, Heyer, & Wyss, 2013). More objective training measures can be obtained by physiological monitoring and direct observation. Oxygen consumption (VO_2), heart rate (HR) and blood lactate concentration ($[La]_{blood}$) have all been extensively used to objectively determine the intensity of training, but each of these methods presents its own limitations. For example, VO_2 is not a practical method to quantify supramaximal training bouts; field-based HR values may be affected by environmental conditions; and $[La]_{blood}$ may not be a suitable measure of intensity above the lactate threshold, and different algorithms or methods of calculation can yield variable results. Direct observation by coaches and/or sport scientists can also provide objective measures of most aspects of training (e.g., measurement of speed/power or physiological measures), but is time-consuming and may introduce a subjective error for each observer. All in all, although physiological monitoring and direct observation can provide valid and reliable measures of training intensity, they can be too expensive and impractical for continuous long-term use for practitioners with limited access to technical and/or financial resources (Hopkins, 1991). In this respect, less frequent physiological monitoring or completion of training test sets under standardised conditions may be an economically viable and practical avenue to evaluate the efficacy of training programs and specific interventions. As an example, submaximal tests such as the Lamberts and Lambert Submaximal Cycle Test (LSCT) are minimally disruptive to planned training and therefore easily included in a training plan, and sensitive to changes in performance as well as fatigue and recovery (Hammes et al., 2016; Lamberts, Swart, Noakes, & Lambert, 2011; Otter, Brink, van der Does, & Lemmink, 2016).

Practical ways of gathering training information are needed to monitor fatigue in an athlete with the goal of adjusting training prescription according to the symptoms that manifest in response to the training program (Lambert & Borresen, 2006; Lambert & Mujika, 2013b). To that end, the information gathered needs to assist the coach to answer the following questions: How hard did the athlete find the session? How hard was the session? How did the athlete recover from the session? How is the athlete coping with the cumulative stress of training? In response to these questions, Lambert and Borresen (2006) suggested to use Training Impulse (TRIMP) and/or session Rating of Perceived Exertion (RPE) in every session, perceived and action recovery scales (Kenttä & Hassmén, 1998), a muscle soreness scale and the Daily Analyses of Life Demands for Athletes (DALDA; Rushall, 1990) on a daily basis, and the Profile of Mood States questionnaire (POMS; McNair, Lorr, & Droppleman, 1971) and the recovery heart rate test (Lamberts, Lemmink, Durandt, & Lambert, 2004) on a weekly basis. A systematic review to assess whether subjective measures accurately reflected changes in athlete well-being (as objectively measured by performance, physiological and biochemical indicators), and whether subjective measures were responsive to acute changes in training load and chronic training, was recently published (Saw et al., 2016). It appears that subjective measures respond to training-induced changes in athlete well-being, which typically worsen with an acute increase in training load and with a chronic training load, but improve with an acute decrease in training load. In addition, there was no consistent association between subjective and objective measures, leading the authors to recommend that athletes report their subjective well-being on a regular basis alongside objective measures (e.g., VO_2max or lactate threshold testing), with the latter being used to quantify physiological and performance capacities in order to guide training prescription. A recent case study described a similar approach of incorporating subjective and objective measures in monitoring elite runners during 21 days of altitude training (Sperlich, Achtzehn, de Marées, von Papen, & Mester, 2016). Training load of the subsequent training session was reduced if two or more of the 11 measured variables were outside the athlete's normal individual range. Running speed at 3 mmol/L blood lactate improved and no athlete showed any signs of a maladaptive response, indicating this approach may have been effective in modulating training as required under conditions of additional physiological stress.

Both external and internal loads contribute to quantifying an athlete's actual training load, and a combination of both is the key for proper training monitoring (Halson, 2014). Monitoring daily training load might contribute to optimising athlete development, given better training regulation and earlier detection of overtraining or injuries (Roos et al., 2013). Assessing the relationship between external loads, internal loads, and competition performance should enhance evaluation of recovery-stress balance and adjustment of individual training programs to optimise adaptation. A recent systematic review indicated the combination of quantitative and qualitative data as the most promising approach to evaluate the training load and athletes' response to the training. Validated questionnaires or RPE, combined with physiological parameters such as HR, are often used on a daily basis and seem to provide the most reliable training-related information. From the coaches' perspective, training duration and mode, RPE, and personal remarks in the athletes' training diaries were considered to be essential information (Roos et al., 2013).

Monitoring the recovery-stress balance for endurance performance

It is generally acknowledged that athletes recover differently. Avoiding overtraining (or underrecovery) and realising peak performance is best achieved when there is an adequate balance between the intensity of training stress and the ability to subsequently recover to continue training (Kellmann, 2010). An imbalance between stress and recovery state is associated with impaired performance and physical recovery, and increased injury risk (Kenttä & Hassmén, 1998; Laux, Krumm, Diers, & Flor, 2015; Van der Does, Brink, Otter, Visscher, & Lemmink, 2017). While physical stress imposed by training is readily quantifiable by the methods described here and elsewhere, there are other factors which may influence an athlete's readiness to train, exercise performance, response to training, and ability to recover, such as psychological stress and mental fatigue, both from training and other aspects of life (Otter et al., 2016; Van Cutsem et al., 2017). Importantly, a recent systematic review (Van Cutsem et al., 2017) found that mental fatigue induced by periods of demanding cognitive activity impaired endurance performance in particular (increased time to completion, decreased self-selected power output/velocity). This was primarily due to a higher perceived exertion, whereas physiological variables traditionally associated with endurance performance (e.g., HR, VO_2, and $[La]_{blood}$) were unchanged by mental fatigue. Consistent with the holistic theme of training monitoring, it is important to monitor these psychological aspects as well, with several perceptual scales and questionnaires [e.g., POMS, DALDA, Recovery-Stress Questionnaire for Athletes (Kellmann & Kallus, 2001, 2016)] readily available for this purpose (Saw et al., 2016). While the prescription of training is the responsibility of coaches and sport science staff, the athlete has a responsibility to engage in effective recovery practises (e.g., sleep, nutrition, social activity, and hydrotherapy) to ensure they are in an adequate state, both physically and mentally, to repeatedly engage in training (Kellmann, 2010). An added benefit of recovery monitoring is the encouragement of self-responsibility among athletes, which should assist their engagement and compliance.

It is well established that most endurance athletes undertake a large volume of training to advance the required psychobiological adaptations and performance in competition (Pinot & Grappe, 2015; Tønnessen et al., 2014). Endurance athletes need to prioritise recovery, both physical and mental, to ensure they meet the demands required of them without overtraining. The distribution of effort, as well as intensity across a training week is an important consideration for coaches when planning training. Training programs need to distribute intensity (measured externally and objectively) as well as exertion/effort (measured subjectively) in a way that facilitates an effective stress/recovery balance for the athlete. Typically, specific high-intensity workouts can be separated by one or more slow long-distance workouts, with the exercise intensity remaining below ventilatory threshold and/or $[La]_{blood}$ of less than 2 mmol (Hydren & Cohen, 2015). Though these extended low intensity (based on speed/power output) training sessions may be considered by practitioners to be a low stress load on an athlete relative to a high-intensity interval session, they could be perceived by an athlete to require a moderate-to-hard level of effort (Sharma et al., 2017). This discrepancy, where the perception of 'easy' and 'hard' days may differ between the athlete and coach, has implications for overall planning and resultant adaptation. Completing an 'easy' day at a greater perceived exertion than planned by the coach may result in an athlete being under-recovered for a subsequent high-quality session and thus be unable to achieve the required training intensities. Coaches of endurance athletes can underestimate session RPE relative to what the athletes expressed (Foster, Helmann, Esten, Brice, & Porcari, 2001; Wallace, Slattery, & Coutts, 2009). For coach-prescribed easy days, athletes can report a higher training load, yet on prescribed harder days, athletes described a lower intensity and load (Foster, Helmann, et al., 2001; Wallace et al., 2009). This intriguing phenomenon suggests potential underrecovery of athletes, a heightened need for global measures of training load which encompass multiple facets of the training dose and response, and the need for monitoring of athlete recovery (Kellmann, 2010). The disconnect between athlete and coach perception of training may lead to undesirable maladaptive responses, and effective monitoring of the load planned by coaches and the actual load completed by athletes is a priority.

The issue of optimal training intensity distribution to enhance physiological adaptation and performance is a perennial one. Based on several studies (Esteve-Lanao, Foster, Seiler, & Lucia, 2007; Guellich & Seiler, 2010; Muñoz et al., 2014; Stöggl & Sperlich, 2014), it appears the polarised model of training is more effective for enhancing endurance performance than traditional threshold training. One explanation for the benefits of polarised training (Seiler, 2010; Seiler & Tønnessen, 2009) is the lower overall stress (both perceptual and physiological) load induced by long-duration, low-intensity exercise compared with highly intensive sessions at/above lactate threshold. This approach facilitates more rapid recovery, which consequently allows more frequent training (twice daily), giving an important long-term adaptive advantage over those completing the similar training volumes but less frequently (Hansen et al., 2005). It would therefore seem an optimal recovery-stress balance is an important factor relating to the effectiveness of polarised training.

Relating external load, internal load, and performance

Both external and internal loads have merit for understanding and athlete's training load and training adaptations, and a combination of both is important for training monitoring and performance prediction (Halson, 2014; Lambert, 2012). The relationships between external load, biological markers of internal load and competition performance have been used to assess training adaptation in highly trained swimmers. In a descriptive longitudinal study, Mujika and coworkers quantified individual external training load during an entire season and tested the swimmers for hormonal, metabolic, immunological and haematological markers of internal load during intensive training and tapering (Mujika, Chatard, & Geyssant, 1996;

Mujika, Chatard, Padilla, Guezennec, & Geyssant, 1996; Mujika, Padilla, Geyssant, & Chatard, 1997). To assess the effects of each training phase on performance, the swimmers participated in competitions held less than one week after each blood sampling session. Hormonal and metabolic indices previously identified as markers of training stress were unaltered by 12 weeks of intensive training and four weeks of tapering, but the testosterone-to-cortisol ratio appeared to be an effective marker of the swimmers' performance capacity (Mujika, Chatard, Padilla, et al., 1996). Improvements in immunological markers correlated with desirable effects of tapering on competition performance (Mujika, Chatard, & Geyssant, 1996). The swimmers' haematological status improved during intensive training, suggesting a positive adaptation to the external load, and competition performance improvement was positively related with the red cell count at the end of taper (Mujika et al., 1997).

Studies of training characterisation describe the training behaviour of athletes in a given sport and/or compare training and competition behaviour (Hopkins, 1991). Interestingly, until the late 1990s sport scientists had neglected to characterise the competition behaviour of professional road cyclists, in terms of both external and internal load. In an attempt to fill such a knowledge gap, Padilla and colleagues published a series of studies in which they described exercise intensity and load during the major three-week professional stage races (i.e., Giro d'Italia, Tour de France, Vuelta a España). Recording distance, time, speed and HR during racing, and based on individual HR – power output curves and exercise intensity thresholds previously determined in the laboratory, competition power outputs were estimated and TRIMPs quantified during short and long individual and team time trials (Padilla, Mujika, Orbañanos, & Angulo, 2000); flat, semi-mountainous and high-mountain stages (Padilla et al., 2001); second-, first-, and off-category mountain passes (Padilla, Mujika, Santisteban, Impellizzeri, & Goiriena, 2008); and physiological and performance capacities of professional road cyclists in relation to their morphotype-dependent speciality were assessed (Mujika & Padilla, 2001; Padilla, Mujika, Cuesta, & Goiriena, 1999). The advent of portable power measuring devices allowed direct determination of the external load (i.e., power output) during cycling racing (Ebert, Martin, Stephens, & Withers, 2006), and this type of measurement can be conducted conveniently in parallel with markers of internal load (e.g., HR, RPE) to make fitness and fatigue assessments, assess stress/recovery balance, ensure adequate performance potential and avoid undesired health outcomes (Halson, 2014).

Concurrent use of these simple internal and external monitoring tools can be effective in determining an individual response to an external stimulus such as hypoxia. It is well established that training intensity is compromised at altitude due to the lower oxygen availability (Chapman, Stager, Tanner, Stray-Gundersen, & Levine, 2011; Saunders, Pyne, & Gore, 2009), however, there is an individual response with some athletes more affected than others (Chapman, 2013; Chapman, Stray-Gundersen, & Levine, 1998). In a recent study of elite runners training at 2100 m altitude, running speed was impaired by up to 6% compared with equivalent sessions performed at sea-level. These effects were dependent on a combination of exercise duration and intensity, with threshold intensity sessions impaired the most (Sharma et al., 2017). While using an external measure of training such as running speed would be useful in determining which athletes were impaired to the greatest degree, and so allow for increased work/rest ratios to facilitate maintenance of training quality, the approach is limited in that it does not account for the level of effort/exertion (i.e., physiological stress) required to produce a given running speed. Accordingly, athletes and coaches should consider including a measure of internal load. In this study, investigators expressed RPE as a function of running speed in order to produce an 'exertion/velocity ratio' (Sharma et al., 2017). The ratio describes the relationship between exertion (in this case on a ten-point RPE scale) and running speed in km/h. An increase in this ratio is indicative of a greater level of exertion to maintain a certain running speed, while a decrease would infer the exertion is easier. As expected, the ratio increased by up to 30% at altitude, suggesting athletes perceive a much higher level of exertion for similar training sessions at altitude compared with sea-level. This relatively simple method of monitoring training could have application longitudinally, e.g., if there was an unexplained increase in the exertion/velocity ratio, this could trigger training modifications. This or related synergistic methods of combining internal and external training quantification require further scientific validation.

Continuing with their assessment of the relationships between external load, internal load, and competition performance, Mujika and colleagues carried out two consecutive experimental studies of potential performance enhancement by way of manipulating training variables during the taper in well-trained middle-distance runners. The first study showed that taper-induced physiological changes were mainly haematological, and distinct physiological changes were elicited from low intensity continuous training and high-intensity interval training during the taper (Mujika et al., 2000). In the second study, training frequency was manipulated during the taper, bringing about increases in immunological, haematological, hormonal, and metabolic markers, indicative that high $[La]_{blood}$ and a hormonal milieu propitious to anabolic processes were necessary for optimum 800 m running performance (Mujika et al., 2002). It is clear that the assessment of relationships between external load, internal load, and performance can help sport scientists, coaches and other practitioners improve training prescription and competition performance.

Conclusion and recommendations for practise

It can be concluded that no single physiological or perceptual marker can accurately quantify the fitness and fatigue responses to training or predict competition performance in endurance athletes. However, their combined use, where quantification of external load provides the context required to interpret the response to training in combination with measures of internal load, permits researchers and practitioners to evaluate recovery-stress balance and adjust individual training programmes. An effective training quantification and monitoring protocol should benefit training adaptation and improve competitive performance.

An important role of sport scientists is to drive innovation in an attempt to gain a fair competitive advantage (Coutts, 2014). However, a drive for innovation and integration of the most recent technologies into daily training quantification and monitoring practises should not take sport science away from personal coaching, effective industry practises, simplicity, validity, reliability, and integrity. In Aaron Coutts' own words, in the age of technology, the principle of Occam's razor still applies (i.e., more things should not be used than are necessary, or it is futile to do with more things that which can be done with fewer). This scientific approach will allow sport scientists to integrate and benefit from technological advancements and hopefully have a positive impact on athletes' training and competition performance (Coutts, 2014). Nevertheless, practitioners should not be led to the wrong conclusion that simple, non-invasive, less-expensive practical methods such as HR are the perfect solution to the training load quantification and athlete adaptation conundrum. For instance, measures of HR cannot inform on all aspects of wellness, fatigue, and performance. Therefore, their use in combination with daily training logs, psychometric questionnaires and non-invasive, cost-effective performance tests may offer a better solution to monitor training status in endurance athletes (Buchheit, 2014).

The key elements of supporting an endurance athlete need to be considered: The level of athlete involvement required, frequency of data collection, speed of data turnover, labour intensity, cost-efficiency, scientific validity, and reliability. Often, such a task becomes a balancing act. Faster-thinking sport science practitioners working directly with athletes and coaches would need to prioritise delivering immediate feedback, ease of use (i.e., minimal disruption to training), coach interest and innovation to gain a competitive advantage, whereas applied researchers working in the background and not directly involved with the training process on a daily basis can provide scientific rigor to methods used in the field (Coutts, 2016). Field-based monitoring of training makes collecting data less controlled compared with laboratory-based research designs. However, using a field-based approach provides higher external validity and valuable information for coaches and practitioners, which may outweigh some of the limitations associated with this approach (Sanders et al., 2017). An effective and sustainable athlete monitoring system incorporates many of these aspects and others, such as remote usability and data translation into simple outcomes such as effect sizes for further interpretation (Halson, 2014).

With respect to endurance sports, the advent of technologies such as power meters and GPS devices have made it relatively straight forward to accurately and reliably quantify external training loads. However, given the importance of providing coherent information to coaches regarding individual athlete responses to training, perceptual and physiological measures of internal load are essential. Combining both approaches to training monitoring should enhance both training prescriptions for endurance athletes and competitive performance.

Acknowledgements

The authors gratefully acknowledge the valuable comments and suggestions provided by Professor David B. Pyne of the University of Canberra and Australian Institute of Sport, Canberra, Australia.

References

Adams, W. C., Bernauer, E. M., Dill, D. B., & Bomar, J. B. (1975). Effects of equivalent sea-level and altitude training on VO_2max and running performance. *Journal of Applied Physiology, 39*(2), 262–266.

Bailey, D. M., Davies, B., Romer, L., Castell, L., Newsholme, E., & Gandy, G. (1998). Implications of moderate altitude training for sea-level endurance in elite distance runners. *European Journal of Applied Physiology and Occupational Physiology, 78*(4), 360–368.

Bonne, T. C., Lundby, C., Jørgensen, S., Johansen, L., Morgan, M., Bech, S. R., ... Nordsborg, N. B. (2014). "Live High – train High" increases hemoglobin mass in Olympic swimmers. *European Journal of Applied Physiology, 114*(7), 1439–1449.

Borresen, J., & Lambert, M. I. (2009). The quantification of training load, the training response and the effect on performance. *Sports Medicine, 39*(9), 779–795.

Boullosa, D. A., Abreu, L., Varela-Sanz, A., & Mujika, I. (2013). Do Olympic athletes train as in the Paleolithic era? *Sports Medicine, 43*(10), 909–917.

Buchheit, M. (2014). Monitoring training status with HR measures: Do all roads lead to Rome? *Frontiers in Physiology, 5*(73). doi:10.3389/fphys.2014.00073

Chapman, R. F. (2013). The individual response to training and competition at altitude. *British Journal of Sports Medicine, 47*(Suppl. 1), i40–i44.

Chapman, R. F., Stager, J. M., Tanner, D. A., Stray-Gundersen, J., & Levine, B. D. (2011). Impairment of 3000-m run time at altitude is influenced by arterial oxyhemoglobin saturation. *Medicine and Science in Sports and Exercise, 43*(9), 1649–1656.

Chapman, R. F., Stickford, A. S. L., Lundby, C., & Levine, B. D. (2014). Timing of return from altitude training for optimal sea-level performance. *Journal of Applied Physiology, 116*(7), 837–843.

Chapman, R. F., Stray-Gundersen, J., & Levine, B. D. (1998). Individual variation in response to altitude training. *Journal of Applied Physiology, 85*(4), 1448–1456.

Coutts, A. J. (2014). In the age of technology, Occam's razor still applies. *International Journal of Sports Physiology and Performance, 9*(5), 741.

Coutts, A. J. (2016). Working fast and working slow: The benefits of embedding research in high performance sport. *International Journal of Sports Physiology and Performance, 11*(1), 1–2.

Ebert, T. R., Martin, D. T., Stephens, B., & Withers, R. T. (2006). Power output during a professional men's road-cycling tour. *International Journal of Sports Physiology and Performance, 1*(4), 324–335.

Esteve-Lanao, J., Foster, C., Seiler, S., & Lucia, A. (2007). Impact of training intensity distribution on performance in endurance athletes. *The Journal of Strength & Conditioning Research, 21*(3), 943–949.

Foster, C., Florhaug, J. A., Franklin, J., Gottschall, L., Hrovatin, L. A., Parker, S., ... Dodge, C. (2001). A new approach to monitoring exercise training. *The Journal of Strength & Conditioning Research, 15*(1), 109–115.

Foster, C., Helmann, K. M., Esten, P. L., Brice, G., & Porcari, J. P. (2001). Differences in perceptions of training by coaches and athletes. *South African Journal of Sports Medicine, 8*(1), 3–7.

Friedmann-Bette, B. (2008). Classical altitude training. *Scandinavian Journal of Medicine & Science in Sports*, *18*(Suppl. 1), 11–20.

Gore, C. J., Hahn, A. G., Burge, C. M., & Telford, R. D. (1997). VO_2max and haemoglobin mass of trained athletes during high intensity training. *International Journal of Sports Medicine*, *28*(6), 477–482.

Gore, C. J., Sharpe, K., Garvican-Lewis, L. A., Saunders, P. U., Humberstone, C. E., Robertson, E. Y., ... Schmidt, W. F. (2013). Altitude training and haemoglobin mass from the optimised carbon monoxide rebreathing method determined by a meta-analysis. *British Journal of Sports Medicine*, 7(Suppl. 1), i31–i39.

Gough, C. E., Saunders, P. U., Fowlie, J., Savage, B., Pyne, D. B., Anson, J. M., ... Gore, C. J. (2012). Influence of altitude training modality on performance and total haemoglobin mass in elite swimmers. *European Journal of Applied Physiology*, *112*(9), 3275–3285.

Guellich, A., & Seiler, S. (2010). Lactate profile changes in relation to training characteristics in junior elite cyclists. *International Journal of Sports Physiology and Performance*, *5*(3), 316–327.

Halson, S. L. (2014). Monitoring training load to understand fatigue in athletes. *Sports Medicine*, *44*(2), 139–147.

Hammes, D., Skorski, S., Schwindling, S., Ferrauti, A., Pfeiffer, M., Kellmann, M., & Meyer, T. (2016). Can the Lamberts and Lambert Submaximal Cycle Test indicate fatigue and recovery in trained cyclists? *International Journal of Sports Physiology and Performance*, *11*(3), 328–336.

Hansen, A. K., Fischer, C. P., Plomgaard, P., Andersen, J. L., Saltin, B., & Pedersen, B. K. (2005). Skeletal muscle adaptation: Training twice every second day vs. training once daily. *Journal of Applied Physiology*, *98*(1), 93–99.

Hopkins, W. G. (1991). Quantification of training in competitive sports. *Sports Medicine*, *12*(3), 161–183.

Hydren, J. R., & Cohen, B. S. (2015). Current scientific evidence for a polarized cardiovascular endurance training model. *The Journal of Strength & Conditioning Research*, *29*(12), 3523–3530.

Impellizzeri, F. M., Rampinini, E., & Marcora, S. M. (2005). Physiological assessment of aerobic training in soccer. *Journal of Sports Sciences*, *23*(6), 583–592.

Jensen, K., Nielsen, T. S., Fiskestrand, A., Lund, J. O., Christensen, N. J., & Sechef, N. H. (1993). High-altitude training does not increase maximal oxygen uptake or work capacity at sea level in rowers. *Scandinavian Journal of Medicine & Science in Sports*, *3*(4), 256–262.

Kellmann, M. (2010). Preventing overtraining in athletes in high intensity sports and stress/recovery monitoring. *Scandinavian Journal of Medicine & Science in Sports*, *20*(Suppl. 2), 95–102.

Kellmann, M., & Kallus, K. W. (2001). *Recovery-Stress Questionnaire for Athletes; User manual*. Champaign, IL: Human Kinetics.

Kellmann, M., & Kallus, K. W. (2016). The Recovery-Stress Questionnaire for Athletes. In K. W. Kallus & M. Kellmann (Eds.), *The Recovery-Stress Questionnaires: User manual* (pp. 86–131). Frankfurt am Main: Pearson Assessment.

Kenttä, G., & Hassmén, P. (1998). Overtraining and recovery. *Sports Medicine*, *26*(1), 1–16.

Lambert, M. I. (2012). Quantification of endurance training and competition loads. In I. Mujika (Ed.), *Endurance training – science and practice* (pp. 211–228). Vitoria-Gasteiz, Basque Country: Iñigo Mujika S.L.U.

Lambert, M. I., & Borresen, J. (2006). A theoretical basis of monitoring fatigue: A practical approach for coaches. *International Journal of Sports Science & Coaching*, *1*(4), 371–388.

Lambert, M. I., & Mujika, I. (2013a). Overtraining prevention. In C. Hausswirth & I. Mujika (Eds.), *Recovery for performance in sport* (pp. 23–28). Champaign, IL: Human Kinetics.

Lambert, M. I., & Mujika, I. (2013b). Physiology of exercise training. In C. Hausswirth & I. Mujika (Eds.), *Recovery for performance in sport* (pp. 3–8). Champaign, IL: Human Kinetics.

Lamberts, R. P., Lemmink, K. A., Durandt, J. J., & Lambert, M. I. (2004). Variation in heart rate during submaximal exercise: Implications for monitoring training. *Journal of Strength & Conditioning Research*, *18*(3), 641–645.

Lamberts, R. P., Swart, J., Noakes, T. D., & Lambert, M. I. (2011). A novel submaximal cycle test to monitor fatigue and predict cycling performance. *British Journal of Sports Medicine*, *45*(10), 797–804.

Laux, P., Krumm, B., Diers, M., & Flor, H. (2015). Recovery–stress balance and injury risk in professional football players: A prospective study. *Journal of Sports Sciences*, *33*(20), 2140–2148.

Levine, B. D., & Stray-Gundersen, J. (1997). "Living high-training low": Effect of moderate-altitude acclimatization with low-altitude training on performance. *Journal of Applied Physiology*, *83*(1), 102–112.

Lundby, C., Millet, G. P., Calbet, J. A., Bärtsch, P., & Subudhi, A. W. (2012). Does 'altitude training' increase exercise performance in elite athletes? *British Journal of Sports Medicine*, *46*(11), 792–795.

McNair, D. M., Lorr, M., & Droppleman, L. F. (1971). *Manual for the Profile of Mood States*. San Diego, CA: Educational and Industrial Testing Service.

Mujika, I. (2013). The alphabet of sport science research starts with Q. *International Journal of Sports Physiology and Performance*, *8*, 465–466.

Mujika, I., Chatard, J. C., Busso, T., Geyssant, A., Barale, F., & Lacoste, L. (1995). Effects of training on performance in competitive swimming. *Canadian Journal of Applied Physiology*, *20*(4), 395–406.

Mujika, I., Chatard, J. C., Busso, T., Geyssant, A., Barale, F., & Lacoste, L. (1996). Use of swim-training profiles and performances data to enhance training effectiveness. *Journal of Swimming Research*, *11*, 23–29.

Mujika, I., Chatard, J. C., & Geyssant, A. (1996). Effects of training and taper on blood leucocyte populations in competitive swimmers: Relationships with cortisol and performance. *International Journal of Sports Medicine*, *17*(3), 213–217.

Mujika, I., Chatard, J. C., Padilla, S., Guezennec, C. Y., & Geyssant, A. (1996). Hormonal responses to training and its tapering off in competitive swimmers: Relationships with performance. *European Journal of Applied Physiology and Occupational Physiology*, *74*(4), 361–366.

Mujika, I., Goya, A., Padilla, S., Grijalba, A., Gorostiaga, E., & Ibañez, J. (2000). Physiological responses to a 6-d taper in middle-distance runners: Influence of training intensity and volume. *Medicine and Science in Sports and Exercise*, *32*(2), 511–517.

Mujika, I., Goya, A., Ruiz, E., Grijalba, A., Santisteban, J., & Padilla, S. (2002). Physiological and performance responses to a 6-day taper in middle-distance runners: Influence of training frequency. *International Journal of Sports Medicine*, *23*(5), 367–373.

Mujika, I., & Padilla, S. (2001). Physiological and performance characteristics of male professional road cyclists. *Sports Medicine*, *31*(7), 479–487.

Mujika, I., Padilla, S., Geyssant, A., & Chatard, J. C. (1997). Hematological responses to training and taper in competitive swimmers: Relationships with performance. *Archives of Physiology and Biochemistry*, *105*(4), 379–385.

Mujika, I., Rønnestad, B. R., & Martin, D. T. (2016). Effects of increased muscle strength and muscle mass on endurance-cycling performance. *International Journal of Sports Physiology and Performance*, *11*(3), 283–289.

Muñoz, I., Seiler, S., Bautista, J., España, J., Larumbe, E., & Esteve-Lanao, J. (2014). Does polarized training improve performance in recreational runners. *International Journal of Sports Physiology and Performance*, *9*(2), 265–272.

Otter, R. T. A., Brink, M. S., van der Does, H. T. D., & Lemmink, K. A. P. M. (2016). Monitoring perceived stress and recovery in relation to cycling performance in female athletes. *International Journal of Sports Medicine*, *37*(1), 12–18.

Padilla, S., Mujika, I., Cuesta, G., & Goiriena, J. J. (1999). Level ground and uphill cycling ability in professional road cycling. *Medicine and Science in Sports and Exercise*, *31*(6), 878–885.

Padilla, S., Mujika, I., Orbañanos, J., & Angulo, F. (2000). Exercise intensity during competition time trials in professional road cycling. *Medicine and Science in Sports and Exercise*, *32*(4), 850–856.

Padilla, S., Mujika, I., Orbañanos, J., Santisteban, J., Angulo, F., & Goiriena, J. J. (2001). Exercise intensity and load during mass-start stage races in professional road cycling. *Medicine and Science in Sports and Exercise*, *33*(5), 796–802.

Padilla, S., Mujika, I., Santisteban, J., Impellizzeri, F. M., & Goiriena, J. J. (2008). Exercise intensity and load during uphill cycling in professional 3-week races. *European Journal of Applied Physiology*, *102*(4), 431–438.

Pinot, J., & Grappe, F. (2015). A six-year monitoring case study of a top-10 cycling Grand Tour finisher. *Journal of Sports Sciences*, *33*(9), 907–914.

Pollock, M. L. (1973). The quantification of endurance training programs. *Exercise and Sport Sciences Reviews*, *1*(1), 155–188.

Roos, L., Taube, W., Brandt, M., Heyer, L., & Wyss, T. (2013). Monitoring of daily training load and training load responses in endurance sports: What do coaches want. *Schweizerische Zeitschrift für Sportmedizin & Sporttraumatologie*, *61*(4), 30–36.

Rushall, B. S. (1990). A tool for measuring stress tolerance in elite athletes. *Journal of Applied Sport Psychology*, *2*(1), 51–66.

Sanders, D., Abt, G., Hesselink, M. K., Myers, T., & Akubat, I. (2017). Methods of monitoring training load and their relationships to changes in fitness and performance in competitive road cyclists. *International Journal of Sports Physiology and Performance*, *12*, 668–675.

Saunders, P. U., Pyne, D. B., & Gore, C. J. (2009). Endurance training at altitude. *High Altitude Medicine & Biology*, *10*(2), 135–148.

Saunders, P. U., Telford, R. D., Pyne, D. B., Cunningham, R. B., Gore, C. J., Hahn, A. G., & Hawley, J. A. (2004). Improved running economy in elite runners after 20 days of simulated moderate-altitude exposure. *Journal of Applied Physiology*, *96*(3), 931–937.

Saw, A. E., Main, L. C., & Gastin, P. B. (2016). Monitoring the athlete training response: Subjective self-reported measures trump commonly used objective measures: A systematic review. *British Journal of Sports Medicine*, *50*(5), 281–291.

Seiler, S. (2010). What is best practice for training intensity and duration distribution in endurance athletes. *International Journal of Sports Physiology and Performance*, *5*(3), 276–291.

Seiler, S., & Tønnessen, E. (2009). Intervals, thresholds, and long slow distance: The role of intensity and duration in endurance training. *Sportscience*, *13*, 32–53.

Sharma, A. P., Garvican-Lewis, L. A., Clark, B., Stanley, J., Robertson, E. Y., Saunders P. U., & Thompson, K. G. (2017). Training at 2100 m altitude affects running speed and session RPE at different intensities in elite middle-distance runners. *International Journal of Sports Physiology and Performance*, *12*(Suppl. 2), S2147–S2152.

Sperlich, B., Achtzehn, S., de Marées, M., von Papen, H., & Mester, J. (2016). Load management in elite German distance runners during 3-weeks of high-altitude training. *Physiological Reports*, *4*(12), e12845.

Stöggl, T., & Sperlich, B. (2014). Polarized training has greater impact on key endurance variables than threshold, high intensity, or high volume training. *Frontiers in Physiology, 5,* 33. doi:10.3389/fphys.2015.00295

Tønnessen, E., Sylta, Ø., Haugen, T. A., Hem, E., Svendsen, I. S., & Seiler, S. (2014). The road to gold: Training and peaking characteristics in the year prior to a gold medal endurance performance. *PloS One, 9*(7), e101796.

Van Cutsem, J., Marcora, S., De Pauw, K., Bailey, S., Meeusen, R., & Roelendts, B. (2017). The effects of mental fatigue on physical performance: A systematic review. *Sports Medicine, 47,* 1569–1588.

van der Does, H. T., Brink, M. S., Otter, R. T., Visscher, C., & Lemmink, K. A. (2017). Injury risk is increased by changes in perceived recovery of team sport players. *Clinical Journal of Sport Medicine, 27*(1), 46–51.

Wallace, L. K., Slattery, K. M., & Coutts, A. J. (2009). The ecological validity and application of the session-RPE method for quantifying training loads in swimming. *Journal of Strength and Conditioning Research, 24*(1), 33–38.

PART III
The impact of sleep on recovery

11
THE ROLE OF SLEEP IN MAXIMISING PERFORMANCE IN ELITE ATHLETES

Johnpaul Caia, Vincent G. Kelly, and Shona L. Halson

Introduction

Sleep is a re-occurring behavioural state of reduced movement and responsiveness. In its simplest form, sleep allows rest from the preceding period of wakefulness. Adequate sleep is distinguished by ample duration, high efficiency (the ratio of sleep duration to time spent in bed), and suitable routine, while following adequate sleep one should feel refreshed and sustain alertness during wake periods. For adults, seven to nine hours of sleep per night is recommended, with less sleep than this considered suboptimal, and likely to compromise health, well-being, and performance (Hirshkowitz et al., 2015). For an athlete, sleeping effectively is a fundamental determinant of preparation for, and recovery from training and competition. This is particularly important given that athletes may require additional sleep to allow adaptation to training stressors and to minimise any residual fatigue from training and competition. Indeed, an imbalance between wake and sleep for an athlete can result in a fatigued state leading to decreased physiological functioning and performance output (Fullagar et al., 2015).

In this chapter we explore the characteristics of sleep and its function before providing insight into what is currently known about sleep in athletes. Rationale and evidence on the influence that reduced sleep quality and quantity have on performance is also presented and to complete the chapter we delve into strategies that have the potential to improve sleep in athletes.

Caia, J., Kelly, V. G., & Halson, S. L. (2018). The role of sleep in maximising performance in elite athletes. In M. Kellmann & J. Beckmann (Eds.), *Sport, Recovery, and Performance: Interdisciplinary Insights* (pp. 151–167). Abingdon: Routledge.

Sleep stages

While sleeping, humans alternate intermittently between two distinct sleep states – rapid eye movement sleep (REM) and non-rapid eye movement sleep (NREM). Comprising up to 20% of sleep in adults per night, REM sleep is spread over several periods and is characteristically defined by rapid eye movements, suppressed skeletal muscle tone, and dreams with perceptual vividness (Crick & Mitchison, 1983). REM sleep is thought of as an activated brain in a paralysed body, and therefore is often referred to as paradoxical sleep.

NREM sleep is subdivided into three stages (stages N1, N2, and N3) related to depth of sleep. A continuum of sleep depth appears to exist, with arousal thresholds lowest in N1, and highest in N3 (Akerstedt & Nilsson, 2003). Stage N3 is often referred to as deep sleep or slow-wave sleep (SWS), with SWS characterised by the presence of high-voltage, slow-frequency brain waves, slow heart and respiratory rates, and low cerebral blood flow (Akerstedt & Nilsson, 2003).

Human adults enter sleep via NREM sleep and rapidly descend from sleep onset through the depths of NREM sleep stages within 15–25 minutes (Figure 11.1). Thereafter, a cycle between NREM and REM sleep is repeated three to four times prior to waking, with each cycle SWS decreases while REM increases (Akerstedt & Nilsson, 2003).

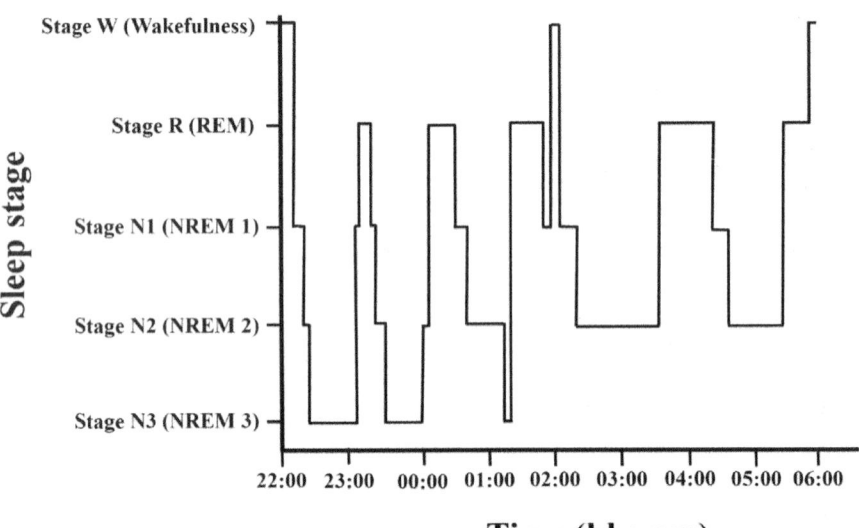

FIGURE 11.1 The progression through sleep stages during a typical night of sleep in adult humans depicted by hypnogram. REM = rapid eye movement; NREM = non-rapid eye movement.

Adapted from Akerstedt and Nilsson (2003).

Sleep function

The function of sleep remains largely unanswered and equivocal, with a lack of consensus existing among the evidence. Theories of REM sleep function have advocated a role for this state in memory and procedural learning, brain stimulation, and localised recuperation processes (Siegel, 2005). Additionally, it has been proposed that REM sleep is vital in encouraging growth and development of the brain and nervous system (Siegel, 2005). This contention is supported by the prevalence of REM sleep in early human life, with newborns sleeping approximately two-thirds of a 24-hour period, and REM sleep occupying half of total sleep time (McCarley, 2007).

It is proposed that NREM sleep is important for somatic function and the replenishment of cerebral glycogen stores that are steadily depleted during waking (Shapiro, Bortz, Mitchell, Bartel, & Jooste, 1981), while recent work shows the importance of SWS for memory consolidation (Rasch & Born, 2013). Furthermore, it is proposed NREM sleep, and in particular SWS, is imperative for recovery in athletes. This contention is supported by observed increases in SWS following a rise in metabolic stress (Shapiro et al., 1981). SWS may also provide an ideal environment for anabolic function, with the release of growth hormone associated with SWS. The release of growth hormone appears rhythmically related to SWS patterns, with secretion rates at their greatest during the deepest periods of SWS. Concurrently, during periods of SWS the release of cortisol is supressed, creating ideal conditions for anabolism (Sassin et al., 1969).

Sleep in athletes

Athletes perceive sleep as an important recovery modality (Venter, 2014); however, elite athletes have often demonstrated compromised sleep. Most recently, the sleep of 175 highly trained male and female athletes from several sporting disciplines was examined using subjective sleep questionnaires. Fifty per cent of athletes were found to be poor sleepers, while daytime sleepiness was prevalent (clinically significant in 28% of athletes) (Swinbourne, Gill, Vaile, & Smart, 2015). Comparable findings have been reported when assessing sleep in athletes using objective measures of sleep. In a recent large-scale study, researchers examined the habitual sleep wake behaviours of 124 elite athletes across a multitude of team and individual sport athletes from the Australian Institute of Sport using wrist actigraphy. On average, athletes obtained only 6.8 hours of sleep per night, at an average sleep efficiency of 86% (Lastella, Roach, Halson, & Sargent, 2015). Notably, athletes from individual sports display shorter sleep durations (6.5 hours) and poorer sleep efficiency (85.9%) when compared to team sport athletes (7.0 hours, 86.4%) (Lastella et al., 2015). Within athletic populations it is important to acknowledge that much of the sleep data presented has been obtained using subjective questionnaires or wrist actigraphy, as opposed to the gold standard polysomnography (Weiss, Johnson,

Berger, & Redline, 2010). However, polysomnography has limitations in that it is labour demanding and time consuming. Consequently, it is largely impractical for field based research involving the monitoring of many athletes, over multiple nights. As such, easy and inexpensive methods such as sleep questionnaires (Samuels, James, Lawson, & Meeuwisse, 2015) and wrist actigraphy (Sargent, Lastella, Halson, & Roach, 2016) offer a non-invasive, and inexpensive means to assess sleep quantity and quality in athletes.

Factors leading to compromised sleep in athletes may be a result of numerous deleterious contributors combined. Furthermore, within elite sport, athletes often encounter circumstances that have the potential to disturb sleep (Table 11.1). Definitive understanding of contributing factors is yet to be reached, while a lack of data exists over prolonged time periods. Notwithstanding, the following paragraphs outline the best supported, and most plausible factors contributing to compromised sleep in athletes.

Within elite sport, scheduling competition events for night time has become commonplace in recent decades. Given the multifaceted demands of post-match routines that exist in elite sport (e.g., medical treatment, media commitments, post-match recovery), it is not improbable that following a night match an athlete may not arrive home or at a hotel until late into the night, following which they may not sleep for several hours given elevated arousal. Such occasions could limit optimal recovery, with this casual sequence having the potential to limit preparation for subsequent training or competitive bouts. Supporting this contention is recent work showing a delayed bedtime in elite male soccer players following a night match that commenced after 18:00 in the German Bundesliga or Dutch Eredivisie (Fullagar, Skorski, Duffield, Julian, et al., 2016). As a result, a reduction in sleep duration ensued, while sleep onset latency (the time taken to transition from full wakefulness to sleep) was lengthened by ten minutes following a night match when compared to a training day (Fullagar, Skorski, Duffield, Julian, et al., 2016). Comparable findings have been reported in elite rugby players, with bedtime delayed following a night match, and a 39% reduction in total sleep time following a Super 15 rugby match (Eagles, McLellan, Hing, Carloss, & Lovell, 2014).

The scheduling of training sessions can also contribute to reduced sleep in athletes. In initial work examining this notion, seven elite Australian swimmers were monitored in the lead up to the 2008 Olympic Games. Clear differences in sleep duration and time in bed were found when athletes were required to train between 06:00 and 08:00 with early morning training resulting in athletes rising from bed approximately four hours earlier when compared to a rest day (Sargent, Halson, & Roach, 2014). Follow up work involving elite Australian athletes across a range of individual and team sports supports these findings, with less than five hours of sleep occurring when training started between 05:00 and 06:00, while training beginning between 07:00 and 10:00 saw six to seven hours of sleep. When training commenced between 10:00 and 11:00, athletes obtained more than seven hours of sleep (Sargent, Lastella, Halson, & Roach, 2014).

TABLE 11.1 Common circumstances faced by athletes in elite sport, their potential to disturb sleep, and potential strategies to maximise sleep in such situations.

Circumstance	Potential Problems	Potential Strategies
Nighttime competition	Reduced time in bed, sleep duration, and sleep efficiency, due to increased arousal and post-competition routines.	Following nighttime competition sleep hygiene practises have benefit in maximising sleep (Fullagar, Skorski, Duffield, & Meyer, 2016). Coaches may also consider the impact of scheduling a morning recovery session the day after nighttime competition, and its potential to further aggravate reductions in time in bed and sleep duration.
Early morning training	Reduced time in bed and sleep duration caused by an early wake time.	If possible, commence training no earlier than 07:00 to maximise time in bed and sleep duration (Sargent et al., 2014). In situations where this is unavoidable, strategic daytime napping should be considered. Further, athletes should look to sleep hygiene practises at night to maximise sleep efficiency.
Prior to important competition	Disrupted sleep on the night(s) prior to a competitive event, caused by arousal from stress, anxiety, and tension.	As part of a sleep hygiene strategy, a pre-bed routine may reduce arousal and promote sleepiness. Athletes may also explore the use of meditation as a form of relaxation prior to bed (Nédélec et al., 2015).
Electronic device use prior to bed	Disturbed sleep patterns, decreased sleep duration and quality, and augmented daytime fatigue caused by exposure to bright light.	In the lead-up to bed, athletes may discontinue the use of electronic devices in an attempt minimise any disruption to sleep (Romyn et al., 2015). Furthermore, if using a smartphone as an alarm, athletes may opt to set their devices to flight mode in an attempt to avoid the sleep disruption.

(*Continued*)

TABLE 11.1 (Continued)

Circumstance	Potential Problems	Potential Strategies
Long-haul travel	Reduced sleep duration and efficiency in-flight. Upon arrival at destination, jet-lag may disrupt sleep for multiple nights.	In-flight, athletes should hydrate regularly, while also moving around the aircraft intermittently. Sleep hygiene practises and bright light exposure timed to the arrival time zone should also be considered (Fowler, Duffield, Morrow, Roach, & Vaile, 2015). Also, where possible, when travelling for competition athletes are encouraged to arrive at their destination with sufficient time prior to competition to minimise the potential of jet-lag to impact performance (Lastella et al., 2015).
Caffeine prior to or during nighttime competition	Sleep is sensitive to evening caffeine intake, with adverse effects on sleep latency, sleep efficiency, and nighttime awakenings.	Sleep hygiene practises encourage limited consumption of caffeine in the hours preceding bed (Irish et al., 2015). In circumstances where caffeine is deemed necessary for performance during nighttime competition, athletes should look to sleep hygiene practises following competition in an attempt to negate the stimulating effects of caffeine consumption.

Athletes are required to deal with an array of psychosocial stressors while competing in elite sport (e.g., poor performance, competition stress, scrutiny from mainstream and social media). The capability of an athlete to handle these pressures can determine the level of stress and anxiety experienced, and may affect ensuing sleep. This may be particularly applicable in times leading up to competition periods or matches, where associated stressors may be elevated. Stress and anxiety can negatively influence sleep behaviour, and accordingly athletes may have a susceptibility to experience disturbed sleep prior to competition (Erlacher, Ehrlenspiel, Adegbesan, & El-Din, 2011). Anecdotally, athletes often report experiencing disrupted sleep on the night(s) prior to a competitive event. Furthermore, some athletes deem competition and its associated demands stressful enough to impact their sleep and resulting performance (Erlacher et al., 2011). In work examining this matter, 632 competitive German athletes across a range of sports completed a questionnaire comprising questions about sleep behaviour prior to an important competition. Sixty-five per cent of athletes slept worse on the night(s) prior to competition, with a considerable portion of these athletes (79%) reporting problems falling asleep on these occasions (Erlacher et al., 2011). Comparable findings have been reported among 283 elite Australian athletes from a variety of sports, with 64% indiciating they had slept worse than usual in the night(s) prior to an important competition over the preceding 12 months (Juliff, Halson, & Peiffer, 2015). Of concern, 51% of all athletes had no strategy to obtain better sleep on the night before an important competition (Juliff et al., 2015).

In modern times, electronic devices (e.g., smartphones, laptops, tablets) have become intrinsically involved in our daily routine. In some cases, the portability of these technologies has seen these devices move into the bedroom environment. The use of smartphones around bed time appears particularly widespread, with smartphones often taken to bed, and used after lights out. This is of considerable concern given that the use of electronic devices prior to sleep is associated with disturbances in regular sleep patterns, poorer sleep quality, sleep loss, and increased daytime fatigue (Exelmans & Van den Bulck, 2016). Exposure to bright light (like that emitted by a smartphone or computer screen) can disrupt circadian rhythms, and suppress melatonin production, leading to an increase in alertness and disturbed sleep (Exelmans & Van den Bulck, 2016). Further, as the use of electronic devices is typically unstructured with no predetermined beginning or end, usage may also delay bed time and reduce sleep duration. This effect could be exacerbated when stimulating and interactive platforms (e.g., social media) are involved, that may cause emotional arousal or disturbances in mood state. To date, a paucity of research exists assessing electronic device use in athletes and its impact on sleep. In the only study presenting such data, eight state-level netball athletes had their sleep and electronic device use monitored via actigraphy and self-report diaries during both a training and competition week. Findings revealed a strong, negative correlation between sleep efficiency and electronic device use, as well as sleep efficiency and time to sleep after electronic device use (Romyn, Robey, Dimmock, Halson, & Peeling, 2015). As such, it appears that electronic device use prior to bed can detrimentally influence sleep in athletes. While further research is needed to fully elucidate this factor, it would seem logical for athletes to avoid or minimise the use of their electronic devices in the lead up to bed.

Regular air travel is common in elite sport, with athletes often required to travel domestically, and on occasion on long-haul international flights across multiple time zones. The effects of short-haul air travel on sleep and recovery in elite athletes appear minimal. While short-haul travel can lead to changes in regular sleep behaviour, fluctuations in sleep quantity and quality appear negligible (Fowler, Duffield, & Vaile, 2015). However, the effect of long-haul air travel on sleep in athletes can be considerable, with both simulated (Fowler, Duffield, & Vaile, 2015) and field based research (Fowler, Duffield, Howle, Waterson, & Vaile, 2015) showing clear detrimental effects on sleep. Indeed, long-haul air travel is associated with multiple negative consequences, collectively referred to as 'travel fatigue', resulting from anxiety about the journey, changes in daily routine, and dehydration from aircraft cabins (Waterhouse, Reilly, & Edwards, 2004).

Caffeine is also a known ergogenic agent effective in enhancing performance in trained athletes when consumed in low to moderate doses (Goldstein et al., 2010). However, it is commonly acknowledged that caffeine encourages wakefulness by antagonising adenosine receptors in the brain (Goldstein et al., 2010), thus it is unsurprising that the consumption of caffeine may interfere with sleep behaviour in athletes. Sleep appears particularly sensitive to evening caffeine intake, with considerable adverse effects on sleep duration, sleep onset latency, sleep efficiency, and awakenings experienced during the night (Drake, Roehrs, Shambroom, & Roth, 2013). This may be particularly applicable when considering athletes who use caffeine as an ergogenic aid prior to, and during competition played in the evening hours. Indeed, moderate doses of caffeine consumed up to six hours prior to bed can have disruptive effects on sleep and therefore intake should be carefully considered, and where possible appropriately timed to minimise any sleep disturbance (Drake et al., 2013).

Sleep loss and performance

When discussing sleep loss, it is important that a distinction is made between sleep reduction, sleep fragmentation and sleep deprivation. Sleep reduction occurs when a human falls asleep later or wakes earlier than usual (Boonstra, Stins, Daffertshofer, & Beek, 2007). Sleep fragmentation is where sleep onset occurs as normal but is followed by intermittent events of waking (Boonstra et al., 2007). Sleep deprivation is an extreme circumstance of sleep reduction, where an individual remains awake for a prolonged period of time, typically involving the loss of one or more nights of sleep (Boonstra et al., 2007). When considering athletes, sleep deprivation research should be interpreted with some caution. While these studies clearly illustrate the importance of sleep to human function, the extent of sleep deprivation used in many research protocols is likely unrealistic for athletes. More refined levels of sleep loss are typically reported in elite athletes, as opposed to total sleep deprivation. The ensuing sections examine the influence that sleep deprivation, reduction, and fragmentation may have on various facets of performance.

Physical performance

It appears that athletes can afford acute sleep loss the night prior to training or competition, without it constituting as a high risk on subsequent performance, although an increased perception of effort may ensue. In field-based tests of aerobic capacity, four hours of sleep loss does not alter intermittent aerobic performance in taekwondo athletes (Mejri et al., 2014). Aerobic capacity also appears resistant to more extreme levels sleep loss with 20-meter shuttle performance maintained following 38 hours of sleep deprivation (Racinais, Hue, Blonc, & Le Gallais, 2004).

The effect of sleep reduction on anaerobic performance appears more complicated, and may depend upon whether sleep loss occurs at the beginning or end of the night. When a night of sleep is reduced to between 3 and 4.5 hours, and this sleep occurs after bedtime is delayed (sleep allowed between 03:00 and 07:00), peak and mean power during Wingate tests is unaffected (Souissi et al., 2013). However, when comparable amounts of sleep occur prior to an early waking (sleep allowed between 22:30 and 03:00), a decrease in performance occurs during the ensuing afternoon (Souissi et al., 2013). The disturbed performance caused by reducing sleep at the end of the night may be explained by a higher level of fatigue resulting from being awake for longer, leading to a decline in peak and mean power. This may be particularly important for athletes who experience sleep difficulties and train or compete in the afternoon.

Collectively, research reporting the effect sleep loss has on muscular strength and power are varied. It appears that efforts of sub-maximal strength requiring sustained exertion has greater vulnerability than a single effort of maximal strength or power. Early work examining this revealed three nights of sleep reduction decreased sub-maximal, and maximal deadlift, bench press, and leg press (Reilly & Piercy, 1994). More recently, effects of 24 hours of sleep deprivation on weightlifting performance were examined in national standard collegiate weightlifters. Maximum weight lifted for the snatch, clean and jerk, and front squat were maintained following sleep deprivation, despite sleepiness, fatigue, mood, and vigour being compromised (Blumert et al., 2007).

Cognitive performance

A loss of sleep can impair cognitive function, mediated through decreased alertness, slowed responses, and diminished attention via lapses (Alhola & Polo-Kantola, 2007). Attentional lapses are brief periods of inattentiveness characterised by sleep-like brain electrical activity (Alhola & Polo-Kantola, 2007). From a performance perspective, the detrimental effects of sleep loss on cognitive function is well established, with decreases observed in reaction time (Jarraya, Jarraya, Chtourou, & Souissi, 2014) and memory performance (Grundgeiger, Bayen, & Horn, 2014). Attentional capacity is also lessened following a period of sleep loss, with the attention of handball goalkeepers compromised following a night where only 4–5 hours of sleep were permitted. Decreases in attentional capacity appear time of day dependent, with performance more affected in the afternoon in comparison to morning (Jarraya et al., 2014).

Sporting performance

Limited research exists examining the effects of sleep loss on sporting performance. Swimmers limited to three consecutive nights of 2.5 hours of sleep experienced no impairment in 50- or 400-meter swim times (Sinnerton & Reilly, 1992). The performance of other sporting tasks may be more susceptible to a decrease in performance. Dart throw performance following 3–4 hours of sleep reduction is compromised, with both accuracy and consistency declining (Edwards & Waterhouse, 2009). Similarly, collegiate tennis players experiencing reduced sleep exhibited impairments in tennis serve accuracy (Reyner & Horne, 2013). These decreases in sport performance may be explained by the high cognitive demands of tasks such as a dart throw or tennis serve, leading to detrimental effects on decision making and executive function.

Immunity, inflammation, and injury

Pro-inflammatory and immune markers interleukin-1 beta, interleukin-6, tumour necrosis factor-alpha, and C-reactive protein all demonstrate sensitivity to changes in sleep. Following a night of 4.5 hours of sleep, plasma concentrations of interleukin-6 and tumour necrosis factor-alpha in footballers are elevated when compared to a baseline night of sleep (Abedelmalek et al., 2013). Given the disruption of immunological and inflammatory function following sleep loss, it is not surprising that sleep behaviour may influence predisposition to the common cold. Research examining this demonstrates that obtaining less than seven hours per night to be associated with lower resistance to infection after being exposed to a rhinovirus (Cohen, Doyle, Alper, Janicki-Deverts, & Turner, 2009).

The amount and quality of sleep obtained by an athlete may also influence their predisposition to injury. Adolescent athletes who reported sleeping less than eight hours per night were 1.7 times more likely to experience injury compared to athletes sleeping eight or more hours (Milewski et al., 2014), with comparable findings reported in elite soccer players (Laux, Krumm, Diers, & Flor, 2015). Inferences about why insufficient sleep is associated with an increase in injury risk is limited from these investigations, with causal relations unable to be established, while sleep data from both studies was derived from self-reported survey responses. A recent study objectively measured sleep in 22 elite Australian footballers across a competitive season, while injury incidence was concurrently tracked. In contrast to previous findings, injury was not affected by sleep duration or efficiency across a competitive season of Australian football (Dennis, Dawson, Heasman, Rogalski, & Robey, 2015). It is worthy to note that while this study used objective measures to assess sleep, sleep monitoring was limited to five nights each week. Subsequently, only injuries sustained during competition, and not during training, were included in the analysis (Dennis et al., 2015).

Strategies to improve sleep in athletes

Napping

For an athlete, naps may aid recovery between multiple training sessions occurring on one day, while also offering a solution to reduce daytime sleepiness, particularly in circumstances of reduced nighttime sleep (e.g., travel, training camp). The timing of nap appears an important factor, with the optimum time for a nap suggested to be during the mid-afternoon hours. This period is typically the midpoint of the day, and corresponds with the afternoon circadian dip (Takahashi, 2003). Subsequently, a nap at this time can improve the ability to function and perform throughout the remainder of the day. In contrast, naps in the late afternoon or evening hours appear less appropriate, and can lead to disruptions on nighttime sleep duration, sleep efficiency, and sleep onset latency (Takahashi, 2003). The duration of a nap also appears important, with naps lasting longer than 30 minutes having the potential to negatively influence nighttime sleep patterns (Nédélec et al., 2015). However, in circumstances of sleep deprivation or accumulated sleep debt, longer naps may be appropriate to allow sufficient rest and recovery. Coaches may consider allowing time in training schedules for athletes to nap; however, any implementation of napping must be controlled in a manner as to not disturb nighttime sleep patterns.

Sleep extension

Sleep extension involves prolonging the time an individual spends at rest in bed, in a deliberate attempt to increase total sleep time. This involves shifting bed time forward or delaying typical wake time, subsequently allowing more time for sleep. Little research has studied the effects of extending sleep, particularly in athletic populations, although initial results are promising.

Extending sleep has been shown to lead to improvements in cognitive functioning, while also eliciting beneficial effects on vigour and feelings of fatigue (Kamdar, Kaplan, Kezirian, & Dement, 2004). Additionally, in recent years, work has emerged addressing how sleep extension may influence athletic performance. This was first examined in five collegiate swimmers who extended their sleep to a minimum of ten hours per night for a six to seven-week period. Following sleep extension, improvements included a faster 15-meter swim sprint, improved turn time, and increased kick strokes. Furthermore, sleep extension saw improved mood and decreased fatigue scores (Mah, Mah, & Dement, 2008). Comparable findings have since followed in collegiate American footballers (Mah, Mah, & Dement, 2010), tennis players (Mah, Mah, & Dement, 2009), and basketballers (Mah, Mah, Kezirian, & Dement, 2011). The initial positive indications on the use of sleep extension in an attempt to improve athletic performance are promising; however, the interpretation of findings is limited given the aforementioned studies have lacked a control group or crossover arm. Furthermore, the magnitude of sleep extension needed per night to bring about positive change in performance remains unclear. Similarly, the cumulative amount of additional sleep required over successive nights or weeks to cause benefit is unknown, with as little as four nights, and as much as eight weeks capable of producing improved performance.

Sleep hygiene practises

Sleep hygiene involves the practise of habits typifying appropriate behavioural and environmental sleep, in an attempt to promote optimal sleep quantity and quality. Sleep hygiene practises are inexpensive, easily accessible, and characterise continuing behaviours that promote ideal sleep. As such, these practises may provide a simple means for athletes looking to maximise their sleep (Figure 11.2).

Sleep hygiene practises advocate stable bed and wake times, in an attempt to promote habitual rhythms of sleepiness and wakefulness. An advancement or delay of regular sleep patterns may disrupt the synchrony of circadian rhythms, and subsequently influence sleep duration and quality (Irish, Kline, Gunn, Buysse, & Hall, 2015). Somewhat inappropriately, due to training and competition demands, the sleep patterns of elite athletes may be irregular at times. For example, during the week an athlete may wake early for training, while conversely they may sleep-in on the morning of a day off (Sargent et al., 2014). During days off from training and competition athletes should be encouraged to be gently engaged in active daytime activity involving exposure to daylight, as opposed to behaviours characterised by idleness (e.g., television, computer games) (Nédélec et al., 2015). Slothful behaviour

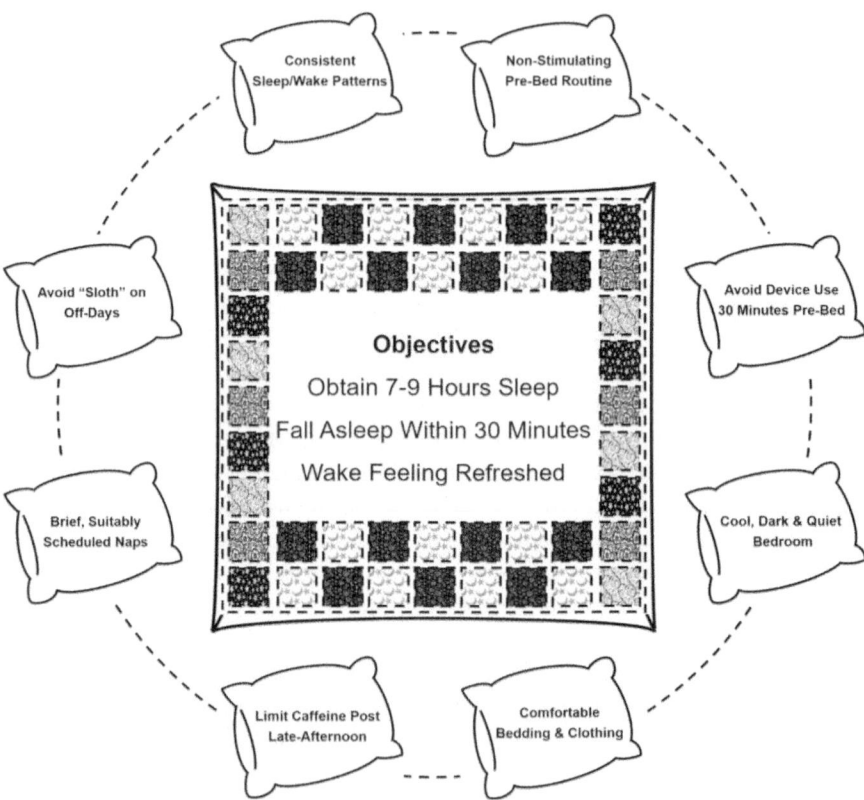

FIGURE 11.2 Considerations and objectives for athletes to maximise sleep. Based on the recommendations of Fullagar et al. (2015), Nédélec et al. (2015), and Irish et al. (2015).

may increase the tendency of daytime sleep periods, potentially disturbing regular sleep patterns (Nédélec et al., 2015).

Sleep hygiene encourages a routine prior to bed that serves as a cue to the body and mind to prepare for sleep. A routine prior to bed provides a period of relaxation between the stressors of the day and nighttime sleep, with stress, tension and anxiety all contributors to cognitive arousal prior to sleep (Venter, 2012). This may be particularly useful in athletes, where stress, anxiety, and arousal can arise in specific circumstances (e.g., prior to an important competition, following late night matches).

Optimal sleep hygiene involves ensuring a cool, quiet, and dark environment within the bedroom. In circumstances with appropriate bed coverings and clothing, exposure to warm environments is most unfavourable, leading to increased wakefulness and decreased REM sleep and SWS (Okamoto-Mizuno & Mizuno, 2012). Noise is also an obvious source of sleep disturbance, given it increases the number of nighttime arousals and suppresses both SWS and REM (Irish et al., 2015). Athletes are advised to limit noise within and around their bedroom environment. When noise sources are not directly modifiable (e.g., traffic) sound reducing tools such as ear plugs should be considered. This may be particularly applicable for athletes sleeping in unfamiliar environments (e.g., hotel rooms) or athletes sleeping in residential dorms (e.g., collegiate athletes). Exposure to light after dark influences circadian rhythms, and subsequent can adversely affect sleep (Dumont & Beaulieu, 2007), and it follows that the bedroom environment should be dark. Practically, darkening curtains may be useful in blocking external sources of artificial light (e.g., street lights), while sleep masks should also be considered. Furthermore, the removal or blocking of artificial light sources from within the bedroom is encouraged (e.g., alarm clock, television standby lights).

Recent work supports the efficacy of sleep hygiene practises in assisting sleep in athletes. Following a late-night match, footballers completing sleep hygiene practises obtained more sleep when compared to footballers who proceeded with their regular post-match routine. Despite this, no differences were observed in physical performance, perceptual recovery or blood-borne markers of muscle damage and inflammation (Fullagar, Skorski, Duffield, & Meyer, 2016). The limited research examining sleep hygiene practises in athletes suggests that there is benefit in athletes adopting simple behaviours that promote good sleep. However, much work is required before the exact utility of sleep hygiene practises for athletes is understood.

Conclusion and recommendation for applied practise

Sleep is an essential element of daily life, and likely serves multiple functions, given that it influences most of our molecular, cellular, physiological, and neurological functions. For athletes, we are now beginning to understand and appreciate the importance of sleep in maximising performance. Sleep loss can lead to decreases in physical output, particularly when considering sub-maximal, sustained efforts. Further, a loss of sleep can affect numerous elements relating to performance, including decision making, mood state, and the potential for illness and injury.

Elite athletes appear vulnerable to losses in sleep, particularly following competition played at night, or when early morning training sessions are scheduled. Similarly, long-haul travel, stress during competition periods, electronic device use prior to sleep, and the use of stimulating ergogenic aids such as caffeine can influence the quantity and quality of sleep obtained by an athlete. We are still unsure of definitive strategies to improve sleep in elite athletes. While multiple potential strategies, including napping, sleep extension, and sleep hygiene practises may have usefulness in improving sleep quantity or quality in athletes, no strategy or combination of strategies has clear evidential basis.

Nevertheless, coaches should be cognisant of the implications of sleep loss for an athlete, particularly over consecutive nights, where debts of sleep may accrue. In such cases, individualised strategies may be devised, which address the issues causing detrimental sleep, while also allowing the athlete an opportunity to obtain adequate sleep.

References

Abedelmalek, S., Chtourou, H., Aloui, A., Aouichaoui, C., Souissi, N., & Tabka, Z. (2013). Effect of time of day and partial sleep deprivation on plasma concentrations of IL-6 during a short-term maximal performance. *European Journal of Applied Physiology, 113*(1), 241–248.

Akerstedt, T., & Nilsson, P. M. (2003). Sleep as restitution: An introduction. *Journal of Internal Medicine, 254*(1), 6–12.

Alhola, P., & Polo-Kantola, P. (2007). Sleep deprivation: Impact on cognitive performance. *Neuropsychiatric Disease and Treatment, 3*(5), 553–567.

Blumert, P. A., Crum, A. J., Ernsting, M., Volek, J. S., Hollander, D. B., Haff, E. E., & Haff, G. G. (2007). The acute effects of twenty-four hours of sleep loss on the performance of national-caliber male collegiate weightlifters. *Journal of Strength and Conditioning Research, 21*(4), 1146–1154.

Boonstra, T. W., Stins, J. F., Daffertshofer, A., & Beek, P. J. (2007). Effects of sleep deprivation on neural functioning: An integrative review. *Cellular and Molecular Life Sciences, 64*(7–8), 934–946.

Cohen, S., Doyle, W. J., Alper, C. M., Janicki-Deverts, D., & Turner, R. B. (2009). Sleep habits and susceptibility to the common cold. *Archives of Internal Medicine, 169*(1), 62–67.

Crick, F., & Mitchison, G. (1983). The function of dream sleep. *Nature, 304*(5922), 111–114.

Dennis, J., Dawson, B., Heasman, J., Rogalski, B., & Robey, E. (2015). Sleep patterns and injury occurrence in elite Australian footballers. *Journal of Science and Medicine in Sport, 19*(2), 113–116.

Drake, C., Roehrs, T., Shambroom, J., & Roth, T. (2013). Caffeine effects on sleep taken 0, 3, or 6 hours before going to bed. *Journal of Clinical Sleep Medicine, 9*(11), 1195–1200.

Dumont, M., & Beaulieu, C. (2007). Light exposure in the natural environment: Relevance to mood and sleep disorders. *Sleep Medicine, 8*(6), 557–565.

Eagles, A., McLellan, C., Hing, W., Carloss, N., & Lovell, D. (2014). Changes in sleep quantity and efficiency in professional rugby union players during home based training and match-play. *Journal of Sports Medicine and Physical Fitness, 56*(5), 565–571.

Edwards, B. J., & Waterhouse, J. (2009). Effects of one night of partial sleep deprivation upon diurnal rhythms of accuracy and consistency in throwing darts. *Chronobiology International, 26*(4), 756–768.

Erlacher, D., Ehrlenspiel, F., Adegbesan, O. A., & El-Din, H. G. (2011). Sleep habits in German athletes before important competitions or games. *Journal of Sports Sciences, 29*(8), 859–866.

Exelmans, L., & Van den Bulck, J. (2016). Bedtime mobile phone use and sleep in adults. *Social Science & Medicine, 148*(1), 93–101.

Fowler, P., Duffield, R., Howle, K., Waterson, A., & Vaile, J. (2015). Effects of northbound long-haul international air travel on sleep quantity and subjective jet lag and wellness in professional Australian soccer players. *International Journal of Sports Physiology and Performance, 10*(5), 648–654.

Fowler, P., Duffield, R., Morrow, I., Roach, G., & Vaile, J. (2015). Effects of sleep hygiene and artificial bright light interventions on recovery from simulated international air travel. *European Journal of Applied Physiology, 115*(3), 541–553.

Fowler, P., Duffield, R., & Vaile, J. (2015). Effects of simulated domestic and international air travel on sleep, performance, and recovery for team sports. *Scandinavian Journal of Medicine and Science in Sports, 25*(3), 441–451.

Fullagar, H., Skorski, S., Duffield, R., Hammes, D., Coutts, A. J., & Meyer, T. (2015). Sleep and athletic performance: The effects of sleep loss on exercise performance, and physiological and cognitive responses to exercise. *Sports Medicine, 45*(2), 161–186.

Fullagar, H., Skorski, S., Duffield, R., Julian, R., Bartlett, J., & Meyer, T. (2016). Impaired sleep and recovery after night matches in elite football players. *Journal of Sports Sciences, 34*(14), 1333–1339.

Fullagar, H., Skorski, S., Duffield, R., & Meyer, T. (2016). The effect of an acute sleep hygiene strategy following a late-night soccer match on recovery of players. *Chronobiology International, 33*(5), 490–405.

Goldstein, E. R., Ziegenfuss, T., Kalman, D., Kreider, R., Campbell, B., Wilborn, C., . . . Antonio, J. (2010). International society of sports nutrition position stand: Caffeine and performance. *Journal of the International Society of Sports Nutrition, 7*(1), 5.

Grundgeiger, T., Bayen, U. J., & Horn, S. S. (2014). Effects of sleep deprivation on prospective memory. *Memory, 22*(6), 679–686.

Hirshkowitz, M., Whiton, K., Albert, S. M., Alessi, C. A., Bruni, O., DonCarlos, L., . . . Katz, E. S. (2015). National Sleep Foundation's sleep time duration recommendations: Methodology and results summary. *Journal of the National Sleep Foundation, 1*(3), 40–43.

Irish, L. A., Kline, C. E., Gunn, H. E., Buysse, D. J., & Hall, M. H. (2015). The role of sleep hygiene in promoting public health: A review of empirical evidence. *Sleep Medicine Reviews, 22*(1), 23–36.

Jarraya, S., Jarraya, M., Chtourou, H., & Souissi, N. (2014). Effect of time of day and partial sleep deprivation on the reaction time and the attentional capacities of the handball goalkeeper. *Biological Rhythm Research, 45*(2), 183–191.

Juliff, L. E., Halson, S. L., & Peiffer, J. J. (2015). Understanding sleep disturbance in athletes prior to important competitions. *Journal of Science and Medicine in Sport, 18*(1), 13–18.

Kamdar, B. B., Kaplan, K. A., Kezirian, E. J., & Dement, W. C. (2004). The impact of extended sleep on daytime alertness, vigilance, and mood. *Sleep Medicine, 5*(5), 441–448.

Lastella, M., Roach, G. D., Halson, S. L., & Sargent, C. (2015). Sleep/wake behaviours of elite athletes from individual and team sports. *European Journal of Sport Science, 15*(2), 94–100.

Laux, P., Krumm, B., Diers, M., & Flor, H. (2015). Recovery-stress balance and injury risk in professional football players: A prospective study. *Journal of Sports Sciences, 33*(20), 2140–2148.

Mah, C., Mah, K. E., & Dement, W. C. (2008). Extended sleep and the effects on mood and athletic performance in collegiate swimmers. *Sleep, 31*(Suppl.), A128.

Mah, C., Mah, K. E., & Dement, W. C. (2009). Athletic performance improvements and sleep extension in collegiate tennis players. *Sleep, 32*(Suppl.), A155.

Mah, C., Mah, K. E., & Dement, W. C. (2010). Sleep extension and athletic performance in collegiate football. *Sleep, 33*(Suppl.), A105–A106.

Mah, C., Mah, K. E., Kezirian, E. J., & Dement, W. C. (2011). The effects of sleep extension on the athletic performance of collegiate basketball players. *Sleep, 34*(7), 943–950.

McCarley, R. W. (2007). Neurobiology of REM and NREM sleep. *Sleep Medicine, 8*(4), 302–330.

Mejri, M., Hammouda, O., Zouaoui, K., Chaouachi, A., Chamari, K., Rayana, M., & Souissi, N. (2014). Effect of two types of partial sleep deprivation on Taekwondo players' performance during intermittent exercise. *Biological Rhythm Research, 45*(1), 17–26.

Milewski, M. D., Skaggs, D. L., Bishop, G. A., Pace, J. L., Ibrahim, D. A., Wren, T. A., & Barzdukas, A. (2014). Chronic lack of sleep is associated with increased sports injuries in adolescent athletes. *Journal of Pediatric Orthopaedics, 34*(2), 129–133.

Nédélec, M., Halson, S., Delecroix, B., Abaidia, A. E., Ahmaidi, S., & Dupont, G. (2015). Sleep hygiene and recovery strategies in elite soccer players. *Sports Medicine, 45*(10), 1387–1400.

Okamoto-Mizuno, K., & Mizuno, K. (2012). Effects of thermal environment on sleep and circadian rhythm. *Journal of Physiological Anthropology, 31*(1), 14.

Racinais, S., Hue, O., Blonc, S., & Le Gallais, D. (2004). Effect of sleep deprivation on shuttle run score in middle-aged amateur athletes. Influence of initial score. *Journal of Sports Medicine and Physical Fitness, 44*(3), 246–248.

Rasch, B., & Born, J. (2013). About sleep's role in memory. *Physiological Reviews, 93*(2), 681–766.

Reilly, T., & Piercy, M. (1994). The effect of partial sleep deprivation on weight-lifting performance. *Ergonomics, 37*(1), 107–115.

Reyner, L. A., & Horne, J. A. (2013). Sleep restriction and serving accuracy in performance tennis players, and effects of caffeine. *Physiology and Behaviour, 120*(1), 93–96.

Romyn, G., Robey, E., Dimmock, J. A., Halson, S. L., & Peeling, P. (2015). Sleep, anxiety and electronic device use by athletes in the training and competition environments. *European Journal of Sport Science, 16*(3), 301–308.

Samuels, C., James, L., Lawson, D., & Meeuwisse, W. (2015). The Athlete Sleep Screening Questionnaire: A new tool for assessing and managing sleep in elite athletes. *British Journal of Sports Medicine, 50*(7), 418–422.

Sargent, C., Halson, S. L., & Roach, G. D. (2014). Sleep or swim? Early-morning training severely restricts the amount of sleep obtained by elite swimmers. *European Journal of Sport Science, 14*(Suppl.), S310–315.

Sargent, C., Lastella, M., Halson, S. L., & Roach, G. D. (2014). The impact of training schedules on the sleep and fatigue of elite athletes. *Chronobiology International, 31*(10), 1160–1168.

Sargent, C., Lastella, M., Halson, S. L., & Roach, G. D. (2016). The validity of activity monitors for measuring sleep in elite athletes. *Journal of Science and Medicine in Sport, 19*(10), 848–853.

Sassin, J. F., Parker, D. C., Mace, J. W., Gotlin, R. W., Johnson, L. C., & Rossman, L. G. (1969). Human growth hormone release: Relation to slow-wave sleep and sleep-walking cycles. *Science, 165*(3892), 513–515.

Shapiro, C. M., Bortz, R., Mitchell, D., Bartel, P., & Jooste, P. (1981). Slow-wave sleep: A recovery period after exercise. *Science, 214*(4526), 1253–1254.

Siegel, J. M. (2005). Clues to the functions of mammalian sleep. *Nature, 437*(7063), 1264–1271.

Sinnerton, S., & Reilly, T. (1992). Effects of sleep loss and time of day in swimmers. In D. Maclaren, T. Reilly, A. Lees, E. London, & F. N. Spon (Eds.), *Biomechanics and medicine in swimming: Swimming science IV* (pp. 399–405). London: E & F Spon.

Souissi, N., Chtourou, H., Aloui, A., Hammouda, O., Dogui, M., Chaouachi, A., & Chamari, K. (2013). Effects of time-of-day and partial sleep deprivation on short-term maximal performances of judo competitors. *Journal of Strength and Conditioning Research*, *27*(9), 2473–2480.

Swinbourne, R., Gill, N., Vaile, J., & Smart, D. (2015). Prevalence of poor sleep quality, sleepiness and obstructive sleep apnoea risk factors in athletes. *European Journal of Sport Science*, *16*(7), 850–858.

Takahashi, M. (2003). The role of prescribed napping in sleep medicine. *Sleep Medicine Reviews*, *7*(3), 227–235.

Venter, R. (2012). Role of sleep in performance and recovery of athletes: A review article. *South African Journal for Research in Sport, Physical Education and Recreation*, *34*(1), 167–184.

Venter, R. (2014). Perceptions of team athletes on the importance of recovery modalities. *European Journal of Sport Science*, *14*(Suppl.), S69–76.

Waterhouse, J., Reilly, T., & Edwards, B. (2004). The stress of travel. *Journal of Sports Sciences*, *22*(10), 946–965.

Weiss, A. R., Johnson, N. L., Berger, N. A., & Redline, S. (2010). Validity of activity-based devices to estimate sleep. *Journal of Clinical Sleep Medicine*, *6*(4), 336–342.

12
SLEEP, DREAMS, AND ATHLETIC PERFORMANCE

Daniel Erlacher and Felix Ehrlenspiel

Introduction

Sleep is generally regarded as a valuable resource for psychological and physiological well-being. In recent years, sleep as a resource of recovery has increasingly been recognised as part of the preparation of peak performance – not only by athletes but also by coaches. In the previous chapter by Caia, Kelly, and Halson (this volume, Chapter 11), the role of sleep in maximizing performance in elite athletes was described. In the first part of this chapter we will review in more detail how sleep is measured and the basic methods of sleep recording. In the second part, interesting areas where sleep medicine and sport science are closely intertwined are presented. Anecdotal evidence about a bad night's sleep prior to a sport event have been reported quite often; however, systematic surveys are scarce. Empirical data on poor sleep and distressing dreams before competition and their relation to competitive anxiety will be discussed. In the third part, the phenomenon of lucid dreaming will be introduced. A lucid dream is a dream in which the dreamer is aware of the dream state, and lucid dreamers are able to execute complex actions within the dream. The possible application of this phenomenon in sports (e.g., motor learning or psychophysiological correlates of dreaming) as well as induction techniques for lucid dreams will be presented.

Measuring sleep in the field and in the laboratory

A normal person sleeps nearly a third of his or her life and sleep is regarded as an essential prerequisite for health, performance, and well-being (Carskadon &

Erlacher, D., & Ehrlenspiel, F. (2018). Sleep, dreams, and athletic performance. In M. Kellmann & J. Beckmann (Eds.), *Sport, Recovery, and Performance: Interdisciplinary Insights* (pp. 168–182). Abingdon: Routledge.

Dement, 2017). However, sleep disturbances are quite common and about 80 different sleep disorders, from obstructive sleep apnoea to sleepwalking, are distinguished (ICSD-3, 2014). The diagnostic methods of sleep medicine show a broad spectrum (Stuck, Maurer, Schredl, & Weeß, 2013) and range from subjective assessments (anamnesis and sleep-questionnaires) to objective methods (actigraphy and polysomnography), whilst sleepiness and fatigue during the day (e.g., multiple sleep test, vigilance test) also serve as diagnostic tools for sleep physicians. These different tools for subjective and objective sleep measures will be described in more detail. Furthermore, some remarks about sleep in athletes will be discussed.

Subjective sleep measures

A good example of a subjective sleep measure is the Pittsburgh Sleep Quality Index (PSQI) by Buysse, Reynolds, Monk, Berman, and Kupfer (1989), which is a self-report questionnaire that evaluates sleep quality and assesses sleep disturbances over the previous month. Nineteen items add up to seven component scores (e.g., subjective sleep quality). The sum of scores for these seven subscales yields one global score of overall sleep quality and ranges from 0 to 21, whereby greater scores indicate higher levels of sleep-related symptoms. According to Buysse and colleagues (1989) a global score higher than 5 (cut-off) divides participants into poor and good sleepers. The PSQI is a widely used instrument and has been applied to athletes in various sports (Swinbourne, Gill, Vaile, & Smart, 2016). Another advantage of the PSQI is there are several validated translations for different languages; e.g., a German adaptation is offered by the German Sleep Society (DGSM).

However, the PSQI assesses sleep in a trait-related perspective over a period of one month and is not able to measure subjective sleep parameter for a single night. This problem is solved, for example, by a German questionnaire: Sleep Questionnaire A and B (Görtelmeyer, 2005). The two versions of the validated self-rating scale of the sleep questionnaire assess the trait component of subjective sleep quality of the previous two weeks (SF-B) and the state component of sleep and sleep quality for the previous night (SF-A; Görtelmeyer, 2005). The SF-A comprises 25 items measuring composite scores of five factors: Sleep quality, feeling of being refreshed in the morning, emotional balance in the evening, psychological exhaustion in the evening, and sleep-related somatic symptoms during sleep. The SF-A has been successfully applied in sport in a time-to-event paradigm, e.g., SF-A were assessed four days before a competition and on the day of the competition to measure changes in sleep quality in athletes (Ehrlenspiel, Erlacher, & Ziegler, in press; Erlacher, Schredl, & Lakus, 2009).

Another possibility to measure subjective sleep variables is to keep a daily sleep diary (Liendl, Lauer, & Hoffmann, 2004). The sleep diary provides an additional source of sleep information with day-to-day variability as well as progress and outcome control. Sleep diaries can comprise either a single item or a different number of questions, while the following variables are quite common (Liendl et al., 2004): Bed time, sleep onset latency, number of awakenings after sleep onset, get-up time, and sleep quality ratings. Applying only a single item (e.g., sleep quality) in a sleep diary might be limited, because it does not allow for the evaluation of reliability or internal consistency. The single questions also do not represent the fact that sleep quality perceptions have been found to be at least two-dimensional; they have been shown to be related to evaluations of nocturnal sleep (e.g., 'calm sleep') and to evaluations of its restorative value, as rated in the morning (e.g., 'feeling well rested'; see examples from Keklund & Åkerstedt, 1997). Subjective sleep measures have been applied successfully in the field of sport; however, for specific questions (e.g., related to sleep stages), objective sleep measures are needed.

Objective sleep measures

As described in the previous chapter by Caia et al. (this volume, Chapter 11), sleep can be divided into four different sleep stages: N1, N2, N3, and R. For the objective classification of those sleep stages, different physiological quantities must be recorded. This is performed in a sleep laboratory by the process of polysomnography. For this purpose, three physiological parameters are derived by means of electroencephalography (EEG), electrooculogram (EOG), and electromyography (EMG): Brain activity, eye movements, and muscle tonus. EEG measure remains the important parameter for determining level of consciousness and allowing determination of sleep stages. Polysomnography is the gold standard in sleep medicine and this method of sleep recording has a long history with governing rules of sleep stages that are over 50 years old (Rechtschaffen & Kales, 1968). In 2007 a revised manual was published by the American Academy of Sleep Medicine (AASM) (Iber, Ancoli-Israel, Chesson, & Quan, 2007); however, since then a debate about established and new methods has developed (Carskadon & Dement, 2017). For the diagnosis and differentiation of sleep disorders, additional physiological measurements are necessary; for example, the respiratory flow for sleep apnoea or the EMG discharge at the legs for recognition of periodic leg movements.

An alternative method for assessing objective sleep data from an individual is actigraphy measured by wrist activity monitors. An activity monitor is a small accelerometer which is sensitive to movement direction and intensity, often worn on the nondominant wrist. The basic idea about actigraphy is that movement is correlated with wakefulness and long periods of inactivity are correlated with sleep (Sargent, Lastella, Halson, & Roach, 2016). Activity monitors have the advantage that they are suitable for use in the field because they are easy to use for participants. However, they are limited as they cannot truly distinguish sleep and wakefulness, and even more so they are not able to distinguish different sleep stages (e.g., Marino et al., 2013). The question about the validity of actigraphy measures have been investigated in different studies with different populations and generally sleep measures with wrist actigraphy compared to polysomnography suffer from specificity, e.g., sleep corresponds to the proportion of epochs PSG-scored as wake epochs that are correctly classified as wake epochs by actigraphy (Marino et al., 2013).

In recent years, an impressive amount on objective sleep data from athletes has been published. Especially, the use of actigraphy opened a new perspective on the sleep of athletes; however, it also brought up some controversial findings which will be discussed in the next paragraph.

Sleep in athletes

Recently, a considerable amount of data on sleep in athletes have been published, reflecting the growing interest of this topic in sports and sport sciences. Most of the studies undertaken in athletes have applied subjective measures and/or actigraphy to collect objective sleep data and therefore the question arises of how valid are those measures in this special population. For example, Lastella, Roach, Halson, and Sargent (2015) reported data of 124 elite athletes over a different number of nights. One interesting result is that athletes from swimming or triathlon have quite low hours of total sleep time (6.4 and 6.1 hours) compared to their bed time (8.5 and 7.9 hours) resulting in low sleep efficiency. Keeping in mind that physical activity is usually promoting sleep (Youngstedt, 2005) it seems almost that elite sport degrades sleep quality and sleep quantity (Gupta, Morgan, & Gilchrist, 2017). However, as mentioned before, actigraphy measures in athletes might be special. In a recent study by Sargent and colleagues (2016), the validity of activity monitors for measuring sleep was tested in elite athletes and results showed that indeed athletes have lower sensitive scores (i.e., ability to detect sleep) than a healthy normal population, e.g., athletes move more often during sleep which leads to underestimation of sleep. Furthermore, the study by Sargent and colleagues (2016) stresses the importance to report exact methodological protocol (e.g., threshold settings for actigraphy) because the outcome on sleep parameters might differ tremendously.

Whereas the sleep/wake behaviour of elite athletes might be well displayed by activity monitors, physiological aspects of sleep which might be related to recovery are not accessible by those measures. In a classical study by Shapiro, Bortz, Mitchell, Bartel, and Jooste (1981), athletes showed after completing a 92-kilometer road race a significant increase in total sleep time and slow-wave sleep. The authors raised the question that slow-wave sleep is important for a recovery period after metabolic stress caused by exercise. Even though the slow-wave hypothesis is not well tested, it shows that sleep parameter might be of value to describe the effectiveness of the recovery process of an athlete. More recent studies stress that this might not only be the case for certain sleep stages but even for local sleep in different brain areas (Huber et al., 2006).

Athletes' sleep and competitions

In every athletic career competition are special highlights and therefore sleep might be of special interest in conjunction with a competition. In particular, the night before an important competition or game might have an impact on an athlete's performance. Besides anecdotal reports and retrospective studies, evidence that indicates athletes might experience poor sleep quality before a competition is quite rare. In this part, we will discuss the question of whether competitions adversely affect subjective experience of sleep quality and, if that is the case, how anxiety is related to the competition and impaired sleep experience. Given anxiety might have effects on different levels of sleep, we will also focus on distressing dreams in the night before a competition.

Sleep before a competition

Caia et al. (this volume, Chapter 11) presented anecdotal and empirical evidence that indicates athletes might experience poor sleep quality before a competition. In large-scale cross-sectional studies, more than 60% of the samples of German (Erlacher, Ehrenspiel, Adegbesan, & Galal El-Din, 2011) and Australian elite athletes answered 'yes' when asked whether they had slept worse than normal before a competition at least once during the previous 12 months. Of the German athletes who had experienced poor pre-competitive sleep, most (60%) reported that their impaired sleep resulted in no effects, with only about 30% reporting that they felt sleepy across the day; that is, they may have perceived less restorative effects of sleep (Erlacher, Ehrenspiel, Adegbesan, et al., 2011). Similar numbers were found in a study examining sleep before a specific event (Lastella, Lovell, & Sargent, 2014). On the morning of a marathon race, 68% of the athletes reported having slept worse during the previous night compared with a normal night. Whereas retrospective self-reports point to impaired sleep quality, studies with repeated measures of self-reported sleep quality did not find support for previous retrospective studies. For example, no differences were found when comparing sleep quality ratings measured by a single item for regular nights with those for nights before competitions in a small sample of female netball players (Romyn, Robey, Dimmock, Halson, & Peeling, 2016) and a sample of road cyclists (Lastella, Roach, Halson, Martin, et al., 2015).

Anxiety could play a moderating role, which might explain why negative effects of competitions on self-reported sleep quality may not be found in all athletes. Savis, Eliot, Gansneder, and Rotella (1997), for example, found that collegiate athletes reported being excited or anxious during the night before important competitions. Accordingly, about 60% in the German and 43.8% in the Australian sample indicated that their 'nervousness about the competition' resulted in poor sleep (Erlacher, Ehrenspiel, Adegbesan, et al., 2011; Juliff, Halson, & Peiffer, 2015). Lastella and colleagues (2014) found that 'anxiety' was the most common reason for disturbed sleep, as it was cited by 21% of marathon runners. Furthermore, netball players (Romyn et al., 2016) and marathon runners (Lastella et al., 2014) showed a negative relation between measures of pre-competitive anxiety and sleep quality ratings. To overcome limitations of retrospective studies, a time-to-event paradigm has also been used to assess competition-related changes in sleep quality and anxiety. Erlacher, Schredl, Ehrlenspiel, and Bosing (2009) found that high school students showed higher states of anxiety in the morning of a sport exam and for the night they reported reduced sleep quality, prolonged sleep latency, and a higher number of nocturnal awakenings in comparison to the baseline measurement one month before the exam. Subjective sleep was assessed by the SF-A and a correlation between the feeling of being refreshed in the morning, cognitive state anxiety, and self-confidence was found for the morning of the exam, e.g., better scores for the feeling of being refreshed in the morning corresponded to lower cognitive state anxiety and higher self-confidence. In future studies performance data is needed to show that subjective sleep interferes with the performance during the sport event.

A similar study design was used in a recent study by Ehrlenspiel and colleagues (in press) but with elite male athletes reporting sleep quality and anxiety before real competitions. Assessments of subjective sleep quality and a multidimensional measure of competitive anxiety (Ehrlenspiel, Brand, & Graf, 2009) took place four days before competition and on the day of competition. As expected, sleep quality deteriorated before the competition, but not perceptions regarding the restorative value of sleep nor reports of sleep problems (measured by SF-A). But beyond group-level effects, intra-individual differences in changes were also found. For example, greater deterioration in sleep quality was reported by athletes who had initially reported more intense worry symptoms. Therefore, the results suggest a strong cognitive component in pre-competitive sleep impairments. Future studies have to tackle the question about whether anxiety precedes impaired sleep quality and thus possibly moderates the relation between competition and poor pre-competitive sleep. It seems that only athletes experiencing pre-competitive anxiety could be prone to experiencing poor sleep quality (Ehrlenspiel et al., in press).

Distressing dreams in the night before a competition

Dreams – characterised as sleep mentation – are defined as all mental experiences (perceptions, thoughts, and emotions) occurring during sleep (Stickgold, 2017). The question of why people dream has fascinated humankind for centuries. Over the years several ideas about the function of dreaming have been formulated, starting from Freud's theory of dreams as guardians of sleep (Freud, 1987) to theories that dreaming is a training field for consciousness (Hobson, 2009). However, the empiric testing of possible functions of dreams encounters certain challenging problems; e.g., to elicit the content of a dream, a participant has to report a dream after awakening. A dream report is therefore biased by the process of sleep-wake transition and the recall of the participant about the dream narrative (Schredl, 2017). Thus the question always arises as to how well the dream report actually depicts the event experienced (Schredl & Erlacher, 2003). A reduction of the nocturnal dream images by the report is inevitable. Besides methodological obstacles most dream researchers agree that nocturnal dreaming is in some way related to waking experience.

Because important sports events cause real-life stress situations as well as sleep problems for athletes, it can be assumed that athletes' dream content may also be altered before competitions. Yet, little is known about how athletes' dreams are affected by competitions or games. In the field of elite sport, no studies have focused on distressing dreams and only some anecdotal evidences can be found in the literature (Mahoney & Avener, 1977). In general, a distressing dream is defined as a frightening dream; whereas, in its extreme form, a nightmare, the sleeper is awakened by frightening dream content (Spoormaker, Schredl, & van den Bout, 2006). Interestingly, examples of distressing dreams in athletes can already be found in the ancient work by the dream interpreter Artemidor from Daldis (ca. 96–180 AC). Male athletes who dreamed about being an infant or having milk in his breast like a woman were bad signs and predicted defeat in an upcoming sporting event (Langenfeld, 1991). In a study by Mahoney and Avener (1977), several psychological variables were measured by a questionnaire from 12 gymnasts, wherea six of them qualified for the Olympic Games and the other six did not. The results indicated that the six qualifiers dreamed more often about gymnastic and sport success than the six gymnasts who failed the Olympic qualification. In addition, the amount of training correlated with the frequency of gymnast dreams and doubts about one's gymnastic abilities correlated with having more tragic dreams. Even though no example for such a tragic dream is given in the article, one might have speculated that such dreams have at least a negative tone.

In a questionnaire study by Erlacher, Ehrlenspiel, and Schredl (2011), 840 German athletes from various sports were asked about distressing dreams on the nights before an important competition or game. About 15% of the athletes stated that they experienced at least one distressing dream before an important competition or game during the preceding 12 months. The content of these distressing dreams referred mainly to athletic failure. Arnulf and colleagues (2014) showed in a non-sport-related sample that in the night before an exam dreaming about this event is quite common. In contrast to the aforementioned studies, the negative dreams (primarily representing problems and failure) predicted better performance on the exam. These results suggest that simulation of waking life situations in dreams is common.

An open question is the question about relationship of cause and effect; so far both interpretations are possible: The negative dream content affects daytime performance or anxiety, or concerns about the upcoming event might alter the dream content in a negative way. It will be a challenge for future studies to test the cause-and-effect relationship in athletes because the systematic manipulation of dream content is quite puzzling.

Lucid dreaming

In contrast to normal dreaming, lucid dreaming is characterised by the reappearance of many wake-like cognitive capabilities within the dream. Minimally defined by the criterion that the sleeper is aware of the current dream state as such, lucid dreaming often leads to full insight into the delusional nature of the dream, access to waking memory, and volitional control over the ongoing dream (Dresler, Erlacher, Czisch, & Spoormaker, 2017). Lucid dreamers are able to execute complex actions within the dream and are able to communicate by eye movements in a sleep laboratory setting to mark specific events within the dream. In this section, different studies will be described which indicate that lucid dream practise increases daytime performance. Furthermore, psychophysiological studies will be presented which point out that lucid dreaming can be seen as a simulation of overt actions. Finally, different techniques to induce lucid dreams will be discussed.

Lucid dream practise

The idea that practise in lucid dreams might be an effective mental strategy to enhance performance during wakefulness was already framed by Tholey (1981). Lucid dream practise is a form of mental practise, which is defined as the cognitive rehearsal of motor activity in the absence of overt physical movement (Driskell, Copper, & Moran, 1994). Meta-analyses show that mental practise has a positive effect on performance (Hinshaw, 1991–92). Apart from anecdotal accounts (Erlacher, 2007), there is limited evidence on the effectiveness of lucid dream practise on performance in wakefulness. In a questionnaire study by Erlacher, Stumbrys, and Schredl (2011–2012), results showed that out of 840 German athletes from different sports, 57% reported to have had at least one lucid dream in their life, while 24% stated to have lucid dreams at least once a month (see Table 12.1). Out of the lucid dreamers, 9% practised motor skills while dreaming lucid, and the majority of this group (about 77%) had the impression that their skills had improved as a result

TABLE 12.1 Lucid dream frequency of a representative sample of German adults ($N = 919$) and a non-representative sample of German athletes ($N = 840$).

Category	Adults $N = 919$		Athletes $N = 840$	
	Frequency	Relative frequency (%)	Frequency	Relative frequency (%)
Never	450	49.0	365	43.5
Less than once per year	143	15.6	78	9.3
About once per year	55	6.0	69	8.2
About 2 to 4 times per year	86	9.4	129	15.4
About once per month	79	8.6	95	11.3
About 2 to 3 times per month	61	6.6	59	7.0
About once per week	34	3.7	20	2.4
Several times per week	11	1.2	25	3.0

of practise within the dream. In a qualitative study by Tholey (1981) six proficient lucid dreamers were asked to perform complex motor skills they were familiar with from waking life in their lucid dreams. Almost all the participants could perform their sports in the lucid dreams and some of the participants reported a better sense of position and movement in waking performance for different sports (trampoline jumping, ski acrobatics, gymnastics).

In a field experiment with a pre-post-design, seven lucid dreamers showed significant improvement after practising a coin tossing task in the lucid dream state in a single night (Erlacher & Schredl, 2010). In an online experiment by Stumbrys, Erlacher, and Schredl (2016), participants of four different groups were asked to rehearse a finger-tapping task either in a lucid dream, awake physically, awake mentally, or not awake. All 68 participants accomplished pre-test in the evening and post-test in the morning, with practise carried out during the night. The results show a significant improvement in all three practise groups, but no improvement in the control group, demonstrating that LDP can indeed enhance simple task performance. In a recent study by Schädlich, Erlacher, and Schredl (2017), the effect of lucid dream practise was studied in a controlled sleep laboratory setting, using a pre-post design with dart throwing in the evening and morning. The lucid dream group practised darts in lucid dreams; however, some participants were distracted during practise, dividing the group into lucid dreamers with few and multiple distractions. Change of performance was compared to a physical practise group and a control group, showing a significant interaction in that only the lucid dreamers with few distractions improved. Even though the results of our studies have to be interpreted with caution, the studies indicate that lucid dream practise can be an effective tool in sports practise if lucid dreamers find ways to minimise distractions during the dream. Moreover, the study emphasises the necessity to investigate lucid dream experiences on a qualitative level, e.g., by analysing the dream reports in detail.

Psychophysiology of lucid dreaming

Two researchers (Hearne, 1978; LaBerge, 1980) independently were able to demonstrate that lucid dreaming occurs during REM sleep and is not the product of brief periods of wakefulness during sleep. Because lucid dreamers have at least partial control of their dream actions, they are able to perform pre-arranged tasks during the dream. In the sleep laboratory study by Hearne (1978) and LaBerge (1980), skilled lucid dreamers were instructed to perform eye movements if they are becoming lucid. In REM sleep, the eye muscles do not underlie the muscle atonic characteristically for REM sleep (Stuck et al., 2013) and thus the eye movements could be detected with the polysomnography and can be easily differentiated from spontaneous eye movements during REM (see Figure 12.1). The results of those studies open the possibility to study psychophysiological correspondence more closely with respect to results from studies from motor imagery. Both dreaming and imagination are a simulation of the real world on a higher cognitive level (Erlacher &

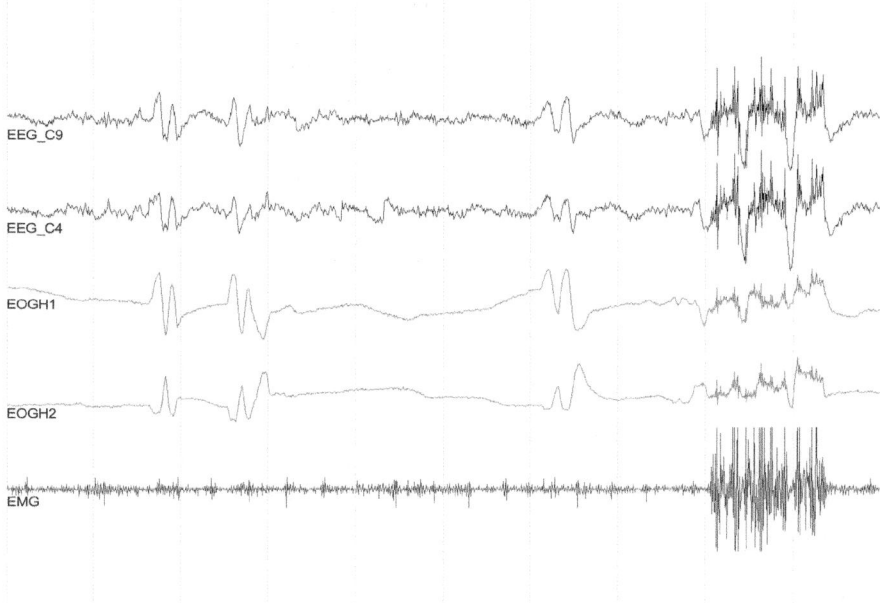

FIGURE 12.1 A sample of one correctly signalled lucid dream with three left-right-left-right (LRLR) eye signals. A waking reaction is seen in the last seconds of the recording.

Schredl, 2008b). This notion is supported by neuroscience studies which suggest that imagined and executed actions share the same neural substrate. Research studies on mental imagery tested this assumption on different levels: Measuring central nervous activity, monitoring autonomic response, and using mental chronometry (Decety, 1996). Jeannerod (2001) integrated these findings into the theory of neural simulation of action. The simulation theory postulates that, in general, covert actions are actual actions, except for the fact that they are not executed, but share for example the same cortical areas. Studies from the field of lucid dream research reveal a strong correlation between dreamed and actual actions and therefore emphasise the assumption that dreamed actions are indeed a neural simulation. Correspondences were found for autonomic responses (Erlacher & Schredl, 2008a), neuronal activation (Dresler et al., 2011; Erlacher, Schredl, & LaBerge, 2003), and temporal aspects (Erlacher, Schädlich, Stumbrys, & Schredl, 2014).

Prevalence and induction of lucid dreams

Although lucid dreaming is considered to be a rare ability, a recent meta-analysis of lucid dream prevalence and frequency shows that 55% of population have experienced lucid dreaming at least once in their lifetime and 23% experience it regularly (once a month or more frequently) (Saunders, Roe, Smith, & Clegg, 2016). Also age-related differences in lucid dreaming prevalence exist, with young children and adolescents reporting lucid dreams more frequently than adults (Voss, Frenzel, Koppehele-Gossel, & Hobson, 2012). The prevalence of lucid dreaming in elite athletes was similar as in general population (Schredl & Erlacher, 2011); however, the percentage of lucid dreams in comparison with all dreams in elite athletes seems to be higher than in general population (see Table 12.1). If lucid dreaming should serve as a possible technique to rehearse sport skill, the question arises as to whether lucid dreaming is a learnable ability (LaBerge, 1980).

A variety of different techniques have been suggested for lucid dream induction (Stumbrys, Erlacher, Schädlich, & Schredl, 2012), which can be loosely classified into three broad categories: Cognitive techniques, external stimulation, and miscellaneous (Stumbrys et al., 2012). The first category encompasses all cognitive activities that are carried out to increase the likelihood of achieving lucidity in a dream state. For this category a great deal of methods have been suggested, which can be further divided into methods where lucidity is initiated from within a dream – i.e., a person becomes lucid during a dream (dream-initiated lucid dreams) – and methods where lucidity is initiated from wakefulness – i.e., a person retains conscious awareness when falling asleep (wake-initiated lucid dreams). The rationale behind the second category is that an external stimulus presented to a sleeping person can be incorporated into their dream (e.g., water spray on sleeping person's face will provoke sudden rainfalls in his or her dream) and that the incorporated stimuli serves as a cue for the dreamer, which reminds him about the dream state (e.g., someone squirting water reminds the dreamer that he or she is dreaming) and therefore triggers dream lucidity (Paul, Schädlich, & Erlacher, 2014). The third category covers miscellaneous aids to gain lucidity like drugs (e.g., Donepezil) but also special sleep/wake patterns, e.g., when a person wakes up in early morning hours and after a certain period of time goes back to bed and takes a nap, is known as Wake-Back-to-Bed (WBTB). WBTB is not a technique per se because it was empirically tested only in combination with other techniques (Mnemonic Induction of Lucid Dreams, MILD) and maybe boosts their effectiveness.

The review of lucid dream induction techniques revealed that none of the induction techniques was verified to induce lucid dreams reliably, consistently and with a high success rate, some methods showed to be promising, e.g., the MILD/WBTB combination (Stumbrys et al., 2012). More recently, non-invasive brain stimulation methods were applied to induce lucid dream; however, transcranial direct current stimulation of the dorsolateral prefrontal cortex during REM sleep showed rather modest success in inducing dream lucidity as assessed by the eye signalling technique (Stumbrys, Erlacher, & Schredl, 2013).

Conclusion and recommendations for practise

In the previous chapter, Caia et al. (this volume, Chapter 11) already pointed out that sleep is an essential state for humans serving multiple functions. Whereas Caia and colleagues focused on research about sleep in athletes and the impact of sleep loss on performance, in this chapter we broadened the view starting from different sleep measures to sleep before a competition and finally to dream and lucid dream research. At first glance those topics seem to be only marginally related to recovery in sport; however, we hope that we still pointed out some important and interesting areas. For example, in the next years it will be a challenge to understand the subjective and objective sleep data of athletes with respect to athletic performance. Especially in the context of recovery it is not only important to collect sleep data but also to understand how sleep is related to recovery processes. One interesting field in which the impact of sleep on athletic performance is directly related is the sleep before an important competition; however, it will be a challenge to collect reliable sleep data in athletes in such important events. Furthermore, we believe that even dream research might provide interesting insights to recovery processes. Therefore, we encourage not only athletes but also coaches to have a closer look at the sleep and dream behaviour.

References

Arnulf, I., Grosliere, L., Le Corvec, T., Golmard, J. L., Lascols, O., & Duguet, A. (2014). Will students pass a competitive exam that they failed in their dreams? *Consciousness and Cognition, 29*, 36–47.

Buysse, D. J., Reynolds, C. F., Monk, T. H., Berman, S. R., & Kupfer, D. J. (1989). The Pittsburgh Sleep Quality Index: A new instrument for psychiatric practice and research. *Psychiatric Research, 28*, 193–213.

Carskadon, M. A., & Dement, W. C. (2017). Normal human sleep: An overview. In M. Kryger, T. Roth, & W. C. Dement (Eds.), *Principles and practice of sleep medicine* (6th ed., pp. 15–24). Philadelphia: Elsevier.

Decety, J. (1996). Do imagined and executed actions share the same neural substrate? *Cognitive Brain Research, 3*, 87–93.

Dresler, M., Erlacher, D., Czisch, M., & Spoormaker, V. I. (2017). Lucid dreaming. In M. Kryger, T. Roth, & W. C. Dement (Eds.), *Principles and practice of sleep medicine* (6th ed., pp. 539–545). Philadelphia: Elsevier.

Dresler, M., Koch, S. P., Wehrle, R., Spoormaker, V. I., Holsboer, F., Steiger, A., . . . Czisch, M. (2011). Dreamed movement elicits activation in the sensorimotor cortex. *Current Biology, 21*(21), 1833–1837.

Driskell, J. E., Copper, C., & Moran, A. (1994). Does mental practice enhance performance? *Journal of Applied Psychology, 79*(4), 481–492.

Ehrlenspiel, F., Brand, R., & Graf, K. (2009). Das Wettkampfangst-Inventar-State [Competitive-Anxiety-Inventory-State]. In R. Brand, F. Ehrlenspiel, & K. Graf (Eds.), *Das Wettkampfangst-Inventar: Manual* [Competitive-Anxiety-Inventory: Manual] (pp. 71–99). Bonn, Germany: BISp.

Ehrlenspiel, F., Erlacher, D., & Ziegler, M. (in press). Changes in subjective sleep quality before a competition and their relation to competitive anxiety. *Behavioral Sleep Medicine.* doi:10.1080/15402002.2016.1253012

Erlacher, D. (2007). *Motorisches Lernen im luziden Traum: Phänomenologische und experimentelle Betrachtungen* [Motor learning in lucid dreams: Phenomenological and experimentel aspects]. Saarbrücken: VDM.

Erlacher, D., Ehrlenspiel, F., Adegbesan, O., & Galal El-Din, H. (2011). Sleep habits in German athletes before important competitions or games. *Journal of Sports Sciences*, *29*(8), 859–866.

Erlacher, D., Ehrlenspiel, F., & Schredl, M. (2011). Frequency of nightmares and gender significantly predict distressing dreams of German athletes before competitions or games. *The Journal of Psychology*, *145*(4), 331–342.

Erlacher, D., Schädlich, M., Stumbrys, T., & Schredl, M. (2014). Time for actions in lucid dreams: Effects of task modality, length, and complexity. *Frontiers in Psychology*, *4*. doi:10.3389/fpsyg.2013.01013

Erlacher, D., & Schredl, M. (2008a). Cardiovascular responses to dreamed physical exercise during REM lucid dreaming. *Dreaming*, *18*, 112–121.

Erlacher, D., & Schredl, M. (2008b). Do REM (lucid) dreamed and executed actions share the same neural substrate? *International Journal of Dream Research*, *1*(1), 7–13.

Erlacher, D., & Schredl, M. (2010). Practicing a motor task in a lucid dream enhances subsequent performance: A pilot study. *The Sport Psychologist*, *24*(2), 157–167.

Erlacher, D., Schredl, M., Ehrlenspiel, F., & Bosing, M. (2009). Subjective sleep quality and state anxiety of high-school students prior to a final sport exam. In A. M. Columbus (Ed.), *Advances in psychology research* (pp. 179–186). New York, NY: Nova Science Publishers.

Erlacher, D., Schredl, M., & LaBerge, S. (2003). Motor area activation during dreamed hand clenching: A pilot study on EEG alpha band. *Sleep and Hypnosis*, *5*(4), 182–187.

Erlacher, D., Schredl, M., & Lakus, G. (2009). Subjective sleep quality prior to home and away games for female volleyball players. *International Journal of Dream Research*, *2*, 70–72.

Erlacher, D., Stumbrys, T., & Schredl, M. (2011–2012). Frequency of lucid dreams and lucid dream practice in German athletes. *Imagination, Cognition and Personality*, *31*(3), 237–246.

Freud, S. (1987). *Die Traumdeutung (1900)* [Dream interpretation]. Frankfurt: Fischer Taschenbuch.

Görtelmeyer, R. (2005). *SF-A/R und SF-B/R. Schlaffragebogen A und B – revidierte Fassung* [SF-A/R and SF-B/R. Sleep questionnaire A and B – revised version]. Göttingen: Hogrefe.

Gupta, L., Morgan, K., & Gilchrist, S. (2017). Does elite sport degrade sleep quality? A systematic review. *Sports Medicine*, *47*, 1317–1333.

Hearne, K. M. (1978). *Lucid dreams: An electrophysiological and psychological study*. Unpublished PhD thesis, University of Liverpool, Liverpool, UK.

Hinshaw, K. E. (1991–92). The effects of mental practice on motor skill performance: Critical evaluation and meta-analysis. *Imagination, Cognition and Personality*, *11*(1), 3–35.

Hobson, J. A. (2009). REM sleep and dreaming: Towards a theory of protoconsciousness. *Nature Reviews Neuroscience*, *10*(11), 803–813.

Huber, R., Ghilardi, M. F., Massimini, M., Ferrarelli, F., Riedner, B. A., Peterson, M. J., & Tononi, G. (2006). Arm immobilization causes cortical plastic changes and locally decreases sleep slow wave activity. *Nature Neuroscience*, *9*(9), 1169–1176.

Iber, C., Ancoli-Israel, S., Chesson, A., & Quan, S. F. (Eds.). (2007). *The AASM manual for the scoring of sleep and associated events: Rules, terminology and technical specifications*. Westchester, IL: American Academy of Sleep Medicine.

ICSD-3 (Ed.). (2014). *International classification of sleep disorders* (3rd ed.). Darien, IL: American Academy of Sleep Medicine.

Jeannerod, M. (2001). Neural simulation of action: A unifying mechanism for motor cognition. *Neuroimage*, *14*, 103–109.

Juliff, L. E., Halson, S. L., & Peiffer, J. J. (2015). Understanding sleep disturbance in athletes prior to important competitions. *Journal of Science and Medicine in Sport*, *18*(1), 13–18.

Keklund, G., & Åkerstedt, T. (1997). Objective components of individual differences in subjective sleep quality. *Journal of Sleep Research, 6*(4), 217–220.

LaBerge, S. (1980). *Lucid dreaming: An exploratory study of consciousness during sleep.* Unpublished PhD thesis, Stanford University Press, Stanford, CA.

Langenfeld, H. (1991). Artemidors Traumbuch als sporthistorische Quelle [Artemidors book of dreams as a resource for the history of sport]. *Stadion, 17*(1), 1–26.

Lastella, M., Lovell, G. P., & Sargent, C. (2014). Athletes' precompetitive sleep behaviour and its relationship with subsequent precompetitive mood and performance. *European Journal of Sport Science, 14*(Suppl. 1), S123–S130.

Lastella, M., Roach, G. D., Halson, S. L., Martin, D. T., West, N. P., & Sargent, C. (2015). Sleep/wake behaviour of endurance cyclists before and during competition. *Journal of Sports Sciences, 33*(3), 293–299.

Lastella, M., Roach, G. D., Halson, S. L., & Sargent, C. (2015). Sleep/wake behaviours of elite athletes from individual and team sports. *European Journal of Sport Science, 15*(2), 94–100.

Liendl, S., Lauer, C. J., & Hoffmann, R. M. (2004). Pre-screening via sleep logs in sleep-disordered patients – adaptational effects, yes or no? *Somnologie, 8*, 67–70.

Mahoney, M. J., & Avener, M. (1977). Psychology of the elite athlete: An exploratory study. *Cognitive Therapy and Research, 1*(2), 135–141.

Marino, M., Li, Y., Rueschman, M. N., Winkelman, J. W., Ellenbogen, J. M., Solet, J. M., ... Buxton, O. M. (2013). Measuring sleep: Accuracy, sensitivity, and specificity of wrist actigraphy compared to polysomnography. *Sleep, 36*(11), 1747–1755.

Paul, F., Schädlich, M., & Erlacher, D. (2014). Lucid dream induction by visual and tactile stimulation: An exploratory sleep laboratory study. *International Journal of Dream Research, 7*(1), 61–66.

Rechtschaffen, A., & Kales, A. (1968). *A manual of standardized terminology, techniques and scoring system for sleep stages of human subjects.* Washington, D.C.: U. S. Public Health Service.

Romyn, G., Robey, E., Dimmock, J. A., Halson, S. L., & Peeling, P. (2016). Sleep, anxiety and electronic device use by athletes in the training and competition environments. *European Journal of Sport Science, 16*(3), 301–308.

Sargent, C., Lastella, M., Halson, S. L., & Roach, G. D. (2016). The validity of activity monitors for measuring sleep in elite athletes. *Journal of Science and Medicine in Sport, 19*(10), 848–853.

Saunders, D. T., Roe, C. A., Smith, G., & Clegg, H. (2016). Lucid dreaming incidence: A quality effects meta-analysis of 50 years of research. *Consciousness and Cognition, 43*, 197–215.

Savis, J. C., Eliot, J. F., Gansneder, B., & Rotella, R. J. (1997). A subjective means of assessing college athletes' sleep: A modification of the morningness/eveningness questionnaire. *International Journal of Sport Psychology, 28*, 157–170.

Schädlich, M., Erlacher, D., & Schredl, M. (2017). Improvement of darts performance following lucid dream practice depends on the number of distractions while rehearsing within the dream – a sleep laboratory pilot study. *Journal of Sports Sciences, 35*(23), 2365–2372.

Schredl, M. (2017). Incorporation of waking experiences into dreams. In M. Kryger, T. Roth, & W. C. Dement (Eds.), *Principles and practice of sleep medicine* (6th ed., pp. 555–560). Philadelphia: Elsevier.

Schredl, M., & Erlacher, D. (2003). The problem of dream content analysis validity as shown by a bizarreness scale. *Sleep and Hypnosis, 5*(3), 129–135.

Schredl, M., & Erlacher, D. (2011). Frequency of lucid dreaming in a representative German sample. *Perceptual and Motor Skills, 112*(1), 104–108.

Shapiro, C. M., Bortz, R., Mitchell, D., Bartel, P., & Jooste, P. (1981). Slow-wave sleep: A recovery period after exercise. *Science*, *214*(4526), 1253–1254.

Spoormaker, V. I., Schredl, M., & van den Bout, J. (2006). Nightmares: From anxiety symptom to sleep disorder. *Sleep Medicine Reviews*, *10*(1), 19–31.

Stickgold, R. (2017). Introduction. In M. Kryger, T. Roth, & W. C. Dement (Eds.), *Principles and practice of sleep medicine* (6th ed., pp. 506–508). Philadelphia: Elsevier.

Stuck, B. A., Maurer, J. T., Schredl, M., & Weeß, H.-G. (2013). *Praxis der Schlafmedizin* [Practice of sleep medicine] (2nd ed.). Heidelberg: Springer Medizin.

Stumbrys, T., Erlacher, D., Schädlich, M., & Schredl, M. (2012). Induction of lucid dreams: A systematic review of evidence. *Consciousness and Cognition*, *21*(3), 1456–1475.

Stumbrys, T., Erlacher, D., & Schredl, M. (2013). Testing the involvement of the prefrontal cortex in lucid dreaming: A tDCS study. *Consciousness and Cognition*, *22*(4), 1214–1222.

Stumbrys, T., Erlacher, D., & Schredl, M. (2016). Effectiveness of motor practice in lucid dreams: A comparison with physical and mental practice. *Journal of Sports Sciences*, *34*(1), 27–34.

Swinbourne, R., Gill, N., Vaile, J., & Smart, D. (2016). Prevalence of poor sleep quality, sleepiness and obstructive sleep apnoea risk factors in athletes. *European Journal of Sport Science*, *16*(7), 850–858.

Tholey, P. (1981). Empirische Untersuchungen über Klarträume [Empirical studies on lucid dreams]. *Gestalt Theory*, *3*, 21–62.

Voss, U., Frenzel, C., Koppehele-Gossel, J., & Hobson, A. (2012). Lucid dreaming: An age-dependent brain dissociation. *Journal of Sleep Research*, *21*(6), 634–642.

Youngstedt, S. D. (2005). Effects of exercise on sleep. *Clinics in Sports Medicine*, *24*(2), 355–365.

13

DOMESTIC AND INTERNATIONAL TRAVEL

Implications for performance and recovery in team-sport athletes

Rob Duffield and Peter M. Fowler

Introduction

Travel has long been synonymous with elite athletic competitions. For example, Australian and English cricket players undertook 45-day steamship journeys for competitive tours as early as the mid-1800s. The increased professionalism of sport and resulting congestion of competition and training demands has further increased the volume and extent of travel. Indeed, the modern professional athlete will have a multitude of travel commitments, ranging from regular short-haul domestic (and international) (< 5 hours) through to long-haul international travel (> 20 hours) for both training and competition needs (Fowler, Duffield, Howle, Waterson, & Vaile, 2015; Fowler, Duffield, & Vaile, 2014). Furthermore, professional teams often organise pre- and mid-season camps in various locations to utilise warm-weather or altitude training to accelerate training adaptations (Buchheit et al., 2013). As a result, travel is an additional stress imposed on professional players' competition and training schedules (Leatherwood & Dragoo, 2012). A vast array of potential stressors are imposed by travel, and accordingly the ability to tolerate and recover from air travel is potentially important for ensuing training or competition success. Accordingly, this chapter will draw upon a collection of recent studies on domestic and international travel in athletes to highlight both the consequences of travel on performance and recovery, whilst outlining strategies to ensure optimal post-flight performance.

Training and competition demands increase the physical and perceptual stress on athletes. Team sports often involve moderate- to long-duration efforts, during

Duffield, R., & Fowler, P. M. (2018). Domestic and international travel: Implications for performance and recovery in team-sport athletes. In M. Kellmann & J. Beckmann (Eds.), *Sport, Recovery, and Performance: Interdisciplinary Insights* (pp. 183–197). Abingdon: Routledge.

which players will undertake many brief, though intense efforts intermixed with rest and low-intensity activity (Bangsbo, Mohr, & Krustrup, 2006). Such demands can supress neuromuscular force and power, increase perceived fatigue and soreness and retard preparation for ensuing training and competition (Nédélec et al., 2012). Accordingly, recovery represents the return to baseline levels of performance, physiological and psychological functioning following competition or training bouts; and for many team sports, an optimal recovery time frame suggested as being upwards of 72 hours (Nédélec et al., 2012). Often this recovery process is expedited by a range of medical, physiological and mental interventions (Hausswirth & Le Meur, 2011). However, of importance is to avoid situations and conditions which may hamper the recovery process, and thus when athletes are required to travel before and after matches, a combination of factors may preclude optimal recovery circumstances.

In regards to recovery during a period requiring extensive travel, given the limited time between matches, short-haul air travel is often a necessity the day after an away match (Goumas, 2014). Time lost to travel and the ensuing disruption of routines and training schedules may inhibit the use of recovery and medical interventions. The preparation and recovery processes prior to and following away matches could therefore be impeded. Furthermore, the magnitude of travel completed by professional teams throughout a season can be substantial. For example, in Australian domestic competitions, football, rugby and soccer teams are required to travel up to ~ 3500 km across three or more time zones following matches (McGuckin, Sinclair, Sealey, & Bowman, 2014; Richmond et al., 2007). Therefore, it has been proposed that frequent travel throughout a season may result in the summation of acute intangible effects of travel (Samuels, 2012). Moreover, since travel is often a requirement for teams the day after an away match, ensuing training loads and recovery may be disrupted, which in turn can affect player preparation. From an international perspective, long-haul travel results in symptoms of jet lag due to the misalignment of endogenous circadian rhythms (e.g., melatonin and body temperature) with the light-dark cycle of the destination (Waterhouse, Reilly, Atkinson, & Edwards, 2007). In addition, symptoms of travel fatigue are induced by the prolonged travel duration and cramped, hypoxic conditions of the cabin (Samuels, 2012). In turn, these conditions create problems with adequate sleep quantity and quality, appropriate hydration and nutritional intake, as well as prevent access to proper medical and physiotherapy practises. Thus, the combination of desynchronisation between internal circadian rhythms with the external environment, as well as impedance of recovery processes make long-haul travel an issue for most athletic groups.

Given travel is often highlighted as a reason for poor performance and recovery, supporting evidence of the effect of travel on recovery and ensuing performance in athletes is minimal. Whilst a collective of laboratory studies exists on non-athletic populations, more recently the effects of various travel demands on sports-specific performance have been reported. Accordingly, this chapter will draw upon a collection of recent studies on domestic and international travel in athletes to highlight both the consequences of travel on recovery and strategies to ensure optimal post-flight performance.

Conditions and effects of air travel

Travel fatigue

Travel fatigue results from exposure to the process and environments related to travel, i.e., the regularity, duration, and conditions of travel. Accordingly, the causes of travel fatigue may be numerous and varied depending on the extent of travel undertaken. For example, causes may include the prolonged exposure to mild hypoxia, cramped conditions and cabin noise (Forbes-Robertson et al., 2012; Waterhouse et al., 2007), and/or the disruption of routines as a result of travel, such as eating and sleeping patterns (Reilly et al., 2007). Symptoms of travel fatigue include, but are not limited to, general fatigue, confusion, irritability and headaches; though these are often rescinded with a sufficient night's sleep (Waterhouse, Reilly, & Edwards, 2004; Waterhouse et al., 2007). More explicit causes of travel fatigue include prolonged sitting in cramped conditions, which may reduce flexibility and mobility, induce deep venous thrombosis (Cesarone et al., 2003; Waterhouse et al., 2004), and together with noise from the plane engines and other passengers, may disrupt sleep during air travel (Forbes-Robertson et al., 2012; Waterhouse et al., 2002). Whilst the symptoms of travel fatigue are reported to be less severe than jet lag, both result in compromised physical and cognitive performance (Reilly et al., 2007).

In addition to the above, it has been suggested that the dry cabin air and low hypobaric pressure may cause hypohydration (Hamada et al., 2002; Reilly et al., 2007), and the reduced quality of the cabin air could impair immune function following prolonged exposure (Coste, Van Beers, Bogdan, & Touitou, 2007; Schwellnus et al., 2012). Furthermore, prolonged exposure to mild hypoxia may reduce oxygen saturation (Geertsema, Williams, Dzendrowskyj, & Hanna, 2008), have a detrimental impact on sleep and exacerbate physiological and perceptual stress (Coste, Van Beers, & Touitou, 2009). A final consequence of travel involves the perceived stress associated with delays and embarking and disembarking formalities, such as checking in, baggage claim and security and customs clearance, which often result in negative perceptual and mood states (Reilly et al., 2007; Waterhouse et al., 2007).

Jet lag

When multiple time zones are rapidly crossed during international air travel, a loss of synchrony occurs between the endogenous circadian rhythms and external cues of the new time zone (Waterhouse et al., 2007). Following transmeridian air travel, circadian rhythms initially retain their habitual rhythms of the place of departure. However, external factors in the new environment, particularly the light-dark cycle, act as zeitgebers (time-givers) and promote resynchronisation of the body clock to align with the new time zone (Forbes-Robertson et al., 2012). As a result, body temperature (Lemmer, Kern, Nold, & Lohrer, 2002; Reilly, Atkinson, & Budgett, 2001; Waterhouse et al., 2002) and hormonal circadian rhythms (Bullock, Martin, Ross, Rosemond, & Marino, 2007; Lemmer et al., 2002), along with the sleep-wake cycle (Beaumont et al., 2004) are disrupted. These changes induce the detrimental symptoms of jet lag, such as increased daytime fatigue and irritability, reduced alertness and negative mood states, gastrointestinal disturbances, together with decreased interest in eating and difficulty sleeping; all of which are likely to suppress physical and cognitive performance (Reilly et al., 2007; Reilly & Waterhouse, 2009).

Symptoms of jet lag occur following long-distance air travel eastward or westward across times zones and tend to be more severe and longer lasting than those of travel fatigue (Reilly et al., 2007). Though this typically occurs when time zones are rapidly crossed during air travel (Waterhouse et al., 2004), symptoms of jet lag have also been noted following simulated time zone changes in the laboratory, highlighting that unlike travel fatigue, jet lag is not caused solely by the demands of travel (Waterhouse et al., 2007). One of the main reported symptoms is poor sleep, especially delayed sleep onset and early awakening after eastward and westward flights, respectively (Beaumont et al., 2004; Takahashi, Nakata, & Arito, 2002). It is proposed that symptoms are worse the greater the number of time zones crossed and if travelling east rather than west (Waterhouse et al., 2004). Indeed, rates of resynchronisation are loosely estimated as half a day per hour of the time difference westwards, or one day per hour of the time difference eastwards (Forbes-Robertson et al., 2012). The predicted faster rate of resynchronisation following westward travel is based on principles of chronobiology, suggesting it is easier to adapt to a phase delay following westward rather than a phase advance after eastward travel (Forbes-Robertson et al., 2012). However, it is accepted the above description is simplistic in nature and high inter-individual variation exists for jet lag symptoms and their severity. Furthermore, evidence of the rates of post-travel resynchronisation of circadian rhythms are also highly variable meaning explicit guides to overcoming jet lag are often generic in nature.

Performance and recovery following domestic or short-haul international travel

Short-haul domestic and international air travel is one of a myriad of factors purported to affect match outcome and the tendency for teams to perform better at home compared to away (Goumas, 2014; Pollard, 2008). Hence, it is frequently highlighted by the media, coaching staff and players as an explanation for poor away match performances (Du Preez & Lambert, 2009). As evidence, crossing a greater number of time zones during domestic air travel for away matches has been correlated with reduced competition performance (Bishop, 2004; Goumas, 2014; Winter, Hammond, Green, Zhang, & Bliwise, 2009). Moreover, the time of competition appears to be influential, with teams gaining an advantage if competition occurs closer to the time of peak physical performance, which is often biased against travelling teams (Leatherwood & Dragoo, 2012). The tendency for teams to perform better at home compared to away, referred to as the 'Home Advantage', is a consistent finding in a range of team sports (Gomez, Pollard, & Luis-Pascual, 2011). For example, situational variables such as match location and status, and opposition quality, together with territoriality, tactics, and the expectancy to perform worse away from home have been identified as the factors most likely to affect competition performance (Lago, Casais, Dominguez, & Sampaio, 2010; Neave & Wolfson, 2003). Whilst difficult to separate Home Advantage from the discreet effects of travel, three specific components of travel are thought to provide an advantage to the home team; including: (i) the disruption of familiar routines; (ii) fatigue from travelling; and (iii) the distance travelled, which may also be inversely associated with crowd support (Smith, Ciacciarelli, Serzan, & Lambert, 2000). In particular, the disruption of familiar routines is the main aspect of travel thought to influence competition performance (Smith et al., 2000). For example, it is speculated that the home team may have physiological and psychological advantages over their opposition because they are able to reside at home rather than in an unfamiliar hotel, can sustain a regular sleep pattern as sleep is not affected by travel demands and/or jet lag, and can maintain normal diet and eating practises (Smith et al., 2000).

Several studies have attempted to determine whether travel is a major factor behind reduced away competition performance in team sports, though to date the evidence is equivocal. For example, separating travel effects through regression analyses on performance data from team sports has revealed that parameters such as distance travelled and number of time zones crossed may account for only 1–2% of the variance in match outcome (Smith et al., 2000). However, in other studies, crossing a greater number of time zones during domestic air travel for away matches has been significantly correlated with reduced competition performance (Bishop, 2004; Winter et al., 2009). For example, a strong positive correlation between Home Advantage and the number of time zones crossed by away teams was observed in professional soccer players in Australia (Goumas, 2014). A limitation of this study was the relatively small number of matches involving away teams that had crossed more than two time zones. Further, in American Major League Baseball, when a match involved a team that had travelled across three time zones it resulted in a winning rate of 61% for the home team (Winter et al., 2009). Furthermore, it was reported that the probability of the home team winning depended on whether the away team had travelled east, and that the home team could expect to score 1.24 (0.79–1.69) more runs than usual when this occurred (Recht, Lew, & Schwartz, 1995). Collectively these findings imply that domestic air travel across time-zones may have a negative impact on competition performance and that west coast teams in Australia and America have the double handicap of playing their away games after travelling east across time-zones. However, no measures other than competition (scoreboard) performance are reported in these studies, and further, more individualised measures of athlete responses are required to better understand the effects of domestic travel.

In order to isolate the effect of travel on physical performance in team sport athletes, Fowler, Duffield, and Vaile (2015) simulated a 5-hour domestic flight with mild hypoxia, seating arrangements, activity, and sleep patterns typically encountered during air travel in a normobaric, hypoxic altitude room. Yo-Yo Intermittent Recovery test performance, sleeping patterns, and mood states remained unchanged following a simulated 5-hour flight in sub-elite team sport athletes. More relevant are studies that investigate the effects of the demands of domestic air travel on technical and tactical performance indicators and team sport physical performance measures (McGuckin et al., 2014; Richmond et al., 2007). During away compared to home matches, professional rugby league players performed more tackles and covered less distance (McGuckin et al., 2014). Conversely, no differences in match statistics, including time between possessions and team assists, were evident in professional Australian Football League players (Richmond et al., 2007). From a physical capacity perspective, no change in grip strength or lower-body power was reported following short-haul air travel (McGuckin et al., 2014). Fowler and colleagues (2014) reported the effects of short-haul air travel on competition performance and subsequent recovery in professional soccer players from home and away matches against the same teams. Whilst oxygen saturation was significantly lower during travel, equivocal differences in sleep quantity and quality, hydration and perceptual fatigue were evident at away compared to home competition. Accordingly, despite poorer away match performances, the short-haul air travel may not explicitly be the reason, and thus situational variables and tactics may be more important.

Whilst the aforementioned studies report acute responses, i.e., within days of a singular bout of travel, it may be the accumulated demands of regular short-haul travel that are of concern for athletes during domestic competitions (Samuels, 2012). Fowler, Duffield, Waterson, and Vaile (2015) reported the effect of home vs. away during early vs. late competition periods on training loads, wellness, and injury in a professional soccer team. Not surprisingly, training load distribution during the weekly microcycle was altered due to the demands of travel, particularly on the day after arrival from an away match. However, no discernible effect of travel was evident on player wellness due to match location (home *vs.* away) or injury occurrence, irrespective of period of the season. Whilst more training sessions were missed at home due to injury, this was a likely artefact of more sessions being completed during home match weeks. Accordingly, regular short-haul travel had negligible accumulative effects on player wellness or injury during a season. Given the previously outlined research in athletes, limited and equivocal evidence exists for the negative effects of domestic short-haul air travel on the recovery timeline of team sport athletes, though a more detailed understanding remains to be elucidated.

Performance and recovery following long-haul international travel

Current data on the performance capacity and timeline of recovery for athletes following long-haul travel is mixed and confusing. Understandably, substantial logistical issues and costs are associated with conducting research into the effects of international air travel on athlete performance and recovery. Consequently, there are limited field-based studies on the effects of an episode of international air travel on sports performance. Reduced grip strength is commonly reported following long-haul transmeridian air travel (Edwards et al., 2000; Reilly et al., 2001). For example, reduced grip strength was reported following 12 hours of eastward air travel across eight time zones (Lemmer et al., 2002), together with nine and 10 hours of westward air travel across five and six time zones in elite gymnasts (Lemmer et al., 2002; Reilly et al., 2001). Though, in contrast to the assumption that eastward has a greater impact on performance than westward travel, no differences in grip strength were reported for four of the athletes when comparing 12 hours of eastward travel across eight time zones to 10 hours of westward travel across six time zones (Lemmer et al., 2002). Admittedly due to its convenient and non-fatiguing nature, hand grip strength is a common measure of the circadian rhythm in muscle performance (Drust, Waterhouse, Atkinson, Edwards, & Reilly, 2005; Reilly et al., 2001). Whilst tests exhibiting these characteristics are preferable when assessing circadian rhythms in physical performance, the ecological validity of hand grip strength to performance in team sport training and competition is questionable.

Accordingly, jump performance is thought to be a non-fatiguing, yet time efficient and more specific team sport action, and thus may be a more appropriate measure. In elite skeleton athletes, reduced velocity, power, eccentric utilisation ratios, box drop jump flight time and contact time to flight time ratio, squat jump velocity and power, and countermovement jump height were observed in the first two days following 24 hours of eastward transmeridian air travel across 15 time zones (Chapman, Bullock, Ross, Rosemond, & Martin, 2012). These results suggest that both skeletal muscle contractile and neuromuscular function, and therefore, jump performance are adversely affected by long-haul transmeridian air travel (Chapman et al., 2012). Conversely, no change in 30 m sprint performance was identified in the same participant population in response to the same travel demands (Bullock et al., 2007). Similarly, minimal disruptions to squat jump height and power output during a 15 s multiple jump test were reported following 10 hours of eastward air travel across seven time zones in an active, but not athletic population (Lagarde et al., 2001). These contrasting results may be due to differences in travel demands, including the duration and distance of travel, and/or the sensitivity, type, and timing of physical performance measures, making meaningful comparisons between studies difficult. These conflicting findings emphasise the equivocal effect of international air travel on physical performance. Such diverse findings could be a result of the varying degrees of success by which study designs have controlled for the multitude of confounding factors that affect sports performance (Leatherwood & Dragoo, 2012; Reilly & Waterhouse, 2009). However, it may also be explained by the inter-individual variation in responses to the different durations and directions of travel, due to age, flexibility of sleeping habits, time of arrival and previous travel experience (Waterhouse et al., 2002).

Recently, Fowler, Duffield, and Vaile (2015) simulated a 24h long-haul international flight in sub-elite team sport athletes. The mild hypoxia, seating arrangements, activity and sleep patterns typically encountered during air travel were replicated in a normobaric, hypoxic altitude room. Both sleep quantity and quality were reduced due to the simulated international flight, resulting in reduced intermittent-sprint performance (Yo-Yo test Level 1) on the day after the simulated flight. Further, negative mood states, perceived fatigue and autonomic function from steady-state heart rate responses were also exacerbated. A similar impact on sleep was reported in an elite team of footballers who undertook 18 hours of westward international air travel with a 4-hour time zone shift (Fullagar et al., 2016). Sleep duration and efficiency were reduced during and following outbound travel. However, these alterations were not dissimilar to the quantity and quality of sleep noted following ensuing night matches. Of interest, perceived jet lag and recovery was not affected by the flight duration or time zone shift, suggesting either the players were habituated to travel, or these travel demands were insufficient to cause significant alterations to player well-being (Fullagar et al., 2016). Therefore, it is possible that they may be able to cope or are familiar with the demands of travel more so than non-athletes, which may assist with explaining the different findings between studies involving different participant populations (Bullock et al., 2007).

Furthermore, a professional soccer team were monitored following 10h northbound air travel across one time zone for sleep, jet lag and wellness (Fowler, Duffield, Howle, et al., 2015). Sleep duration was reduced on the night prior to travel due to the early awakening to get to the airport; however, it was not unduly affected in the days thereafter. Subjective jet lag was increased and player wellness reduced during the days post-travel. Accordingly, despite minimal time zone change, some evidence for disrupted sleep and fatigue was evident. Such a response may be due to misinterpretation by younger, less experienced players who reported higher jet lag and lower wellness than their more experienced colleagues. Similarly, National team footballers who undertook eastward long-haul air travel across 11 time zones reported increased perceived jet lag for four days, poorer self-reported sleep duration both during travel and in the four days post-travel and a reduction in mean wellness during the week following travel (Fowler, McCall, Jones, & Duffield, 2017). These results in National team footballers highlight the reduction in player preparedness for ensuing training and competition, despite the lack of explicit physical performance data. Finally, Fowler, Duffield, Lu, Hickmans, and Scott (2016) also reported the effects of 24-hour travel westward across 11 time zones on subjective jet lag, sleep and wellness responses, together with self-reported upper-respiratory tract infection (URTI) symptoms in professional rugby league players. Self-reported sleep onset times and wake up times were earlier in the days following travel. Of interest, no effects of travel on wellness and muscle strength or range of motion were evident. However, an increase in URTI symptoms existed in the week after travel. The increase in URTI symptoms and severity conforms to earlier reports that athletes are at greater risk of URTI's when crossing more than five time zones away from their place of residence (Schwellnus et al., 2012). Accordingly, protection of athletes from foreign pathogens and immune system infection is integral for the health of travelling players. Again though, limited sport-specific performance measures were collected, so it remains unknown as to whether such factors from international travel reduce competition performance.

Interventions to improve post-travel readiness

As previously outlined, the demands of long-haul transmeridian air travel, combined with the detrimental consequences of jet lag, may induce adverse physiological, perceptual and sleep responses and in turn suppress physical performance (Chapman et al., 2012; Coste et al., 2009). Interventions to overcome these individual or collective effects would be advantageous for travelling team sport athletes. However, a paucity of interventions has been confirmed as beneficial to travelling athletes. Instead, based on an understanding of chronobiology from laboratory-based experiments (Deacon & Arendt, 1996; Revell et al., 2006), generic recommendations have been published to promote the resynchronisation of circadian rhythms and thus, minimise the negative effects of jet lag following international air travel in athletes (Arendt, 2009; Forbes-Robertson et al., 2012; Reilly et al., 2007). However, it is yet unclear whether these recommendations have any effect on the recovery of physical performance following travel, particularly in elite athletes.

Following long-haul transmeridian air travel, external cues referred to as zeitgebers (time-givers), are reported to gradually resynchronise endogenous circadian rhythms (Forbes-Robertson et al., 2012). Though natural light is the strongest of these external cues, exercise, meal timing and exogenous melatonin can also contribute to resynchronisation (Arendt, 2009; Forbes-Robertson et al., 2012). Jet lag symptoms persist until the circadian rhythms are aligned with the external cues of the destination, which theoretically takes approximately one day per time zone crossed (Forbes-Robertson et al., 2012). Whilst it has been recommended that athletes allow a sufficient number of days in a new time zone for the body clock to fully adjust prior to competition (Reilly et al., 2007), this is often not plausible due to training and competition schedules. As a result, travel frequently occurs relatively close prior to and/or following competition. A faster rate of adaptation to a new time zone would reduce the duration of jet lag symptoms and therefore, the possible suppression of physical performance (Arendt, 2009). Consequently, improving the rate of adaptation, which is the goal of the majority of travel interventions, within the logistics of travel could be beneficial for team sport athletes. Despite the lack of evidence, to accelerate the resynchronisation of the sleep-wake cycle, previous recommendations propose that during travel, sleep should be scheduled according to when it is night at the destination, and must be avoided when it is daytime at the destination (Reilly & Edwards, 2007; Waterhouse et al., 2004).

In contrast, several studies have investigated the use of specific pharmacological interventions including caffeine, short-acting benzodiazepine hypnotics and melatonin (Beaumont et al., 2004; Edwards et al., 2000; Reilly et al., 2001). Considering the suggested unwanted side-effects (Beaumont et al., 2004; Reilly et al., 2001) and medical concerns over the use of many pharmacological interventions, the appropriate timing of bright light and exercise is currently advocated as the simplest, most appropriate and effective method of adjusting circadian rhythms in athletes (Forbes-Robertson et al., 2012). Consequently, the commercial availability of portable artificial bright light sources, such as light boxes and light glasses, as a treatment for jet lag has recently increased. Whilst evidence suggests these devices may adjust circadian rhythms in well controlled laboratory studies (Wright, Lack, & Kennaway, 2004), their effectiveness at enhancing the recovery of physical performance following transmeridian air travel is limited (Boulos et al., 2002), particularly in elite team sport athletes (Thompson et al., 2013). Furthermore, as sleep disruption is likely during and following long-haul transmeridian air travel (Beaumont et al., 2004; Takahashi et al., 2002; Waterhouse et al., 2002), which may itself reduce ensuing physical performance, sleep interventions that minimise this disruption may also enhance performance recovery, though this remains to be investigated.

A further complication is the decision on whether to attempt to resynchronise circadian rhythms to the new time zone following international air travel. For short stays (one to two days), attempts to resynchronise the body clock are not recommended (Forbes-Robertson et al., 2012). Instead, individuals are encouraged to stay on home time and schedule important events at the time of maximum alertness in the departure time zone (Arendt, 2009; Forbes-Robertson et al., 2012). However, this is logistically difficult in an applied setting, given it is not possible to adjust competition times to suit team sport athletes and the annoyance of not aligning behaviour with local times. Hence, the use of hypnotics (e.g., melatonin and benzodiazepines) and stimulants (e.g., caffeine) are sometimes advocated to reduce sleep disruption and maintain alertness and performance (Waterhouse et al., 2007). For longer stays (≥ four to five days) light exposure and/or exogenous melatonin administration are recommended to promote adaptation of circadian rhythms prior to departure and upon arrival to alleviate jet lag symptoms (Arendt, 2009; Forbes-Robertson et al., 2012). Indeed, a 'travel management program', which is a comprehensive approach to the management of jet lag and travel fatigue that includes pre-, during and post-travel periods (see Table 13.1), has been advocated for longer stays (Fowler, 2015; Samuels, 2012).

TABLE 13.1 Practical applications for optimal recovery following travel as adapted from those published by Fowler (2015).

---

1. Pre-travel
    i. Undertake sleep hygiene practises prior to travel to minimise sleep debt.
    ii. If feasible, replace long-duration, moderate-intensity training (which may be immunosuppressive) with shorter, high-intensity, high-quality sessions.
    iii. Consider immune-booster supplements, i.e., vitamin C, zinc acetate, or gluconate, to reduce the risk of illness.
2. During Travel
    i. Attempt to sleep whenever possible, but particularly when it is night time at the place of destination.

ii. Practise good sleep hygiene.
   –Minimise the use of light emitting electronic equipment.
   –Avoid caffeine.
   –Utilise eye masks, neck pillows, ear plugs, and/or noise-cancelling headphones.
   –Wear comfortable, loose-fitting clothing.
  iii. The airplane cabin is a 'high-risk' environment for infection/illness, therefore:
   –Don't self-inoculate by touching eyes, nose, and mouth.
   –Avoid contact with most frequently touched area of door handles and avoid using the whole hand.
   –Cough and sneeze into the elbow, not hands.
   –Practise good hand hygiene by washing them frequently and using a hand sanitiser with residual activity.
3. Post-travel
  i. Physical performance may be reduced in the first few days ($\leq$ 72 hours) following arrival and adjust training load as appropriate.
  ii. Practise good sleep hygiene.
   –Minimise the use of electronic equipment and dim room lights 1 hour prior to bed.
   –Avoid caffeine approximately 4–5 hours prior to sleep (this may vary between individuals).
   –Ensure cool (~19–21°C), quiet, and dark conditions throughout the sleep period. Eye masks and ear plugs may be helpful, particularly with reinitiating sleep onset if early waking occurs.
   –Napping can be useful to counteract nighttime sleep disruption. However, naps should be kept to $\leq$ 1 hour and not too close to bed time as this may interfere with sleep.
  iii. Light exposure and training times.
   –Westward travel (phase-delay required) – seek light/exercise for the 2–3 hours prior to core body temperature minimum (T_{min}; ~05:00 local time) & avoid light/exercise for the 2–3 hours following T_{min}.
   –Eastward travel (phase-advance required) – avoid light/exercise for the 2–3 hours prior to T_{min} & seek light/exercise for the 2–3 hours following T_{min}.
   –If the timing of light exposure is outside daylight hours or it is an overcast day, supplementing natural with artificial light may be beneficial.
   –Be wary of light exposure and training too close to bed time as this may interfere with sleep.
  iv. Melatonin administration (3–5 mg has typically been used in field studies). Westward travel – administration in the morning (body clock time) around the T_{min}. Eastward travel – administration in the evening (body clock time).
  v. Caffeine administration.
   –Could be utilised to reduce sleepiness/increase alertness around training and competition.
  vi. Take care with the dose and pharmacokinetics of pharmacological interventions as they can induce negative side-effects and/or phase-shifts in the wrong direction.
  vii. Due to potential side-effects, behavioural interventions (i.e., light exposure) should be preferred and prioritised over pharmacological, though use as is required under medical supervision.

Conclusion and recommendations for practise

Travel is an unavoidable stress for many high-performance athletes, whether it consists of regular short-haul or occasional long-haul travel. Accordingly, the ability to tolerate and recover from air travel is potentially important for ensuing training or competition success. Discounting the effect of Home Advantage, limited and equivocal evidence exists for the negative effects of domestic short-haul air travel, though the regularity of high volumes of such travel likely induce symptoms of travel fatigue across a season. A multitude of mechanisms result in long-haul international travel affecting ensuing physical performance and recovery, alongside exacerbated physiological, immunological and sleep responses. Regardless, appropriate planning and availability of strategies should be part of the practitioners' tool kit to deal with either the perceptual aspects of domestic travel fatigue, or the more physiologically onerous demands of long-haul travel. Either way, improving athlete perceptions, tolerance and preparation for travel is a must to ensure optimised post-travel performance and recovery.

References

Arendt, J. (2009). Managing jet lag: Some of the problems and possible new solutions. *Sleep Medicine Reviews*, 13(4), 249–256.

Bangsbo, J., Mohr, M., & Krustrup, P. (2006). Physical and metabolic demands of training and match-play in the elite football player. *Journal of Sports Sciences*, 24, 665–674.

Beaumont, M., Batejat, D., Pierard, C., Van Beers, P., Denis, J. B., Coste, O., . . . Lagarde, D. (2004). Caffeine or melatonin effects on sleep and sleepiness after rapid eastward transmeridian travel. *Journal of Applied Physiology*, 96(1), 50–58.

Bishop, D. (2004). The effects of travel on team performance in the Australian national netball competition. *Journal of Science and Medicine in Sport*, 7(1), 118–122.

Boulos, Z., Macchi, M. M., Sturchler, M. P., Stewart, K. T., Brainard, G. C., Suhner, A., . . . Steffen, R. (2002). Light visor treatment for jet lag after westward travel across six time zones. *Aviation, Space, and Environmental Medicine*, 73(10), 953–963.

Buchheit, M., Simpson, B. M., Garvican-Lewis, L. A., Hammond, K., Kley, M., Schmidt, W. F., . . . Roach, G. D. (2013). Wellness, fatigue and physical performance acclimatisation to a 2-week soccer camp at 3600 m (ISA3600). *British Journal of Sports Medicine*, 47(1), 100–106.

Bullock, N., Martin, D. T., Ross, A., Rosemond, D., & Marino, F. E. (2007). Effect of long haul travel on maximal sprint performance and diurnal variations in elite skeleton athletes. *British Journal of Sports Medicine*, 41(9), 569–573.

Cesarone, M. R., Belcaro, G., Errichi, B. M., Nicolaides, A. N., Geroulakos, G., Ippolito, E., . . . Stuard, S. (2003). The lonflit4-concorde deep venous thrombosis and edema study: Prevention with travel stockings. *Angiology*, 54(2), 143–154.

Chapman, D. W., Bullock, N., Ross, A., Rosemond, D., & Martin, D. T. (2012). Detrimental effects of west to east transmeridian flight on jump performance. *European Journal of Applied Physiology*, 112(5), 1663–1669.

Coste, O., Van Beers, P., Bogdan, A., & Touitou, Y. (2007). Human immune circadian system in prolonged mild hypoxia during simulated flights. *Chronobiology International*, 24(1), 87–98.

Coste, O., Van Beers, P., & Touitou, Y. (2009). Hypoxia-induced changes in recovery sleep, core body temperature, urinary 6-sulphatoxymelatonin and free cortisol after a simulated long-duration flight. *Journal of Sleep Research, 18*(4), 454–465.

Deacon, S., & Arendt, J. (1996). Adapting to phase shifts. An experimental model for jet lag and shift work. *Physiology & Behaviour, 59*(4), 665–673.

Drust, B., Waterhouse, J., Atkinson, G., Edwards, B., & Reilly, T. (2005). Circadian rhythms in sports performance – an update. *Chronobiology International, 22*(1), 21–44.

Du Preez, M., & Lambert, M. (2009). Travel fatigue and home ground advantage in South African super 12 rugby teams. *South African Journal of Sports Medicine, 19*(1), 20–22.

Edwards, B. J., Atkinson, G., Waterhouse, J., Reilly, T., Godfrey, R., & Budgett, R. (2000). Use of melatonin in recovery from jet-lag following an eastward flight across 10 time-zones. *Ergonomics, 43*(10), 1501–1513.

Forbes-Robertson, S., Dudley, E., Vadgama, P., Cook, C., Drawer, S., & Kilduff, L. (2012). Circadian disruption and remedial interventions: Effects and interventions for jet lag for athletic peak performance. *Sports Medicine, 42*(3), 185–208.

Fowler, P. (2015). Performance recovery following long-haul international travel in team sport athletes. *Aspetar Sports Medicine Journal, 4*(3), 502–509.

Fowler, P., Duffield, R., Howle, K., Waterson, A., & Vaile, J. (2015). Effects of northbound long-haul international air travel on sleep quantity and subjective jet lag and wellness in professional Australian soccer players. *International Journal of Sports Physiology & Performance, 10*(5), 648–654.

Fowler, P., Duffield, R., Lu, D., Hickmans, J. A., & Scott, T. J. (2016). Effects of long-haul transmeridian travel on subjective jet-lag and self-reported sleep and upper respiratory symptoms in professional Rugby League players. *International Journal of Sports Physiology & Performance, 11*(7), 876–884.

Fowler, P., Duffield, R., & Vaile, J. (2014). Effects of domestic air travel on technical and tactical performance and recovery in soccer. *International Journal of Sports Physiology & Performance, 9*(3), 378–386.

Fowler, P., Duffield, R., & Vaile, J. (2015). Effects of simulated domestic and international air travel on sleep, performance, and recovery for team sports. *Scandinavian Journal of Medicine and Science in Sports, 25*(3), 441–451.

Fowler, P., Duffield, R., Waterson A., & Vaile, J. (2015). Effects of regular away travel on training loads, recovery, and injury rates in professional Australian soccer players. *International Journal of Sports Physiology & Performance, 10*(5), 546–552.

Fowler, P., McCall, A., Jones, M., & Duffield, R. (2017). Effects of long-haul transmeridian travel on player preparedness: Case study of a national team at the 2014 FIFA World Cup. *Journal of Sports Science and Medicine, 20*(4), 322–327.

Fullagar, H. H., Duffield, R., Skorski, S., White, D., Bloomfield, J., Kölling, S., & Meyer, T. (2016). Sleep, travel, and recovery responses of national footballers during and after long-haul international air travel. *International Journal of Sports Physiology & Performance, 11*(1), 86–95.

Geertsema, C., Williams, A. B., Dzendrowskyj, P., & Hanna, C. (2008). Effect of commercial airline travel on oxygen saturation in athletes. *British Journal of Sports Medicine, 42*(11), 877–881.

Gomez, M. A., Pollard, R., & Luis-Pascual, J. C. (2011). Comparison of the home advantage in nine different professional team sports in Spain. *Perceptual and Motor Skills, 113*(1), 150–156.

Goumas, C. (2014). Home advantage in Australian soccer. *Journal of Science and Medicine in Sport, 17*(1), 119–123.

Hamada, K., Doi, T., Sakurai, M., Matsumoto, K., Yanagisawa, K., Suzuki, T., . . . Okoshi, H. (2002). Effects of hydration on fluid balance and lower-extremity blood viscosity during long airplane flights. *Journal of the American Medical Association, 287*(7), 844–845.

Hausswirth, C., & Le Meur, Y. (2011). Physiological and nutritional aspects of post-exercise recovery: Specific recommendations for female athletes. *Sports Medicine, 41*(10), 861–882.

Lagarde, D., Chappuis, B., Billaud, P. F., Ramont, L., Chauffard, F., & French, J. (2001). Evaluation of pharmacological aids on physical performance after a transmeridian flight. *Medicine and Science in Sports and Exercise, 33*(4), 628–634.

Lago, C., Casais, L., Dominguez, E., & Sampaio, J. (2010). The effects of situational variables on distance covered at various speeds in elite soccer. *European Journal of Sport Science, 10*(2), 103–109.

Leatherwood, W. E., & Dragoo, J. L. (2012). Effect of airline travel on performance: A review of the literature. *British Journal of Sports Medicine, 47*(9), 561–567.

Lemmer, B., Kern, R. I., Nold, G., & Lohrer, H. (2002). Jet lag in athletes after eastward and westward time-zone transition. *Chronobiology International, 19*(4), 743–764.

McGuckin, T. A., Sinclair, W. H., Sealey, R. M., & Bowman, P. (2014). The effects of air travel on performance measures of elite Australian rugby league players. *European Journal of Sport Science, 14*(1), S116–122.

Neave, N., & Wolfson, S. (2003). Testosterone, territoriality, and the 'home advantage'. *Physiology & Behaviour, 78*(2), 269–275.

Nédélec, M., McCall, A., Carling, C., Legall, F., Berthoin, S., & Dupont, G. (2012). Recovery in soccer: Part I – post-match fatigue and time course of recovery. *Sports Medicine, 42*(12), 997–1015.

Pollard, R. (2008). Home advantage in football: A current review of an unsolved puzzle. *The Open Sports Sciences Journal, 1*(1), 12–14.

Recht, L. D., Lew, R. A., & Schwartz, W. J. (1995). Baseball teams beaten by jet lag. *Nature, 377*, 583.

Reilly, T., Atkinson, G., & Budgett, R. (2001). Effect of low-dose temazepam on physiological variables and performance tests following a westerly flight across five time zones. *International Journal of Sports Medicine, 22*(3), 166–174.

Reilly, T., Atkinson, G., Edwards, B., Waterhouse, J., Åkerstedt, T., Davenne, D., . . . Wirz-Justice, A. (2007). Coping with jet-lag: A position statement for the European College of Sport Science. *European Journal of Sport Science, 7*(1), 1–7.

Reilly, T., & Edwards, B. (2007). Altered sleep-wake cycles and physical performance in athletes. *Physiology & Behaviour, 90*(2–3), 274–284.

Reilly, T., & Waterhouse, J. (2009). Sports performance: Is there evidence that the body clock plays a role? *European Journal of Applied Physiology, 106*(3), 321–332.

Revell, V. L., Burgess, H. J., Gazda, C. J., Smith, M. R., Fogg, L. F., & Eastman, C. I. (2006). Advancing human circadian rhythms with afternoon melatonin and morning intermittent bright light. *Journal of Clinical Endocrinology & Metabolism, 91*(1), 54–59.

Richmond, L. K., Dawson, B., Stewart, G., Cormack, S., Hillman, D. R., & Eastwood, P. R. (2007). The effect of interstate travel on the sleep patterns and performance of elite Australian rules footballers. *Journal of Science and Medicine in Sport, 10*(4), 252–258.

Samuels, C. H. (2012). Jet lag and travel fatigue: A comprehensive management plan for sport medicine physicians and high-performance support teams. *Clinical Journal of Sport Medicine, 22*(3), 268–273.

Schwellnus, M. P., Derman, W. E., Jordaan, E., Page, T., Lambert, M. I., Readhead, C., . . . Kara, S. (2012). Elite athletes travelling to international destinations > 5 time zone differences from their home country have a 2–3-fold increased risk of illness. *British Journal of Sports Medicine, 46*(11), 816–821.

Smith, D. R., Ciacciarelli, A., Serzan, J., & Lambert, D. (2000). Travel and the home advantage in professional sports. *Sociology of Sport Journal, 17*(4), 364–385.

Takahashi, M., Nakata, A., & Arito, H. (2002). Disturbed sleep – wake patterns during and after short-term international travel among academics attending conferences. *International Archives of Occupational and Environmental Health, 75*(6), 435–440.

Thompson, A., Batterham, A., Jones, H., Gregson, W., Scott, D., & Atkinson, G. (2013). The practicality and effectiveness of supplementary bright light for reducing jet-lag in elite female athletes. *International Journal of Sports Medicine, 34*(7), 582–589.

Waterhouse, J., Reilly, T., Atkinson, G., & Edwards, B. (2007). Jet lag: Trends and coping strategies. *The Lancet, 369*(9567), 1117–1129.

Waterhouse, J., Reilly, T., & Edwards, B. (2004). The stress of travel. *Journal of Sports Sciences, 22*(10), 946–965.

Waterhouse, J., Edwards, B., Nevill, A., Carvalho, S., Atkinson, G., Buckley, P., . . . Ramsay, R. (2002). Identifying some determinants of "jet lag" and its symptoms: A study of athletes and other travellers. *British Journal of Sports Medicine, 36*(1), 54–60.

Winter, W. C., Hammond, W. R., Green, N. H., Zhang, Z., & Bliwise, D. L. (2009). Measuring circadian advantage in major league baseball: A 10-year retrospective study. *International Journal of Sports Physiology and Performance, 4*(3), 394–401.

Wright, H. R., Lack L. C., & Kennaway, D. J. (2004). Differential effects of light wavelength in phase advancing the melatonin rhythm. *Journal of Pineal Research, 36*(2), 140–144.

PART IV
Transfer to related areas

14
WHAT DO SPORT COACHES KNOW ABOUT RECOVERY?

Christine Nash and John Sproule

Introduction

A key skill of the sports coach is to deliver effective training sessions to develop the performer and/or team and enhance competition, and the monitoring of athletes is vital in this process. Traditionally sports coaches have little formal education or training in this area. Much appears to be learned through trial and error and experience; however, the sports coaches' lack of education or expertise in this area can lead to both short- and long-term issues that can be detrimental to performance or more seriously, dangerous to the health and well-being of the athletes.

This chapter examines the knowledge of sports coaches from a variety of sports on the theory and practical applications of recovery techniques. Coaches, especially at the performance level, are searching for any advantage for their teams or individual performers. This drive for performance enhancement in elite sports requires that the coach and athlete find a balance between training and recovery to avoid negative consequences, such as underperformance and the onset of an overtraining syndrome. The use of scientific knowledge and a systematic approach can enhance the training and recovery process, especially as the goal of recovery should be to restore psychological and physiological resources; however, in many sports the coaches do not possess this level of scientific knowledge around recovery processes.

As a result of increasing professionalism, elite athletes' training loads have increased and this has manifested in a number of athletes experiencing negative instead of positive training responses (Kellmann, 2002). This could be explained by an increase in professional training by the athletes but a lack of similar increase in

---

Nash, C., & Sproule, J. (2018). What do sport coaches know about recovery? In M. Kellmann & J. Beckmann (Eds.), *Sport, Recovery, and Performance: Interdisciplinary Insights* (pp. 201–220). Abingdon: Routledge.

professional knowledge and understanding on the part of the coach. The development of the Recovery-Stress Questionnaire for Athletes (RESTQ-Sport; Kellmann & Kallus, 2001, 2016) could provide much needed information for both coach and athlete. However, this would pre-suppose that the coach was aware of this, able to administer, analyse and then interpret the results, unless there was a suitably qualified individual who could take on this task.

Much of the available literature surrounding recovery tends to be from three perspectives:

1. Recovery from injury/trauma.
2. Recovery modalities from a scientific perspective.
3. Recovery enhancement for the athlete.

To date very little is known and understood about the sports coaches' knowledge, understanding and application of recovery techniques.

Coaches' knowledge of recovery

There is a wide variety of opinion anecdotally when talking to sport coaches not just around the notion of recovery but also what sports coaches understood by the concept of recovery and where they gained this knowledge. The majority of coaches were of the opinion that recovery was only necessary after hard training or competition and the overwhelming feeling was that sports coaches were able to accurately gauge the recovery necessary. There was very little understanding of any specific modalities that coaches could use to monitor or enhance the recovery process. However, it must be stressed that this was not the opinion of all the coaches.

In order to objectively determine coaches' knowledge of recovery in early 2016 an online survey was designed using elements of the RESTQ-Sport mentioned earlier as well as collecting demographic and evidence of practical application of recovery techniques within coaching environments. Coaches from Europe and North America were asked both their understanding and usage of elements of recovery, using the summary definitions provided in the RESTQ-Sport. For example, emotional stress was defined as exhibition of frequent irritation, aggression, anxiety and inhibition and lack of energy was explained as inability to concentrate and lack of energy and decision. This survey was available online and distributed to coaching groups.

Given the introductory conversations with sports coaches about their knowledge – or perhaps lack of knowledge – of recovery, it was important to establish the level of their coaching education and the main sport they coached. Figure 14.1 shows the range of sports coached as well as the self-determined level of the responding coaches, novice, developmental and elite. In total, there were 1,237 responses to this 2016 survey (novice = 624; developmental = 457; elite = 156).

Responding coaches were asked to provide their understanding of the term recovery. In general, the novice coaches considered recovery to be the ability to

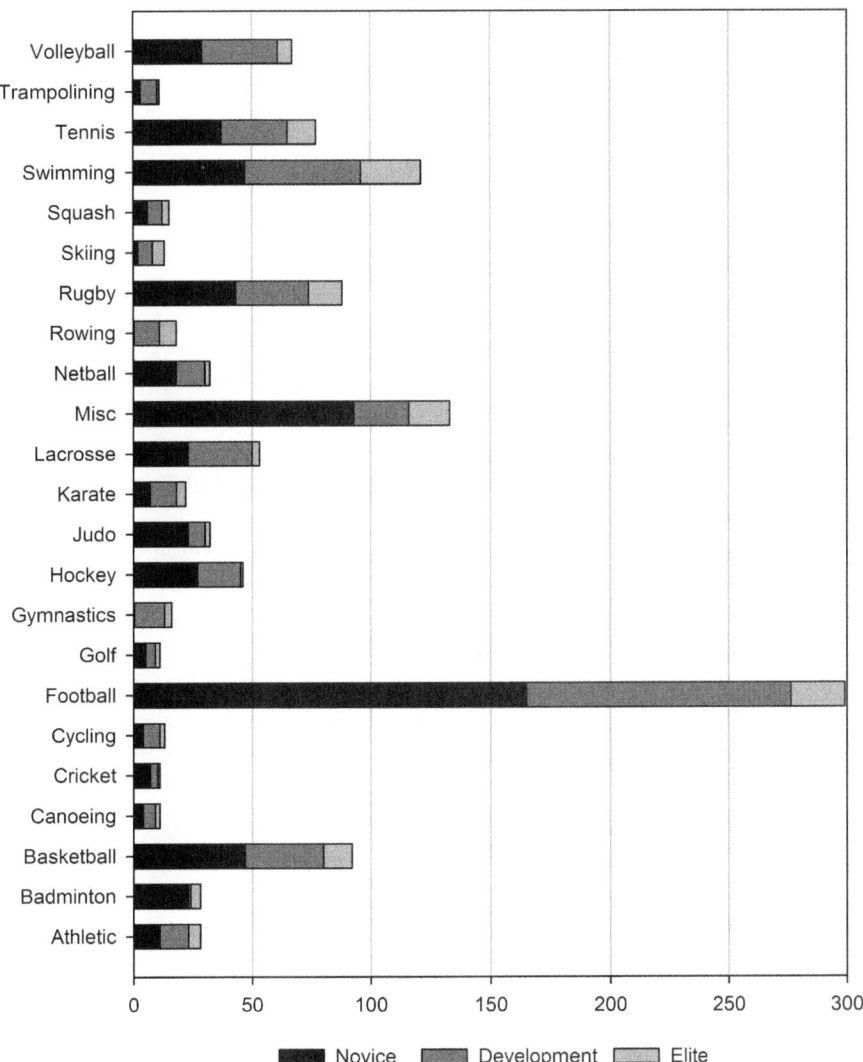

FIGURE 14.1 Demographics of responding sports coaches showing sport and level of coaching qualifications.

keep performing, whereas developmental coaches considered recovery to be a response to training and competition. The elite level coaches were much more effusive in their definitions, for example:

> They need enough time to recuperate from training and competition. Because it is during rest that their bodies adapt to the stress placed upon them during intense workout sessions and competitions.

It is important to plan recovery the same way you would plan training and competition. It is so important.

Recovery is not just about training, our guys travel regularly and that is very debilitating to performance. So everything needs to be managed very carefully and precisely.

Figure 14.2 shows the attributes and concepts the responding elite coaches felt were important about recovery. Words such as training, plan, important, essential and competition were all mentioned by a significant number of these coaches.

From this basic question, it can be seen that there is a large range of knowledge and understanding around the concept of recovery, which does not bode well for some of the athletes under these coaches' care. When this knowledge gap was examined more closely by the 2016 survey in the context of recovery, it became clear that with this mixed group of coaches there was little difference in knowledge between the novice and developmental coaches. Figure 14.3 shows the responding coaches' perceptions of the importance of elements of the RESTQ-Sport in the recovery of athletes (Kellmann & Kallus, 2001, 2016).

Closer inspection of Figure 14.3 shows the elite coaches considered these elements to be significant although some, for example, self-regulation, self-efficacy, and success, were more important than others. Sport coaching plays significant roles in the development of elite athletes as well as in the promotion of physical activity for all. We suggest that successful sports coaching may be more likely to happen when a coach has the ability to monitor and regulate his or her own behaviour; for example, both goal-setting and developmental planning are core components of effective sports coaching. Coaches at all levels need an understanding of all factors as they can affect recovery. Hence, research on interventions to enhance self-regulation skills and strategies that could be used by coaches is warranted.

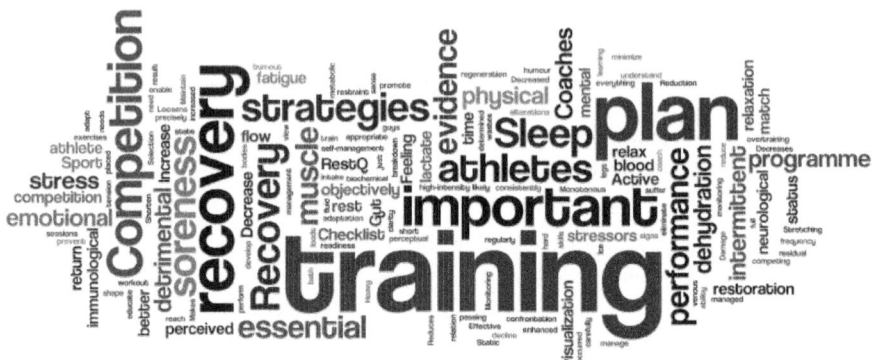

FIGURE 14.2 Wordle created from elite coaches (*N* = 156) responses to their understanding of the term *recovery*.

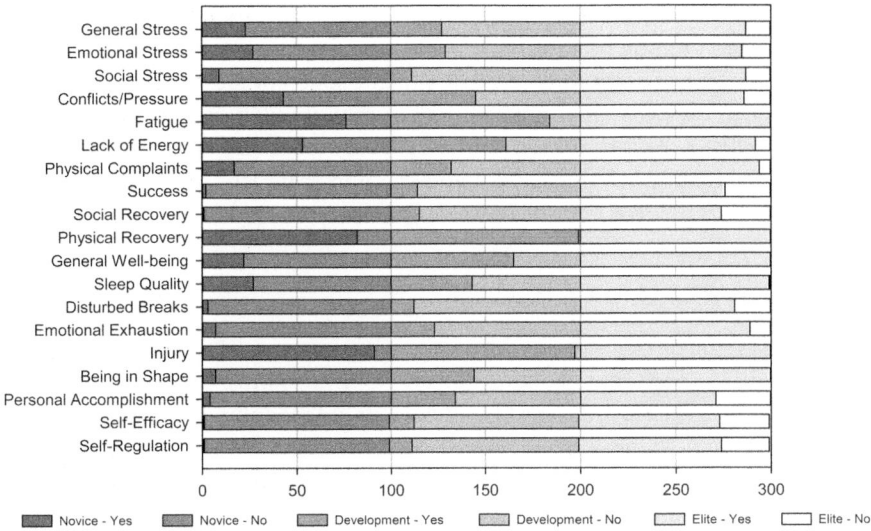

FIGURE 14.3 Awareness of recovery concepts by coaching level.

The novice and developmental coaches, not surprisingly, all rated injury, physical recovery, and fatigue as very important for recovery. Perhaps this related to their limited understanding of the concept of recovery and the reference to health and safety aspects connected with their limited formal coach education experiences. Recently, the different, but related, subject of fatigue was investigated within swimming, examining coaches' practises within swim training, specifically breaststroke (Thow, Nash, & Turner, 2015). Elite coaches indicated that they understood and made allowances for fatigue within swimming training. Again, the findings showed that the more experienced and educated the coaches the more methods and strategies they used to monitor fatigue. However, an intervention study, designed to highlight markers of fatigue and point out key components in breaststroke showed no significant differences between the intervention and control group. This indicated that coaches at all levels required further knowledge surrounding fatigue (Thow et al., 2015). Even if coaches and athletes usually determine recovery subjectively, based on experience, monitoring markers that are used to avoid overtraining syndrome can provide valuable information about the recovery process (Gastmann & Lehmann, 1999). This information will be useful for coaches and athletes when deciding whether the athlete has fully recovered and if training can be resumed.

Use of specific recovery interventions

After the analysis of the 2016 online survey, novice, developmental and elite level coaches from the sports of football and swimming were questioned to gather further information regarding their specific recovery practises. This was done individually and face-to-face, aiming to elicit more in-depth information to add richness of the information gathered from the online survey. The sports of football and swimming were chosen as they were the sports with the largest number of respondents to the survey, as well as representing team and individual sports. The order of the specific recovery interventions is predicated upon the importance placed upon it by the coaches.

Sleep and rest

Insomnia is defined by difficulty initiating or maintaining sleep, and this can be exacerbated by commonly encountered situations in sports, such as training and competing at night, enduring travel, and congested scheduling (e.g., playing three highly competitive hockey matches in seven days). Athlete sleep disturbances can affect their performance in training and competition and potentially compromise recovery (Fullagar, Duffield, Skorski, Julian, & Meyer, 2015). Insomnia is high among elite athletes, with sleep quality appearing most vulnerable prior to major competitive events, during periods of high-intensity training and following long-haul travel to competitions (Gupta, Morgan, & Gilchrist, 2017). Recently, Nédélec, Halson, Abaidia, and Ahmaidi's (2015) review on stress, sleep and recovery in elite soccer players concluded that because sleep provides psychological and physiological functions considered critical to optimal recovery, the increased frequency of sub-optimal sleeping patterns in elite soccer players means this is a common cause of impaired recovery in these athletes. These coaches acknowledged that lack of sleep for any level of athlete can be the difference between winning and losing a competition or being able to commit fully to a practise session. One novice football coach expressed the sentiments of his contemporaries saying that:

> *It stands to reason. If you don't get enough sleep how can you possibly train the way we want them to.*

However, none of these football coaches actually had any idea of the sleep quality of any of their players. When asked, these coaches generally felt that motivating players to try harder was the best way to overcome a perceived lack of sleep.

The elite coaches in both football and swimming discussed the importance of rest as well as quality sleep. One elite swimming coach highlighted some of the difficulties associated with swimming training, saying:

> *We have to fit around the pool availability a lot of times and that is not always ideal for the swimmers. Early mornings are not conducive to great sleeping patterns but the top swimmers get used to it. They can usually sleep anywhere but it would be better if they did not have to.*

Similarly, the elite football coaches highlighted the relentless nature of the game and the league structures, thinking:

> Early on in the season players can cope but the situation is cumulative. Players don't seem to be able to get sufficient rest, especially at certain times during the season. The worrying thing is, the more successful you are, the more you win, the more games you have to play and the tireder you get. I suppose the only positive is that everyone else is in the same position.

There seems to be a recognition that the structure of some sports does not appear to support the coaches or athletes in training and competition. The elite coaches were clearly aware of the needs of their athletes but seemed unable to organise both training and competition to allow adequate sleep and rest. Traditionally the benefits of sleep have not been well understood by all sports coaches and sleep is probably the most important form of recovery an athlete can have, providing invaluable adaptation time to the physical, neurological, immunological and emotional stressors that they experience during training (Erlacher, Ehrlenspiel, Adegbesan, & El-Din, 2011). In summary, sleep is important for recovery of both physiological and cognitive function.

Stretching

These swimming and football coaches all considered stretching to be an integral component of the recovery process, but had varying explanations of how they incorporated stretching into their sessions. The novice and developmental swimming coaches all oversaw stretching sessions on a regular basis and were highly aware of the importance of stretching within swimming. This stretching was generally carried out prior to the swimmers entering the water, sometimes in the showers as the warm water was seen to aid this process.

There was a debate between novice and developmental football coaches around the type of stretching that should be utilised but little strategy or management as to how stretching was incorporated effectively into their training sessions. These coaches felt that giving the players some time to stretch was sufficient, a developmental coach saying:

> Some players like to do dynamic stretching and others like to do static stretching and some more like to do a mixture of both. I'm not sure what is best – I think it is very individual – but whatever gets the blood flowing. We use it during warm ups and cool downs – it helps prepare the players for the up-coming game.

Although stretching is anecdotally one of the most used recovery strategies, the literature examining the effects of stretching as a recovery method is sparse, for example, in football, Kinugasa and Kilding (2009) discussed the effects of a short burst of static stretching following a match. This was found to be less effective than other methods such as water immersion or active recovery.

An elite swimming coach explained the use of stretching within swimming, saying:

> *We have a very structured practise, so what we do is put it into place at competitions and training. During competitions, we use it to speed up post-race recovery and help pre-race warm ups. We use dynamic stretches before we get into the water and static stretches after the swim down.*

Research has reported that static stretching can have a negative effect upon performance whereas a dynamic warm up may enhance performance. However, the effects upon recovery have not been adequately researched so this is perhaps based upon the swimming coaches' intuition after years of experience (Aguilar et al., 2012). To date there is little evidence to support stretching as a recovery strategy. Two separate reviews of recovery methods have concluded that there was no benefit for stretching as a recovery modality (Barnett, 2006; Vaile, Halson, & Graham, 2010). Thus, it would appear that stretching alone is not generally effective as a recovery method to improve performance indicators, such as rate of force development or time to exhaustion. Nevertheless, it can have a positive effect of *perceived* pain and fatigue, which why it is advised to use stretching in association with other recovery methods for optimal performance in the context of competitions (Rabita & Delextrat, 2013).

Cool down

The majority of these interviewed swimming and football coaches agreed that the cool down is used to promote recovery and return the body to a pre-training level. A developmental swimming coach explained that:

> *During a hard session your body is subject to a number of stressors. Muscle fibres, tendons and ligaments get damaged, even if you are in the water, and waste products build up within your body. If you do the cool down at the correct intensity that will help your body in its repair process.*

The elite football coaches agreed with this but were insistent that football players should be responsible for their own cool-down activities. When pushed there was a feeling that it was to develop some responsibility in the group of players, to be accountable for some aspect of their performance. Nevertheless, after further probing it emerged that this was what had happened when these coaches had been players and they appeared to be maintaining the status quo.

Another swimming coach admitted that the practise may vary for pragmatic reasons:

> *Actually I absolutely agree that the cool down is important, especially after a hard session but I really have to say that sometimes I don't have time. We are very limited in*

> *our pool time and at the end the public are coming in to use the pool. We have had the situation where the lane ropes are coming out and the swimmers are completing their cool-down while dodging the dive-bombers.*

Cool down, or active recovery, is used within sports regularly as a means to enhance the recovery process, traditionally involving periods of low intensity exercise performed between heavy training sessions or between competitions. Research into the efficacy of cool down has shown it to speed up the removal of lactate (Watts, Daggett, Gallagher, & Wilkins, 2000). However, others (e.g., Barnett, 2006) have questioned the validity of the removal of lactate as a predictor of training recovery.

Massage

The inclusion of massage at this stage may be misleading, as customarily massage treatment is available at swimming competitions, ostensibly to enhance recovery between events during a long day of racing. As a result, the swimming coaches were all very enthusiastic about the use of massage as a recovery, a developmental swimming coach stating:

> *Massage is a kind of tradition within swimming and the swimmers really say it helps them – it relaxes them, removes the lactic acid and just generally puts them in a better frame of mind.*

An elite swimming coach was more circumspect saying:

> *I'm not sure what the evidence shows. I've heard mixed reports although I haven't actually read anything about it myself. On reflection I'm not sure if it really matters. The swimmers like it and it certainly makes them more positive, they feel like the meet matters if there is massage available.*

The football coaches did not actually use the term massage but rub down, and this usually happened after a knock during training or competition. One elite football coach, admitting that he had some massage training, was quite effusive on the subject, explaining:

> *Well there are different types of massage techniques that help with different things, for example Swedish massage helps with blood pressure and friction massage helps relieve anxiety. There is also evidence that massage helps prevent DOMS, increases blood flow to the extremities and also flushes out lactate acid – all very useful for recovery.*

A recent systematic review investigating the effect of massage on Delayed Onset Muscle Soreness (DOMS) suggested massage reduces perceived levels of DOMS (Nelson, 2013). However, another study, Wiltshire and colleagues (2010) reported that massage impaired blood flow and lactate removal. Practically coaches should be aware that there is evidence that massages: Do not affect range of motion; can improve perceived recovery and hence increased investment and tolerance for subsequent efforts; help to relieve low-to-moderate-intensity pain contributing to a feeling of well-being; reduce cramps and stiffness (Couturier, 2013).

Nutrition

To maintain optimal performance, it is necessary to refuel with carbohydrate supply during exercise. This is because mechanisms of neuromuscular fatigue are associated with a reduced the drive to exercise during extremely prolonged training bouts by drawing on muscular fuel reserves, or by the accumulation of fatigue-inducing metabolites. Thus, the duration that training or exercise can be maintained decreases as the power requirements increase. During moderate intensity training (below the lactate threshold), fatigue develops slowly and is predominantly of central nervous system origin. In the heavy training domain (above lactate threshold but below critical power), both central and peripheral (muscle) fatigue are observed. Fatigue is frequently correlated with the depletion of muscle glycogen. In their recent review of the power-duration relationship, Burnley and Jones (2016) evidenced that severe-intensity exercise is associated with progressive derangements of muscle metabolic homeostasis and consequent peripheral fatigue. For many athletes, glycogen is the primary source of fuel during moderate to high-intensity training or competition. Depletion of glycogen will cause fatigue and thus performance may be compromised by an athlete's inability to replenish glycogen stores. One principle aim of recovery nutrition can be to optimise muscle and liver glycogen status, and this is dependent on exogenous carbohydrate intake, before during and after a training bout or competition, enhancing insulin sensitivity and muscle permeability to glucose through increase GLUT-4 activation (Ojuka & Goyaram, 2014). The timing of carbohydrate ingestion is important, with the rate of muscle glycogen storage 33% greater with earlier CHO feeding (< 1 hour) compared to delayed feeding (> 2 hours) (Ivy et al., 2002). However, it is important to note that glycogen synthesis continues up to 72 hours post-exercise. An elite swimming coach explained the difficulties, saying:

> The difficulty with our top swimmers is to try and get them to eat enough – especially of the right stuff. They need to eat 6,500–7,000 calories per day – that is a lot of food. On top of that I would like them to eat little and often but when I suggest snacks that would be good they don't like them – they want McDonalds or something like that. As well as the immediate refuelling we also want to think about muscle repair and the immune system – you can't get that from a burger and fries.

Protein is an essential macronutrient in connective tissue, cell membranes and muscle cells. It is also beneficial for athletes to consume dietary protein post-exercise to compensate for protein loss during exercise because: 1. exercise causes a substantial breakdown of muscle protein; and 2. the rate of protein turnover in skeletal muscle increases in the 30 minutes post-training (Moore et al., 2009). A novice football coach highlighted his understanding, saying:

> *We also try and make sure that the players eat something as soon as they finish training.*

Indeed, a combination of protein and carbohydrate post-exercise improves glycogen repletion, protein balance, and markers of muscle damage, and this is clearly beneficial for recovery and future performance. Also, there is some evidence to suggest vitamins A, B6, B12, C, D, E and folic acid and the trace elements iron, zinc, copper and selenium work in synergy to support the protective activities of the immune cells to help maintain health and performance during periods of heightened stress (e.g., He et al., 2013). Recovery is a particular challenge for athletes who are undertaking two or more sessions each day, such as the norm for top swimmers, training for prolonged periods, such as some footballers, as highlighted by this developmental football coach:

> *At the Academy we make sure they eat properly. We give them breakfast, lunch and dinner. The menus have all been checked by the nutritionists. If we want them to be able to give 100% to training, we need to make sure they have the right fuel.*

Water immersion

There were several different types of water immersion techniques mentioned by this group of coaches but the most common was the ice bath, although hot water immersion, hydrotherapy and contrast therapy were also mentioned. The football coaches were advocates of hot baths after competitions but also used ice baths after training. A developmental coach explained:

> *We have heard a lot about this but it is hard to get the players to give up the warm bath. I think it has a lot to do with comfort. Training quite often happens in the cold so there is little motivation for players to get into freezing water – they much prefer a warm bath as it helps soothe the muscles and wash away the tiredness.*

However, an elite football coach provided a more informed explanation:

> *We train in the cold and nowadays pitch technology has evolved to keep grass on the pitch throughout the year. This makes the pitch very hard which has a knock on effect. It places stress and strain on legs and lower backs – ice baths can help with this.*

The novice football coaches had not considered using ice baths, one saying:

> *I saw a video of Andy Murray using them but he trains in hot countries. Don't think we need them here.*

It appears that there are a number of differing views surrounding the efficacy of water immersion in football from these coaches. These coaches gave the impression that there was little coordinated and informed knowledge source that allowed coaches to develop their knowledge base around this area of current practise.

An elite swimming coach offered this view, saying:

> *We know that ice baths constrict blood vessels, remove waste products and reduce swelling so the increased blood flow speeds circulation and the recovery process gets a head start. It's hard to get ice baths in swimming pools though difficult to keep them as cold as they need to be.*

Research suggests that swimmers competing in a competition will not necessarily see any physiological benefits from an ice bath, as the races lack the level of eccentric contractions needed to elicit muscle damage (Jakeman, Macrae, & Eston, 2009). Bieuzen, Bleakley, and Costello (2013) carried out a review of the effects of cold water therapy, contrast baths and warm water therapy on both muscle soreness and on markers of exercise-induced muscle damage. Both cold water and contrast baths had a significant effect on reducing muscle soreness post-exercise but warm water was not as effective.

Periodisation

Failure to induce optimal training adaptations will result in either undertraining or overtraining. Periodisation, considered a planning strategy for athlete preparation, a way to plan systematically to reduce the risk of injury, avoid overtraining and to maximise training sessions. Thus, a key responsibility of a coach is to provide a better chance of increasing athletes' readiness for further training and attain peak performance in competition. Coaches are advised to use periodised training approaches when designing training plans. An important aspect for short and long-term training is to ensure accelerated recovery after training. However, a novice football coach reflected:

> *I'm not sure about periodisation – I don't really think about long-term – it's more about the players you have in front of you and what they want to do. Does it have anything to do with recovery?*

With periodisation, athletes vary the type, amount, and intensity of training for several weeks, a month, a whole year, or a four-year cycle for example. A swimming coach explained how this worked in her club:

> *We have a very structured programme. Because of all the different competitions, young swimmers can be competing every weekend at some points of the year.*

Evidence based models of periodisation have been presented, including for example, two variations of the block periodised approach. The concentrated unidirectional training design means enhancement of one leading fitness component, and is suited to athletic disciplines requiring one fitness component (e.g., jumping performance). Whereas the multi-targeted design involves the development of many targeted abilities within sequenced block mesocycles containing a minimal number of compatible training modalities. This multi-targeted system is suited to sports and disciplines, such as endurance, team, combat, and aesthetic sports that require the application of many athletic abilities (Issurin, 2016). This was further explained by an elite football coach, saying:

> *We stop the players playing for school and other clubs. The programme that we use is geared around all the training and competition that we have scheduled. It is really important that the players are not doing more – we need to manage the recovery process.*

A goal of a training programme can be to disrupt homeostasis, based around the principle of overload from cycles of progressively intensified training separated by reduced volume or intensity or both, as highlighted by an elite swimming coach:

> *At certain times of the year we need to watch. The distance gets greater with increasing intensity and we need to make sure that the swimmers are coping. Generally, we can tell by the way they look in the water and their general demeanour. We don't want them to get ill either.*

To be effective in achieving optimal performance in their athletes, coaches must use appropriate recovery strategies to return psychological, physiological, and performance variables to conditions identified in the absence of fatigue. Rugby union is a team sport that places metabolic, physical and mental stresses on the body (West et al., 2014). Interestingly, it has been reported that activity levels in rugby union can be higher in adolescents compared to elite adults, supporting that coaches require age-specific evidence in order to implement appropriate recovery within adolescent rugby population (Henderson, Cook, Kidgell, & Gastin, 2015). A recent study (Brown, 2016) involved 129 coaches from five countries (England, Scotland, Wales, Ireland, Australia) of adolescent rugby players ($N = 407$) aged 10–19 years with coaching experience ranging from less than one year (1.6%) to more than nine years (44.2%). The three post-training and post-match modalities with highest overall use were static stretching (32.2%), passive recovery (27.0%) and foam rolling (11.6%). Figure 14.4 below shows player and coach reasons for performing recovery, with experience the most supported reason in both coaches (39.3%) and players (41.6%). However, it was surprising to find that only about one in five coaches (19.3%) based their recovery interventions on (research) evidence. Indeed, in this University of Edinburgh study two-fifths of the coaches of

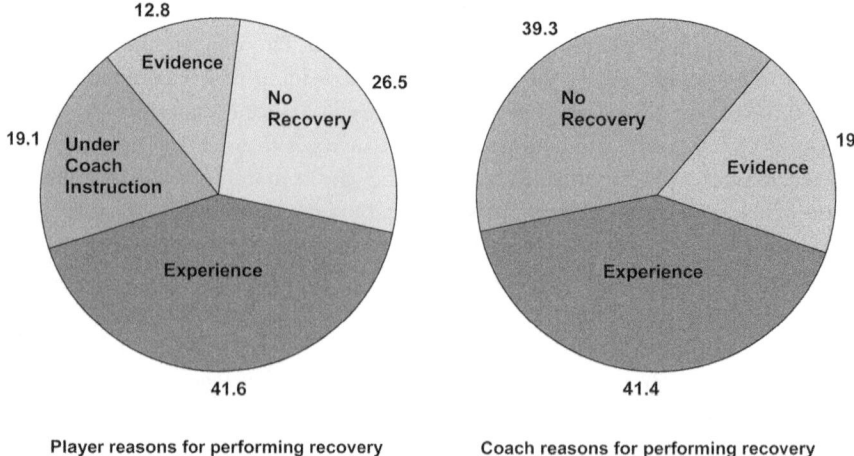

FIGURE 14.4 The reasons for using recovery modalities, according to players and coaches of adolescent rugby union.

adolescent rugby players reported that they did not know when their players had recovered!

Thus, recovery is one of the basic training principles. It relates to that part of the training and competition process where the benefits of training are maximised through practises concerned with the management and minimisation of fatigue. Recovery strategies enhance receptivity to training stimuli, and reduce the incidence of illnesses and injuries experienced through disproportionate workloads and stress. Therefore, it is important that coaches know – and know how to monitor and assess – when their athletes have recovered.

Compression garments

Recently athletes have been using some form of external compression to improve performance, often in the form of compression clothing (e.g., may improve the energy cost). This is not just prevalent in performance sport as recreational runners wearing compression garments have been found to have a reduction in delayed onset muscle soreness after wearing compression garments during a continuous 10K run (Ali, Caine, & Snow, 2007). Studies have shown evidence that compression may enhance exercise performance by altering muscle force, muscle power, or muscle contraction efficiency (Davies, Thompson, & Cooper, 2009). With regards to recovery there have been mixed findings, but it has been shown that compression clothing can enhance perceived (pain and fatigue) recovery (Duffield, Cannon, & King, 2010). Within swimming the wearing of compression garments has become the norm, whilst competing and while waiting between races. An elite swimming coach explained,

> It has become a bit of a norm for swimmers to wear compression gear during meets. I haven't seen any evidence that suggests it actually does the job. My swimmers saw Adam Peaty wearing it so if it is good enough for him then why not?

A developmental coach added,

> Our junior swimmers see the older swimmers wearing compression gear so they want to wear it too. I'm not sure if the parents are keen – it is expensive stuff but there is so much copying on the poolside. I'm glad this seems to be a sensible thing to copy this time – some of the others haven't been so great!

In football, Hill, van Someren, Leeder, and Pedlar (2014) ascertained that wearing a compression garment after an intense match or difficult training session can improve recovery by decreasing muscle soreness and muscle damage. However, Nédélec and colleagues (2013) considered that scientific evidence for strategies, such as compression garments, and their ability to accelerate the recovery process is still lacking. A developmental football coach said,

> I don't think this is really big in football. We tend to wear our training gear and then get back into our suits for travel. Not much place for compression wear.

There have been a number of studies on the effects of compression clothing on recovery after exercise. In 2011 MacRae, Cotter, and Laing, concluded that while compression clothing generally reduced DOMS little else was clear. Born, Sperlich, and Holmberg (2013) conducted a later review showing there were reductions in muscle swelling and DOMS, blood lactate removal, and increases in body temperature when compression garments were worn after exercise.

Relaxation techniques

Relaxation techniques have been traditionally used in sport primarily to enhance recovery from training and competition, manage anxiety, and improve performance. They have been suggested to increase concentration, enhance motor skills, and improve ability to handle arousal and stress. There are several psychological strategies that could be could be used that these coaches did not mention during the discussions, such as visualisation and imagery. Coaches need to ensure that athletes maximise the benefits from demanding training sessions and remain robust enough to cope with competitive performances at major events, so it is vital that individual athletes' have the ability to recognise when and how they need to recover. Athletes who fail to recover efficiently can, over time, show symptoms of underperformance syndrome that may lead to burnout. Burnout is defined as a state of mental, emotional, and physical exhaustion brought on by persistent devotion to a goal whose achievement is dramatically opposed to reality. Recent research has found that burnout is more prevalent in individual sport than team sport, which was confirmed by these coaches (Frank, Nixdorf, & Beckmann, 2013). One elite football coach said:

> *Our players generally manage to relax very well – we have a clear definition between training and not training. We find that works well – players know when they have to concentrate and pay attention but then we encourage them to just chill and do nothing. That's why so many play golf!*

This was a recurring theme with these football coaches – players knew how to relax and did not need to use any strategies or techniques for recovery – in fact all these football coaches were against using any psychological techniques or relaxation approaches with players.

The swimming coaches, on the other hand, mentioned several relaxation techniques that they considered assisted with the recovery process, for example, meditation, centring and progressive muscular relaxation. One developmental swimming coach thought,

> *We start by teaching them skills they can use during competitions, like concentration for starts, but it develops from there. Relaxation is really important – there is a lot of hanging around at swim meets and sometimes at training.*

An elite swimming coach added,

> *I encourage swimmers to inhale and exhale deeply while they are on the starting blocks but actually it is really good for them to just think about relaxing and start by a deep inhale and deep exhale. If they can manage to lie down and close their eyes at the same time – great.*

None of these coaches appeared to consider psychological strategies as being useful specifically for the recovery process. The football coaches did not appear to use any relaxation techniques at all and the swimming coaches suggested that they had initially taught them to swimmers for other reasons but found they could be utilised for use in recovery.

What is the role of the coach in recovery?

Adequate recovery has been shown to result in the restoration of physiological and psychological processes, so that the athlete can compete or train again at an appropriate level. Recovery from training and competition is complex and typically dependent on the nature of the exercise performed and any other outside stressors. An effective coach needs to understand not only what is being stimulated through prescribed training sessions, but also what is being fatigued. The challenge is to recognise the type of fatigue and then select specific strategies to reduce and minimise this fatigue as soon as possible after the training or performance situation. Most of the coaches discussed within this chapter admitted that they had little or no input during formal coaching courses about the recovery process. As a result, they felt that their knowledge of the recovery process needed improvement. When asked who should provide this information they really had no answer.

Given this admitted lack of knowledge these coaches were hesitant about being able to implement or manage a recovery strategy for their athletes or teams. There was a perception that a more knowledgeable individual, possibly a sports scientist should be responsible for this area. This would also cause issues for the coaches as they considered that a recovery strategy would impact on all other aspects of their programme therefore they felt they should be able to at least oversee the process.

Halson (2014) suggested that coaches and support staff are taking an increasingly scientific approach to both designing and monitoring training programs, using objective measures, such as time-motion analysis or more subjective measures such as perceptions. Some coaches have taken this a step further by using online technology to monitor specific aspects, for example, share and save training programmes, manage load, monitor wellness, sleep, soreness, assess fitness and chart recovery.

Conclusion and recommendations for practise

In the past years, there has been a significant increase in research examining both the effects of recovery on performance and potential mechanisms with recent research suggesting that a number of mechanisms can enhance performance when utilised appropriately. Many high-performance athletes have become professional, resulting in heavier training loads; however, the support services provided have not always kept up to date with advances in research, knowledge, and technology. This is especially noticeable in some of the smaller sports.

Professionalism in sport has provided the foundation for elite athletes to focus purely on training and competition. Furthermore, high-performance sport and the importance of successful performances have led athletes and coaches to continually seek any advantage that may improve performance. It follows that the rate and quality of recovery are extremely important for the high-performance athlete and that optimal recovery may provide numerous benefits during repetitive high-level training and competition. Therefore, investigating different recovery interventions and their effects on fatigue, muscle injury, recovery and performance is important.

Given the findings in this chapter if knowledge and application of recovery strategies is to be considered important for performance within both individual and team sport then coaches need to have further information and support within their coaching practise. For athletes to achieve optimal (and repeatable) performance, with reduced risk of injury, coaches must engage in planning for both training *and* recovery. Therefore, coaches must be able to:

- Understand the principles of recovery and how this affects training.
- Identify responses to training and stress.
- Monitor and assess training responses.
- Recognise how various types of fatigue that affect training and performance.
- Apply a range of recovery strategies and techniques.
- Plan recovery strategies within individual sessions as well as longer term training plans.
- Individualise recovery programmes in response to the needs of individual participants and the needs of the sport.
- Evaluate the short- and long-term effectiveness of recovery strategies and techniques within periodised training programmes.

In light of the knowledge gap highlighted by the majority of coaches consulted for this chapter if the recovery process is to be enhanced then sports coaches need to be able to access this type of knowledge easily. When considering the essential knowledge highlighted above a systematic review of the informal and formal methods by which coaches can become better informed on the importance of recovery seems overdue.

References

Aguilar, A. J., DiStefano, L. J., Brown, C. N., Herman, D. C., Guskiewicz, K. M., & Padua, D. A. (2012). A dynamic warm-up model increases quadriceps strength and hamstring flexibility. *Journal of Strength and Conditioning Research*, 26(4), 1130–1141.

Ali, A., Caine, M. P., & Snow, B. G. (2007). Graduated compression stockings: Physiological and perceptual responses during and after exercise. *Journal of Sports Sciences*, 25, 413–419.

Barnett, A. (2006). Using recovery modalities between training sessions in elite athletes: Does it help? *Sports Medicine*, 36, 781–796.

Bieuzen, F., Bleakley, C. M., & Costello, J. T. (2013). Contrast water therapy and exercise induced muscle damage: A systematic review and meta-analysis. *PLoS One*, 8(4), 62356.

Born, D. P., Sperlich, B., & Holmberg, H. C. (2013). Bringing light into the dark: Effects of compression clothing on performance and recovery. *International Journal of Sports Physiology and Performance*, 8, 4–18.

Brown, N. (2016). *The practices, beliefs and benefits of recovery in adolescent rugby union*. Unpublished Dissertation, University of Edinburgh, Edinburgh.

Burnley, M., & Jones, A. M. (2016). Power-duration relationship: Physiology, fatigue, and the limits of human performance. *European Journal of Sport Science*, 3, 1–12.

Couturier, A. (2013). Massage and physiotherapy. In C. Hausswirth & I. Mujika (Eds.), *Recovery for performance in sport* (pp. 111–132). Champaign, IL: Human Kinetics.

Davies, V., Thompson, K. G., & Cooper, S. M. (2009). The effects of compression garments on recovery. *Journal of Strength & Conditioning Research*, 23(6), 1786–1794.

Duffield, R., Cannon, J., & King, M. (2010). The effects of compression garments on recovery of muscle performance following high-intensity sprint and plyometric exercise. *Journal of Science & Medicine in Sport*, 13(1), 136–140.

Erlacher, D., Ehrlenspiel, F., Adegbesan, O. A., & El-Din, H. G. (2011). Sleep habits in German athletes before important competitions or games. *Journal of Sports Sciences, 29*, 859–866.

Frank, R., Nixdorf, I., & Beckmann, J. (2013). Depressionen im Hochleistungssport: Prävalenzen und psychologische Einflüsse [Depression in elite athletes: Prevalence and psychological factors]. *Deutsche Zeitschrift für Sportmedizin, 64*, 320–326.

Fullagar, H. H. K., Duffield, R., Skorski, S., Julian, R., & Meyer, T. (2015). Sleep and recovery in team sport: Current sleep-related issues facing professional team-sport athletes. *International Journal of Sports Physiology and Performance, 10*(8), 950–957.

Gastmann, U. A. L., & Lehmann, M. J. (1999). Monitoring overload and regeneration in cyclists. In M. Lehmann, C. Foster, U. Gastmann, H. Keizer, & J. M. Steinacker (Eds.), *Overload, performance incompetence and regeneration in sport* (pp. 131–137). New York, NY: Kluwer Academic.

Gupta, L., Morgan, K., & Gilchrist, S. (2017). Does elite sport degrade sleep quality? A systematic review. *Sports Medicine, 47*, 1317–1333.

Halson, S. L. (2014). Monitoring training load to understand fatigue in athletes. *Sports Medicine, 44*, 139–147.

He, C.-S., Handzlik, M. K., Fraser, W. D., Muhamad, A. S., Preston, H., Richardson, A., & Gleeson, M. (2013). Influence of vitamin D status on respiratory infection incidence and immune function during 4 months of winter training in endurance sport athletes. *Exercise Immunology Review, 19*, 86–101.

Henderson, B., Cook, J., Kidgell, D. J., & Gastin, P. B. (2015). Game and training load differences in elite junior Australian football. *Journal of Sports Science and Medicine, 14*, 494–500.

Hill, J., van Someren, K., Leeder, J., & Pedlar, C. (2014). Compression garments and recovery from exercise-induced muscle damage: A meta-analysis. *British Journal of Sports Medicine, 48*, 1340–1346.

Issurin, V. B. (2016). Benefits and limitations of block periodized training approaches to athletes' preparation: A review. *Sports Medicine, 46*, 329–338.

Ivy, J. L., Goforth, H. G., Damon, B. M., McCauley, T. R., Parsons, E. C., & Price, T. B. (2002). Early postexercise muscle glycogen recovery is enhanced with a carbohydrate-protein supplement. *Journal of Applied Physiology, 93*(4), 1337–1344.

Jakeman, J. R., Macrae, R., & Eston, R. (2009). A single 10-min bout of cold-water immersion therapy after strenuous plyometric exercise has no beneficial effect on recovery from the symptoms of exercise induced muscle damage. *Ergonomics, 52*(4), 456–460.

Kellmann, M. (2002). Underrecovery and overtraining: Different concepts – similar impact? In M. Kellmann (Ed.), *Enhancing recovery: Preventing underperformance in athletes* (pp. 3–24). Champaign, IL: Human Kinetics.

Kellmann, M., & Kallus, K. W. (2001). *Recovery-Stress Questionnaire for Athletes: User manual*. Champaign, IL: Human Kinetics.

Kellmann, M., & Kallus, K. W. (2016). The Recovery-Stress Questionnaire for Athletes. In K. W. Kallus & M. Kellmann (Eds.), *The Recovery-Stress Questionnaires: User manual* (pp. 86–131). Frankfurt am Main: Pearson Assessment.

Kinugasa, T., & Kilding, A. E. (2009). A comparison of post-match recovery strategies in youth soccer players. *Journal of Strength & Conditioning Research, 23*, 1402–1407.

MacRae, B. A., Cotter, J. D., & Laing, R. M. (2011). Compression garments and exercise: Garment considerations, physiology and performance. *Sports Medicine, 41*, 815–843.

Moore, D. R., Robinson, M. J., Fry, J. L., Tang, J. E., Glover, E. I., Wilkinson, S. B., ... Phillips, S. M. (2009). Ingested protein dose response of muscle and albumin protein synthesis after resistance exercise in young men. *American Journal of Clinical Nutrition, 89*(1), 161–168.

Nédélec, M., Halson, S., Abaidia, A.-E., & Ahmaidi, S. (2015). Stress, sleep and recovery in elite soccer: A critical review of the literature. *Sports Medicine, 45*, 1387–1400.

Nédélec, M., McCall, A., Carling, C., Legall, F., Berthoin, S., & Dupont, G. (2013). Recovery in soccer: Part II-Recovery strategies. *Sports Medicine, 43,* 9–22.

Nelson, N. (2013). Delayed onset muscle soreness: Is massage effective? *Journal of Bodyworks & Movement Therapies, 17*(4), 475–482.

Ojuka, E. O., & Goyaram, V. (2014). Mechanisms in exercise-induced increase in glucose disposal in skeletal muscle. *Medicine and Sports Science, 60,* 71–81.

Rabita, G., & Delextrat, A. (2013). Stretching. In C. Hausswirth & I. Mujika (Eds.), *Recovery for performance in sport* (pp. 55–69). Champaign, IL: Human Kinetics.

Thow, J., Nash, C., & Turner, T. (2015). *The application of 2-dimensional video analysis by competitive swimming coaches to monitor fatigue in breaststroke technique during training.* Unpublished PhD Thesis, University of Edinburgh, Edinburgh.

Vaile, J., Halson, S., & Graham, S. (2010). Recovery review: Science vs. practice. *Journal of Australian Strength and Conditioning, 2*(Suppl.), 5–21.

Watts, P. B., Daggett, M., Gallagher, P., & Wilkins, B. (2000). Metabolic response during sport rock climbing and the effects of active versus passive recovery. *International Journal of Sports Medicine, 21*(3), 185–190.

West, D., Finn, C., Cunningham, D., Shearer, D., Jones, M., Harrington, B., . . . Kilduff, L. P. (2014). Neuromuscular function, hormonal, and mood responses to a professional rugby union match. *Journal of Strength and Conditioning Research, 28*(1), 194–200.

Wiltshire, E.V., Poitras, V., Pak, M., Hong, T., Rayner, J., & Tschakovsky, M. E. (2010). Massage impairs postexercise muscle blood flow and "lactic acid" removal. *Medicine & Science in Sports and Exercise, 42,* 1062–1071.

15
STRESS AND RECOVERY IN EXTREME SITUATIONS

Michel Nicolas, Marvin Gaudino, and Philippe Vacher

Introduction

The psychological impacts of extreme situations are a great concern and have become an issue of major importance for performance, well-being and the outcome of missions (Kanas, 1998). A situation is considered as extreme when an individual is subjected to exceptional physical or psychosocial circumstances demanding adaptive responses which could overwhelm its physiological and psychological resources (Rivolier, 1992). Thus, extreme situations represent unfamiliar conditions (risks, hazards, and ultimately death) confronting persons with their limits and consequently with their adaptive capacities. Extreme situations are for example extreme sports, long-duration spaceflights, wintering in polar stations or polar expeditions, submarine missions, solitary navigation, deep diving, very high terrestrial altitude, and military missions.

Danger is more limited to experimental situations and extreme analogues[1] such as space, high-altitude simulations or polar stations, but these simulated situations delineate an interesting paradigm for the examination of physical and psychosocial stress experienced by the participants in these specific conditions. Thus, extreme situations have provided researchers with a unique opportunity to investigate stress and recovery dimensions. This appears to be essential because these dimensions can jeopardise the success of extreme missions and threaten the survival of crewmembers. The present chapter aims at the examination of the impact of extreme situations on the psychological constructs of stress and recovery.

Nicolas, M., Gaudino, M., & Vacher, P. (2018). Stress and recovery in extreme situations. In M. Kellmann & J. Beckmann (Eds.), *Sport, Recovery, and Performance: Interdisciplinary Insights* (pp. 221–232). Abingdon: Routledge.

The role of stress in extreme situations

Stress factors in polar stations

The specific peculiarities of extreme situations pose unique challenges depending on the type of condition (Kanas & Manzey, 2008; Suedfeld, 2005). During a winter in polar stations, winterovers (participants remaining in a polar station during winter) must face unfamiliar psychological challenges arising from physical, occupational, and psychosocial origins. The physical environment is unusual and unique, especially in the Antarctic where emergency medical evacuation is impossible a large part of the year because of the climatic conditions. The natural environment is hazardous characterised by unusual light-dark cycles, low levels of atmospheric oxygen, low humidity, extreme cold, and sudden storms (Salam, 2012). The indoor environment focuses on efficiency, ease of transport, and costs. Thus, the facilities are monotonous, offer limited mobility, comfort, and stimulation.

Occupational stressors are marked by monotony and boredom, time pressure, autonomy, high/low workloads, lack of separation between living and working spaces and, thus, work and leisure. Crew members exhibit little control over their own schedules, which tend to fluctuate between periods of idle boredom and periods of intense work (Nicolas & Gushin, 2014; Sandal, Leon, & Palinkas, 2006; Suedfeld, 2005). Social stressors encompass family/home-life disruption caused by physical separation and limited telecommunications, as well as forced social interaction within the same limited small and unchanging crew. Above all, the crew members are isolated and confined in a site far from their accustomed surroundings. These stressors are specific characteristics of Isolated and Confined Extreme environments (ICEs). More specifically in the Concordia polar station, teams are composed of different nationalities and cultures. Consequently, communication is hampered by the lack of a common culture and native language. Additionally, multicultural issues may increase levels of stress. These physical, occupational and psychosocial stressors have been shown to induce dysfunctional stress responses resulting in detrimental interpersonal tensions and decrements in performance (e.g., Kanas & Manzey, 2008; Leon, Sandal, & Larsen, 2011; Nicolas, Bishop, Weiss, & Gaudino, 2016).

Stress factors in space missions

In space missions, the most severe stressors arise from microgravity and other environmental stress such as risks of meteorites and radiations, as well as monotony, lack of comfort, boredom, confinement, isolation, and restricted social contacts (Kanas & Manzey, 2008). In addition, long-duration and long-distance space flights to Mars involve the so-called 'Earth-out-of-view phenomenon', high degree of autonomy, changing workload ranging from underloading to overloading. Increases in both durations of flight and the distance from the Earth augment the impact of these stressors on affective states, initiate interpersonal conflicts and foster work problems (Kanas & Manzey, 2008). The effects of microgravity long-term exposure have mainly focused on physiological aspects (cardiovascular deconditioning, bone weakening and decrease in muscular strength). However, the psychosocial outcomes have clearly been shown to significantly impact human behaviour and performance (Bishop, 2004; Gushin, 1995; Manzey & Lorenz, 1998). Thus, a better understanding of the affective processes is fundamental to ensure both the participants' well-being and their successful adaptation (Palinkas, 2003).

Stress and recovery responses in extreme situations

The scarce previous research in human sciences has indicated that extreme situations can induce adverse effects including dysfunctional responses to stress in real life situations such as prolonged spaceflights (Grigoriev & Fedorov, 1996; Kanas & Manzey, 2008; Kass & Kass, 1999; Suedfeld & Steel, 2000), ground-based studies such as bed rest (Choukèr et al., 2001; Grigoriev & Fedorov, 1996; Ishizaki et al., 2002; Nicolas & Weiss, 2009), space simulation in the Arctic (Bishop, Kobrick, Battler, & Binsted, 2010), or in the Antarctic (Leon et al., 2011; Nicolas, Bishop, et al., 2016; Nicolas, Suedfeld, Weiss, & Gaudino, 2015).

It is important to bear in mind that a certain level of stress is considered necessary for adapting both biologically (Selye, 1950) and psychologically (Lazarus & Folkman, 1984). However, an excessive level of stress with regard to intensity, frequency, accumulation and duration could generate impaired stress outcomes affecting both well-being and performance especially in extreme situations (Geuna & Brunelli, 1995; Nicolas & Gushin, 2014; Nicolas & Weiss, 2009).

Thus, an optimal level of stress that is related to the individual resources should improve the safety of the mission and the survival chances of the crew (Marsh & Rygalov, 2008; Palinkas, 1992). The recovery process is defined as the restoration of physiological and psychological resources which can counterbalance negative effects of stress and thus help crew members to adjust to the situation (Kellmann & Kallus, 2001; Meeusen et al., 2013). Recognised as one of the most interesting developments on recovery in sport psychology (Davis, Orzeck, & Keelan, 2007), the recovery-stress model of Kellmann and Kallus (2001), indicate the impact of perceived stress levels to the person's own capabilities to recover in several dimensions (social, emotional, physical and behavioural). Unbalanced recovery-stress states can lead to dysfunctional outcomes such as chronic fatigue and its concomitant overtraining and psychological exhaustion and consequently, compromise the participant's adaptation to sport training and competition (for a review, see Kellmann, 2010; Nicolas, Banizette, & Millet, 2011), and to space analogue environments (Nicolas & Weiss, 2009; Nicolas et al., 2015).

Stress and recovery responses in polar stations

Space analogues such as Antarctic stations are acknowledged as natural laboratories for the study of the effects of extreme situations on human behaviour (Suedfeld,

2010). The international Antarctic Concordia Station offers one of the most severe environments on earth to study the effects of stress and recovery states on healthy participants. The French-Italian Concordia Station is one of the permanent Antarctic facilities dedicated to scientific research to study human adaptation to isolated, confined extreme environments. Geographically remote at a high altitude on Dome C in the middle of Antarctica, Concordia is located among the coldest, windiest, and driest areas on earth.

Our team investigates the affective, social, cognitive, and personality aspects of the psychological adaptation process in this extreme situation of polar wintering in Concordia. Among these psychological factors, stress and recovery states play a central role with other indicators of adaptation like perceived stress and control, and defence mechanisms. Few, if any research has addressed the time patterns and the relationships between perceived stress, recovery, control, attention lapses, and defence mechanisms during a 12-month wintering in Concordia polar station with an international crew of 14 volunteers. The main findings indicated that a wintering in Concordia induced some stress mainly in the social dimension and showed relationships between stress and recovery states and perceived stress and control (Nicolas et al., 2015). On the one hand, strong significant positive correlations were found between stress states and perceived stress. On the other hand, recovery states were strongly and positively associated with perceived control. These results highlight the role of stress and recovery in psychological adaptation and offer additional insights into the affective, social and cognitive processes involved in adaptation.

The importance of the social dimension

One of the interesting findings of the study by Nicolas et al. (2015), is linked to the multidimensional assessment of stress and recovery states with the Recovery-Stress Questionnaire for Athletes (RESTQ-Sport; Kellmann & Kallus, 2001) indicating in such severe and prolonged conditions, it is not the physical or environmental factors that disrupt the adaptation, but the social dimension. The scale *Social Stress* was the only dimension which was significantly impacted by the strict ICE condition imposed by a wintering in Concordia with a significant continuous increase across the 12-month wintering. Small group studies in other isolated environments suggest that long-term isolation and confinement could provoke interpersonal issues and social tension (for reviews, see Leon et al., 2011; Palinkas & Suedfeld, 2008; Zimmer, Cabral, Borges, Côco, & Hameister, 2013). These findings are also in accordance with other recent studies in space analogues, the Women International Space Simulation for Exploration (WISE) 2005 study, a 60-day head-down tilt bed rest (HDTBR; Nicolas, 2009), and the Mars 105 experiment (Nicolas & Gushin, 2014). Both showed that the social dimension is the key factor in adaptation, especially during prolonged ICE missions that cause difficulties for the participants during the later stages, when psychosocial problems become increasingly likely. However, contrary to expectations it is found that these psychosocial issues are expected to develop even more as human beings travel further from Earth on long-term space missions. However, empirical findings suggest that people living and working in space orbital missions do not routinely experience increased tension or decreased cohesion during the second half of the mission (Kanas et al., 2006).

Even though no increased tension or reduced cohesion is observed, social interactions with the same few persons over a long duration of time are linked to a decrease in professional performance which could jeopardise adaptation to isolated and confined extreme environments (Nicolas, Bishop, et al., 2016). These psychosocial issues have important implications for pre-mission selection and training, monitoring and support of crews during the mission, but are often neglected during post-mission readaptation. Another interesting issue consists of the relationship between total recovery and perceived control. Perceived control was originally defined as one's need to demonstrate competence and mastery over the environment (White, 1959). It may be a function of the extent to which the individual perceives that its personal resources are adequate to deal with adaptation demands (for a review, see, Armitage & Conner, 2001). It was found that individuals who feel that they have the resources to face the demands of ICE life would recover better from this constraining situation (Nicolas et al., 2015).

Stress and recovery responses in space missions

Long-term manned spaceflights are certainly one of the most challenging issue for space organisations. Space simulation provides a good psychological analogue to explore multidimensional patterns of change in both stress and recovery over time. The WISE-2005 study (Women International Space Simulation for Exploration) was designed to simulate a microgravity situation with long-term head-down tilt bed rest (HDTBR) at -6° for a duration of 60 days in healthy women. The complete experiment consisted of three stages: A 20-day baseline control period (BDC), a 60-day HDTBR and a 20-day post-HDT ambulatory recovery period (R+). Our team investigated the time-course of stress and recovery states and their relations to perceived social support and personality traits. A significant increase in stress was found for all the participants between the beginning and the end of the HDT period, indicating that simulated microgravity involving immobilisation, isolation, and confinement induces stress.

Among the five major personality factors (NEO-PI-R; Costa & McCrae, 1992), only neuroticism was linked to stress and recovery with a positive association with stress and a negative association with recovery. These findings show the impact of simulated microgravity on stress and recovery states, and the relations of these affective states to a personality trait. Neuroticism has been found to be negatively associated with the adaptive profiles identified in longitudinal studies of American astronaut candidate performance (McFadden, Helmreich, Rose, & Fogg, 1994). Low neuroticism proved to be favourable for dealing with high-stress components in extreme environments (Palinkas & Suedfeld, 2008). Thus, it can be derived that HDT induces impairments in psychological states leading to subsequent alterations in stress and decreases in recovery.

Human spaceflights to Mars

Human spaceflights to Mars certainly represent the most important challenge and beyond, the next 'great step for humanity'.[2] We investigated another space analogue with the Mars 500 study in 2010–2011 funded by the European (ESA) and Russian (Roscosmos) Space Agencies. The isolation facility located at the Institute for Biomedical Problems (IBMP) in Moscow comprised four hermetically sealed interconnected habitat modules (habitable, medical, utility, and Martian landing simulator modules), plus one external module simulating the Martian surface.

Contrary to our hypothesis and to several previous studies, the main finding of the present study was the significant decrease in stress throughout the experimentation (Nicolas & Gushin, 2014). The modifications in the psychological states provoked by the ICE experiment showed that despite a global reduction, the social stress dimension was yet again the most affected by the ICE conditions with an increase in the mid-ICE period. As opposed to the *Social Stress* scale of the RESTQ-Sport, the *Social Recovery* scale showed a strong tendency to increase. In addition, fatigue was reported by all the participants with a significant global decrease marked by an increase during the post-ICE period. However, the physical dimension showed no variation either in its stress component (*Lack of Energy, Physical Complaints*) or in its recovery component (*Physical Recovery, Being in Shape*). These unexpected results can be explained by the high motivation of the participants rigorously selected for these long-term experimentations (Palinkas & Browner, 1995; Palinkas & Houseal, 2000). Furthermore, environmental conditions and physical factors were different from an actual spaceflight with possible sanitary evacuations in case of emergency and no physical dangers such as radiation or meteorites. The findings showed that ICE environments might not systematically induce stress leading to subsequent disadaptation in these specific contexts. The stressors and consequences observed in the environment of space analogues offer insights into recovery and stress states that may have an impact not only in long-term space flights but also in the general population.

Stress and recovery responses in extreme sport

Monitoring of both psychological stress and recovery are a key issue for increasing athletes' health, well-being, and performance (Nicolas, Gaudreau, & Franche, 2011). Due to its intense induced mental and physical fatigue, ultramarathons represent an interesting field of investigation of stress and recovery processes. Ultramarathons are considered as one of the most demanding challenges in ultra-endurance events, pushing the athletes to the outer limits of their resources to perform beyond ordinary limits (Pearson, 2006).

These extreme endurance races are characterised by an extremely long distance, intensity, elevation, and duration considerably higher than a marathon. The peculiarities of strenuous endurance exercise are often associated with cold temperatures, humidity and wind involving unique challenges which can jeopardise adaptation (Millet & Millet, 2012).

The research team (Nicolas et al., 2011) monitored stress and recovery states in ultramarathoners before and after a 24-hour ultramarathon and at one-month follow-up. The demand of continuous effort over a 24-hour period could generate competitive stress and a deficit in recovery for a long time after the competition. As expected, the various components of stress and recovery were affected in their physical, emotional, and social dimensions by the 24-hour race. These alterations in psychological states did not return to their initial levels for several days. Stress decreased significantly six days after the race on the contrary, recovery returned to pre-race values 15 days after the race. Thus, a period of two weeks is critical for both stress and recovery despite differences in time-courses during the one-month monitoring (Nicolas et al., 2011). The findings suggest that an ultra-endurance race induces perceived stress and leads to subsequent alterations in perceived recovery on psychological, physical, emotional, and social dimensions with specific temporal patterns. Practically, these findings underline the importance of regular monitoring of stress and recovery in ultra-endurance athletes during the training process and the early stages after a race.

The short RESTQ-Sport version

These several studies in extreme situations confirm that the Recovery-Stress Questionnaire for Athletes (RESTQ-Sport) can be applied not only in sport but also in extreme situations. This self-report measure encompasses physical, psychological, and social dimensions of both stress and recovery to indicate the extent to which someone is stressed, as well as which recovery strategies are used in response. Several studies have indicated the effectiveness of the RESTQ-Sport in monitoring individuals and teams during training camps or over an entire season (Brink, Nederhof, Visscher, Schmikli, & Lemmink, 2010; Coutts, Slattery, & Wallace, 2007; Di Fronso, Nakamura, Bortoli, Robazza, & Bertollo, 2013; Filho et al., 2015). However, criticism about the factorial structure and the administration length for the 76-item version of this quantitative tool has been raised (Davis et al., 2007).

Recently Kellmann and Kallus (2016) proposed a more economic, 36-item version of the instrument. A recent study revealed good fits for the factorial structure of the 12-scales representing 36 items with internal consistency coefficients and item analyses indicating acceptable reliability for the French version (Nicolas, Vacher, Martinent, & Mourot, in press). In addition, changes and relationships between the RESTQ-Sport-36, HRV and training load in elite athletes supplied external validity of the short French version of the RESTQ-Sport. These findings provided evidence for the usefulness of the short version of the RESTQ-Sport-36 to procure a comprehensive and multidimensional profile of athletes' perceptions of stress and recovery.

Monitoring is well-known as one of the best prevention strategies regarding maladaptive psychological and physiological states (Meeusen et al., 2013). Effective monitoring should enable coaches to adapt training loads to athlete's recovery capacities and for sport psychologists to propose individualised interventions.

However, a quantitative tool cannot substitute supportive relationships between coaches and athletes which are the key to improve coping abilities and goal attainments in sport performance (Nicolas et al., 2011). Furthermore, the recovery-stress model offers the possibility to specify the impact of different sources of stress and to compare perceived stress levels to the person's own capabilities to recover. However, it is important to bear in mind that the sources of stress are not only due to athletic influences, but also to academic or occupational demands which have to be taken into account to propose a complete recovery-stress states profile.

Conclusion and recommendations for practise

A better understanding of stress and recovery processes might have practical implications in psychological countermeasures for dealing with the human factor in extreme situations. Preventive countermeasures and interventions would prevent pathogenic psychological outcomes on both the well-being of the participants and their adaptation to such constraining environments, and would contribute to the success of missions in extreme environments. Further improvements in countermeasures may be possible by striking a balance between recovery-stress states in order to enhance adaptation to such constraining situations, thereby increasing salutogenic experiences in ICE environments. Interventions can be trained through regular exercises and especially practises during short simulated missions.

The role of psychologists should consist in the development and validation of interventions to expand the repertoire of coping strategies of the participants to stimulate psychological adaptation processes and consequently participants' performance and well-being (Nicolas, 2010). These psychological skills concern the different stages of a mission: Before, during and after the exposition to extreme situations. Interventions concern pre-mission selection and training (e.g., stress management, training in interpersonal relations, leadership skills, coping strategies), monitoring and support of crews during the mission (telepsychology), but also and often neglected, during post-mission re-adaptation (psychological follow-up).

Regarding improvement in the recovery-stress balance, recovery activities should be based on individual preferences and fully integrated in the schedule of working or training program. Leisure time and distraction should not be neglected particularly in tedious and repetitive situations. Findings reported that distraction has beneficial effects on psychological states in the general population (Gleser & Mendelberg, 1990; Leith, 2010) or participants in space analogue (Ishizaki, Fukuoka, Ishizaki, Tanaka, & Ishitobi, 2004).

Our studies confirm and give further insight into the role of recovery-stress states in adaptation to ICE environments. Our previous works indicated that deviations from the recovery-stress balance may lead to failed adaptation in extreme situations. The function of a recovery activity is to restore the balance between recovery and stress states in order to support the individual's adaptation to potentially stressful situations. Thus, to optimise adaptation in extreme situations, stress and recovery states should be addressed in order to monitor the balance between these states. As practitioners, we considered preventive measures and interventions such as close monitoring of the recovery-stress balance of participants and the planning of recovery including leisure time and distraction as important facets. These procedures may help to obtain a positive outcome on psychological states in extreme environments. Although not yet fully investigated, efficient psychological preparation may reduce stress, promote recovery, and support adaptive responses to such extreme environments.

Acknowledgements

We wish to thank all the participants, teams, researchers, and collaborators who contributed to these experiments. These studies were sponsored by the European Space Agency (ESA), the National Aeronautics and Space Administration of the USA (NASA), the Canadian Space Agency (CSA), the Russian space agency (Roscosmos), the French space agency Centre National d'Etudes Spatiales (CNES) and the French Polar Institute IPEV (Institut Paul Emile Victor) and received the support of the Terres Australes et Antarctiques Françaises (TAAF) and the University and the Region of Bourgogne Franche-Comté.

Notes

1 An existing field setting could be analogue with respect to one or more of the following characteristics similar to the environment to be investigated: (1) Analogue missions are an integrated set of activities in support of, or simulating future exploration missions (e.g., Moon or Mars); (2) Analogue environments are environments sharing one or more salient features (e.g., temperature, remoteness, topology, mineralogy) with the target environment; and (3) Analogue populations includes the same characteristics of the targeted population (e.g., selection, motivation, demographics, occupation, personality) (European Space Agency, 2010).
2 In reference to Neil Armstrong, the first man to walk on the moon: 'That's one small step for man, one giant leap for mankind'.

References

Armitage, C. J., & Conner, M. (2001). Efficacy of the theory of planned behaviour: A meta-analytic review. *British Journal of Social Psychology, 40*(4), 471–499.
Bishop, S. L. (2004). Evaluating teams in extreme environments: From issues to answers. *Aviation, Space, and Environmental Medicine, 75*(7), 14–21.
Bishop, S. L., Kobrick, R., Battler, M., & Binsted, K. (2010). FMARS 2007: Stress and coping in an arctic Mars simulation. *Acta Astronautica, 66*(9–10), 1353–1367.
Brink, M. S., Nederhof, E., Visscher, C., Schmikli, S. L., & Lemmink, K. A. (2010). Monitoring load, recovery, and performance in young elite soccer players. *Journal of Strength & Conditioning Research, 24*(3), 597–603.
Choukèr, A., Thiel, M., Baranov, V., Meshkov, D., Kotov, A., Peter, K., . . . Christ, F. (2001). Simulated microgravity, psychic stress, and immune cells in men: Observations during 120-day 6° HDT. *Journal of Applied Physiology, 90*(5), 1736–1743.
Costa Jr., P. T., & McCrae, R. R. (1992). *Revised NEO Personality Inventory (NEOPI-R) professional manual*. Odessa, FL: Psychological Assessment Resources.

Coutts, A. J., Slattery, K. M., & Wallace, L. K. (2007). Practical tests for monitoring performance, fatigue and recovery in triathletes. *Journal of Science and Medicine in Sport, 10*(6), 372–381.

Davis, H., Orzeck, T., & Keelan, P. (2007). Psychometric item evaluations of the Recovery-Stress Questionnaire for Athletes. *Psychology of Sport and Exercise, 8*(6), 917–938.

Di Fronso, S., Nakamura, F. Y., Bortoli, L., Robazza, C., & Bertollo, M. (2013). Stress and recovery balance in amateur basketball players: Differences by gender and preparation phase. *International Journal of Sports Physiology and Performance, 8*(6), 618–622.

European Space Agency. (2010, August 31). *Human spaceflight and exploration seminar*. Noordwijk, Netherlands: ESTEC.

Filho, E., Di Fronso, S., Forzini, F., Murgia, M., Agostini, T., Bortoli, L., . . . Bertollo, M. (2015). Athletic performance and recovery – stress factors in cycling: An ever changing balance. *European Journal of Sport Science, 15*(8), 671–680.

Geuna, S., & Brunelli, F. (1995). Stressors, stress and stress consequences during long-duration manned space missions a descriptive model. *Acta Astronautica, 36*(6), 347–356.

Gleser, J., & Mendelberg, H. (1990). Exercise and sport in mental health: A review of the literature. *Israel Journal of Psychiatry and Related Sciences, 27*, 99–112.

Grigoriev, A. I., & Fedorov, B. M. (1996). Stresses under conditions of a normal mode of life, during hypokinesia (simulating effects of weightlessness) and in space flights. *Fiziologiia Cheloveka, 22*(2), 10–19.

Gushin, V. I. (1995). Problems of psychological control in prolonged spaceflight. *Earth Space Review, 4*(1), 28–31.

Ishizaki, Y., Fukuoka, H., Ishizaki, T., Tanaka, H., & Ishitobi, H. (2004). The implementation of game in a 20-day head-down tilting bed rest experiment upon mood status and neurotic levels of rest subjects. *Acta Astronautica, 55*(11), 945–952.

Ishizaki, Y., Ishizaki, T., Fukuoka, H., Kim, C.-S., Fujita, M., Maegawa, Y., . . . Gunji, A. (2002). Changes in mood status and neurotic levels during a 20-day bed rest. *Acta Astronautica, 50*(7), 453–459.

Kanas, N. (1998). Psychosocial issues affecting crews during long-duration international space missions. *Acta Astronautica, 42*(1), 339–361.

Kanas, N., & Manzey, D. (2008). *Space psychology and psychiatry* (2nd ed.). Dodrecht, Netherlands: Springer.

Kanas, N., Salnitskiy, V. P., Ritsher, J. B., Gushin, V. I., Weiss, D. S., Saylor, S. A., . . . Marmar, C. R. (2006). Human interactions in space: ISS vs. Shuttle/Mir. *Acta Astronautica, 59*(1–5), 413–419.

Kass, R., & Kass, J. (1999). Psycho-social training for man in space. *Acta Astronautica, 45*(2), 115–118.

Kellmann, M. (2010). Preventing overtraining in athletes in high-intensity sports and stress/recovery monitoring: Preventing overtraining. *Scandinavian Journal of Medicine & Science in Sports, 20*, 95–102.

Kellmann, M., & Kallus, K. W. (2001). *Recovery-Stress Questionnaire for Athletes: User manual*. Champaign, IL: Human Kinetics.

Kellmann, M., & Kallus, K. W. (2016). The Recovery-Stress Questionnaire for Athletes. In K. W. Kallus & M. Kellmann (Eds.), *The Recovery-Stress Questionnaires: User manual* (pp. 86–131). Frankfurt am Main: Pearson Assessment.

Lazarus, R. S., & Folkman, S. (1984). Coping and adaptation. In W. D. Gentry (Ed.), *The handbook of behavioral medicine* (pp. 282–325). New York, NY: Guilford.

Leith, L. M. (2010). *Foundations of exercise and mental health*. Morgantown, WV: Fitness Information Technology.

Leon, G. R., Sandal, G. M., & Larsen, E. (2011). Human performance in polar environments. *Journal of Environmental Psychology, 31*(4), 353–360.

Manzey, D., & Lorenz, B. (1998). Mental performance during short-term and long-term spaceflight. *Brain Research Reviews, 28*(1), 215–221.

Marsh, M. S., & Rygalov, V. Y. (2008). Conceptual approach for stress estimates among astronauts and cosmonauts. *Combustion, 2015,* 6–22.

McFadden, T. J., Helmreich, R. L., Rose, R. M., & Fogg, L. F. (1994). Predicting astronaut effectiveness: A multivariate approach. *Aviation, Space, and Environmental Medicine, 65*(10), 904–909.

Meeusen, R., Duclos, M., Foster, C., Fry, A., Gleeson, M., Nieman, D., . . . Urhausen, A. (2013). Prevention, diagnosis, and treatment of the overtraining syndrome: Joint consensus statement of the European College of Sport Science and the American College of Sports Medicine. *Medicine and Science in Sports and Exercise, 45*(1), 186–205.

Millet, G. P., & Millet, G. Y. (2012). Ultramarathon is an outstanding model for the study of adaptive responses to extreme load and stress. *BMC Medicine, 10*(1), 77.

Nicolas, M. (2009). Personality, social support and affective states during simulated microgravity in healthy women. *Advances in Space Research, 44*(12), 1470–1478.

Nicolas, M. (2010, August 31). *Social, occupational, environmental and psychological adaptation in ICE situations.* Human Spaceflight and Exploration, Concordia Station, ESA (European Space Agency)/ESTEC, Noordwijk, Netherlands.

Nicolas, M., Banizette, M., & Millet, G. Y. (2011). Stress and recovery states after a 24 h ultra-marathon race: A one-month follow-up study. *Psychology of Sport and Exercise, 12*(4), 368–374.

Nicolas, M., Bishop, S. L., Weiss, K., & Gaudino, M. (2016). Social, occupational, and cultural adaptation during a 12-month wintering in Antarctica. *Aerospace Medicine and Human Performance, 87*(9), 781–789.

Nicolas, M., Gaudreau, P., & Franche, V. (2011). Perception of coaching behaviors, coping, and achievement in a sport competition. *Journal of Sport & Exercise Psychology, 33*(3), 460–468.

Nicolas, M., & Gushin, V. (2014). Stress and recovery responses during a 105-day ground-based space simulation: Stress and recovery during mars 105. *Stress and Health, 31*(5), 403–410.

Nicolas, M., Suedfeld, P., Weiss, K., & Gaudino, M. (2015). Affective, social, and cognitive outcomes during a 1-year wintering in Concordia. *Environment and Behavior, 48*(8), 1073–1091.

Nicolas, M., Vacher, P., Martinent, G., & Mourot, L. (in press). Monitoring stress and recovery states: Structural and external stages of the short version of the RESTQ-Sport in elite swimmers before championships. *Journal of Sport and Health Science.* doi:10.1016/j.jshs.2016.03.007

Nicolas, M., & Weiss, K. (2009). Stress and recovery assessment during simulated microgravity: Effects of exercise during a long-term head-down tilt bed rest in women. *Journal of Environmental Psychology, 29*(4), 522–528.

Palinkas, L. A. (1992). Going to extremes: The cultural context of stress, illness and coping in Antarctica. *Social Science & Medicine, 35*(5), 651–664.

Palinkas, L. A. (2003). The psychology of isolated and confined environments: Understanding human behavior in Antarctica. *American Psychologist, 58*(5), 353–363.

Palinkas, L. A., & Browner, D. (1995). Effects of prolonged isolation in extreme environments on stress, coping, and depression. *Journal of Applied Social Psychology, 25*(7), 557–576.

Palinkas, L. A., & Houseal, M. (2000). Stages of change in mood and behavior during a winter in Antarctica. *Environment and Behavior, 32*(1), 128–141.

Palinkas, L. A., & Suedfeld, P. (2008). Psychological effects of polar expeditions. *The Lancet, 371*(9607), 153–163.

Pearson, H. (2006). Physiology: Freaks of nature? *Nature, 444*(7122), 1000–1001.

Rivolier, J. (1992). *Facteurs humains et situations extremes*. Paris: Masson.

Salam, A. P. (2012). Exploration class missions on earth: Lessons learnt from life in extreme Antarctic isolation and confinement. In A. Chouker (Ed.), *Stress challenges and immunity in space* (pp. 425–439). Heidelberg: Springer.

Sandal, G. M., Leon, G. R., & Palinkas, L. A. (2006). Human challenges in polar and space environments. In R. Amils, C. Ellis-Evans, & H. Hinghofer-Szalkay (Eds.), *Life in extreme environments* (pp. 399–414). Dodrecht, Netherlands: Springer.

Selye, H. (1950). *Stress*. Montreal, Canada: Acta. Inc.

Suedfeld, P. (2005). Invulnerability, coping, salutogenesis, integration: Four phases of space psychology. *Aviation, Space, and Environmental Medicine, 76*(Suppl. 1), B61–B66.

Suedfeld, P. (2010). Historical space psychology: Early terrestrial explorations as Mars analogues. *Planetary and Space Science, 58*(4), 639–645.

Suedfeld, P., & Steel, G. D. (2000). The environmental psychology of capsule habitats. *Annual Review of Psychology, 51*(1), 227–253.

White, R. W. (1959). Motivation reconsidered: The concept of competence. *Psychological Review, 66*(5), 297–333.

Zimmer, M., Cabral, J. C. C. R., Borges, F. C., Côco, K. G., & Hameister, B. da R. (2013). Psychological changes arising from an Antarctic stay: Systematic overview. *Estudos de Psicologia (Campinas), 30*(3), 415–423.

16
STRESS AND RECOVERY IN APPLIED SETTINGS

Long working hours, recovery, and breaks

K. Wolfgang Kallus and Kerstin Gaisbachgrabner

Introduction

Recovery is still a Cinderella of psychological and psychophysiological research in sports, work, and related settings such as clinic, school, or family. It has been agreed that recovery is much more than a passive process which occurs more or less automatically between two performances. In sports, recovery takes place within and between competitions, training sessions, between training and competition and is intelligently structured across the different phases of the season. The interplay between stress and recovery is even more complex than on the first sight. Recovery takes place with complex interlinked time dynamics on different functional levels – ranging from activation processes in the central and vegetative systems via muscular, metabolic, and humoral processes to psychological processes and social processes with partners and coworkers, in teams and families. Some processes are biologically determined and work automatically, some processes can be influenced by cognitions and behaviour and some recovery processes are motivated and action oriented or even socially oriented behaviours. Recovery has received much more attention in sports in the past decades. Thus, models from sports have been transferred to work settings (Allmer, 1996). The transfer is quite difficult from time to time, as breaks in sports (e.g., half-times, time-outs) are well structured in most cases. The sluice model for breaks (Eberspächer, Hermann, & Kallus, 1993) is a good example. Breaks in sports are often defined by rules and need less preparation compared to breaks in work settings, which are only formally structured in case of coffee break and lunch break. In work settings breaks often need a proper planning,

Kallus, K. W., & Gaisbachgrabner, K. (2018). Stress and recovery in applied settings: Long working hours, recovery, and breaks. In M. Kellmann & J. Beckmann (Eds.), *Sport, Recovery, and Performance: Interdisciplinary Insights* (pp. 233–246). Abingdon: Routledge.

good preparation, and an appropriate setting to fit into the multitasking 'all time available' mode of modern work.

In the following sections some results from the recovery-stress interplay at work will be outlined, which might allow a transfer to sport settings. In work settings resources have to be recovered within a working day, between working days, on weekends and on vacations. Data from laboratory and field studies show that intelligent work-break-schedules are very effective to provide a high performance level throughout the working day, in addition to reducing negative mood changes and the appearance of physical stress symptoms (Buchegger, 2017). A high risk of depleting resources due to 'underrecovery' (Kellmann, 2010) can be shown in work psychology by an analysis of the effects of overtime work (so-called long working hours; Gaisbachgrabner, 2014). Increased risks for a broad range of symptoms are reported in the literature, ranging from hypertension, and myocardial infarction, diabetes mellitus, musculoskeletal diseases and overweight to more psychological symptoms like fatigue, daily sleepiness, and reduced sleep quality. These results on long working hours might also be relevant for different fields in high-performance sports.

Definition of long working hours

Daily and weekly working hours are a core topic in discussions between unions and employers and have been subject to political regulations in the European Union and the member states. There is no scientific agreement how many hours constitute the threshold of long working hours, especially as weekly working time is only one factor among others, which determines the weekly workload (Kallus, Boucsein, & Spanner, 2009). Breaks and daily working schedules as well as the type of job have to be taken into account as well. However, long working hours are beyond normal working hours, which have been defined by the European commission in the Directives 93/104/EC (1993), 2000/34/EC (2000), 2003/88/EC (2003) as follows:

- Maximum average working week (including overtime) of 48 hours over a 17-week reference period [which is well in line with classical and recent empirical evidence (Spurgeon, Harrington, & Cooper, 1997; Tucker & Folkard, 2012)].
- Minimum daily rest period of 11 consecutive hours in every 24 hours.
- Breaks when the working day exceeds 6 hours.
- Minimum weekly rest period of 24 hours plus the 11 hours daily rest period in every seven-day period.
- Minimum of four weeks' paid annual leave.
- Night work restricted to an average of 8 hours in any 24-hour period.

Empirical results use different cut-offs to define long working hours. Sudden death from heart attacks were observed in Japanese workers 'Karoshi', whose working hours exceeded 60 hours per week (Iwasaki, Takahashi, & Nakata, 2006). Spurgeon and colleagues (1997) as well as Knauth (2007) conclude that long working hours between 50 and 55 hours per week are associated with serious health problems. Dex, Clark, and Taylor (1995) argue that long working hours may be considered differently for men (over 60 hours per week) and women (over 40 hours per week). Caruso, Hitchcock, Dick, Russo, and Schmit (2004) report that simple overtime of over 40 hours per week shows negative effects like elevated risk for neck, shoulder, and back disorders, more cardiovascular and musculoskeletal complaints, fatigue, and impaired performance according to Nachreiner, Rädiker, Janßen, and Schomann (2005). Psychovegetative complaints show a steep linear increase from 40 hours on, while musculoskeletal disorders and other show increased risks especially beyond 60 hours per week.

Long working hours are difficult to define because working schedules, hours in main job and other jobs, commuting time, business travel time, as well as other obligations must be considered as well. At the same time, the relation between hours worked and the resulting stress levels can vary considerably for daily, weekly, or annual working hours with different ways to compensate peaks in working hours. Overtime can be viewed as the area between regular working schedules and long working hours.

Overtime hours are defined as ". . . work performed by an employee in excess of the normal hours of work which has been officially requested and approved by management. It is work that is not part of an employee's regularly scheduled working week and for which an employee may be compensated" (Eurofound, 2007, p. 2).

Reduced options for recovery connected with long working hours are explicitly or at least implicitly included in the models (e.g., Tucker & Folkard, 2012), which try to explain the broad range of adverse effects of long working hours. An excessive use of resources should normally be compensated by more and not by less recovery. This critical situation, which should be avoided in work and sports is well reflected in recent data obtained with the Recovery-Stress Questionnaire (Kallus & Kellmann, 2016) in a sample of blue collar workers.

Recovery-stress state, overtime, and long working hours

With respect to the recovery-stress profile overtime showed only marginal effects compared to normal working hours in a study with Austrian blue collar workers (Gaisbachgrabner, 2014), while long working hours resulted in significant ($p < .05$) effects in stress as well as recovery scales like *General Stress*, *Fatigue*, *Social Recovery*, and *Sleep Quality* in the basic areas of the Recovery-Stress Questionnaire for Work (RESTQ-Work; Jiménez, Dunkl, & Kallus, 2016) (Figure 16.1). In addition, a couple of effects in the work-specific scales turned out to be significant ($p < .05$; *Spillover, Loss of Meaning, Efficient Breaks, Leisure*).

The effects of long working hours on both stress and recovery as indicated in the RESTQ-Work were also visible in physical stress markers. A very striking effect occurred for thyroid functions.

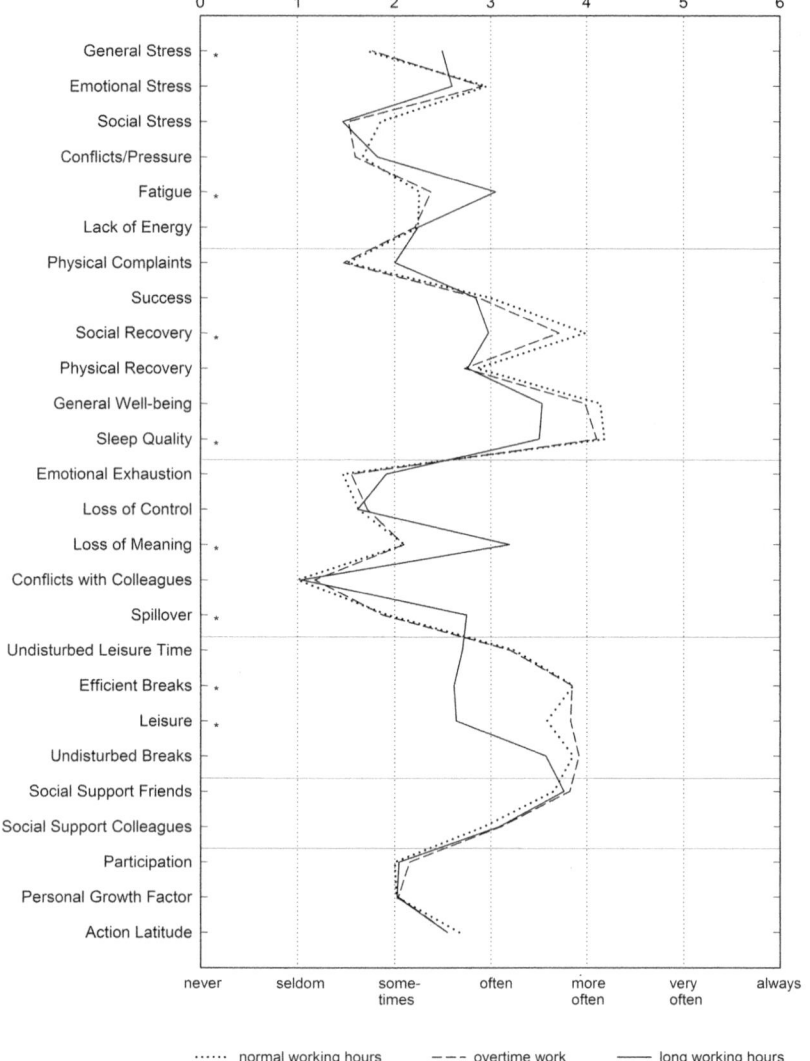

FIGURE 16.1 RESTQ-Basic scales and different groups of working time (Manova: $F[2, 199]) = 4.285, p < .0001, \eta_p^2 = .215$). ★= $p < .05$.

Working hours and thyroid function

In a first study Gaisbachgrabner (2014) detected an odds ratio of 8.5 for thyroid dysfunction (clinical diagnosis) in the group of long working hours compared to normal working hours, in a study with an overall sample size of $N = 173$. The study was conducted with an Austrian sample of blue collar workers sample for normal and long working hours.

In a replication study ($N = 203$) the overall risk was a bit lower. However, the significant increased risk of thyroid dysfunction in the long working hours' group was replicated with an odds ratio of 4.5 (Gaisbachgrabner, 2014).

Finally, the above found relationship was tested in a small prospective study, when a new period of long working hours was announced in the company. No experimental data could be collected, but repeated measures of physiological stress markers were obtained. Data indicate that long working hours affect thyroid functions and other stress markers. A significant drop in a marker of thyroid functioning (ft3) occurred only when p-values were interpreted as one sided, indicating, that thyroid function changed in the period of long working hours. No recovery in ft3 was observed in the (short) recovery period of 14 days. However, corresponding changes were found in the area of the classical stress hormone cortisol.

Working hours and cortisol

Long-term stress or more severe stress reactions lead to changes in the morning values of cortisol, which is termed the cortisol awakening response (CAR; Kirschbaum, 1991) and can be measured from salvia samples. Salvia samples after waking up were collected during phases of normal working hours and long working hours for the seven subjects of the above-mentioned sample. Shifts with long working hours are accompanied by a significant increase in cortisol awakening values, which declines in the recovery phase (Figure 16.2).

The study adds evidence to the problem, that long working hours disrupt the recovery-stress balance and disturb psychophysiological functions (stress-cortisol, stress-thyroid-functions).

The problem of long working hours is often overlooked in high-performance amateurs, who have intensive training blocks before and after their normal working hours on several days. All in all, 60h per week plus intensive competition weekends are an underestimate of effort for most of them. For the high-performance sports area, which is concerned with young athletes and adolescents the findings recommend to include thyroid function in the sport-medical monitoring as the thyroid gland plays a central role in the regulation of metabolism, growth and skeletal maturation (Bettendorf et al., 2016). At least, the overall work plus training time should be considered.

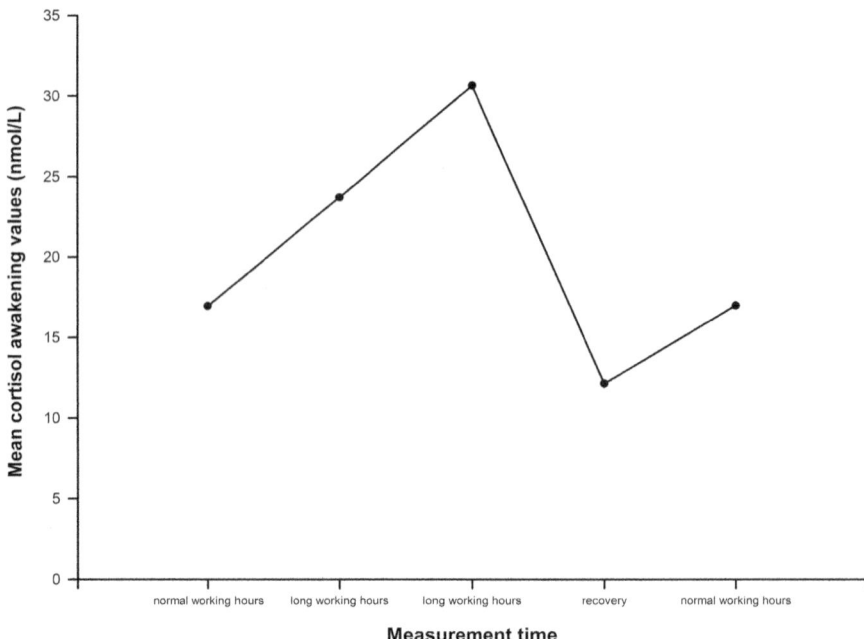

FIGURE 16.2 Cortisol awakening value over different working periods ($F[1, 5] = 32.610, p = .030, \eta_p^2 = .985$).

Working hours and subjective critical situations

The RESTQ is an easy to use tool for a good training monitoring. An even more parsimonious tool has been developed to assess the occurrence of stress during a working period. This might easily be transferred to a competition period or a training period. The Rating of Subjective Critical Situations (SCS; Kallus et al., 2014) is a 'quick' measure to catch stressful events during a working period, SCS scores seem to be quite sensitive to indicate the occurrence of subjective stress events. However, SCS ratings give no indication of how to intervene, which balances advantages and disadvantage between SCS scaling and a RESTQ-profile.

Time course of SCS ratings in the above mentioned sample of Gaisbachgrabner (2014) parallel those of cortisol in Figure 16.3. However, effect sizes turned out to be even higher with SCS ratings ($F[2, 4] = 6.800, p \leq .0001, \eta_p^2 = .850$). This has an interesting methodological consequence as SCS-rating seem to vary with physiologically measured stress levels. At the same time results indicate that stronger deviations from routine appear during long working hours.

In a study with air traffic controllers Kallus and colleagues (2014) assessed cortisol levels before, during, and after full-shift observations. For those controllers with high SCS-ratings on the observed day cortisol awakening values (Kirschbaum, 1991) were obtained on three consecutive days together with afternoon and night values. For controllers with high SCS ratings (more than 30

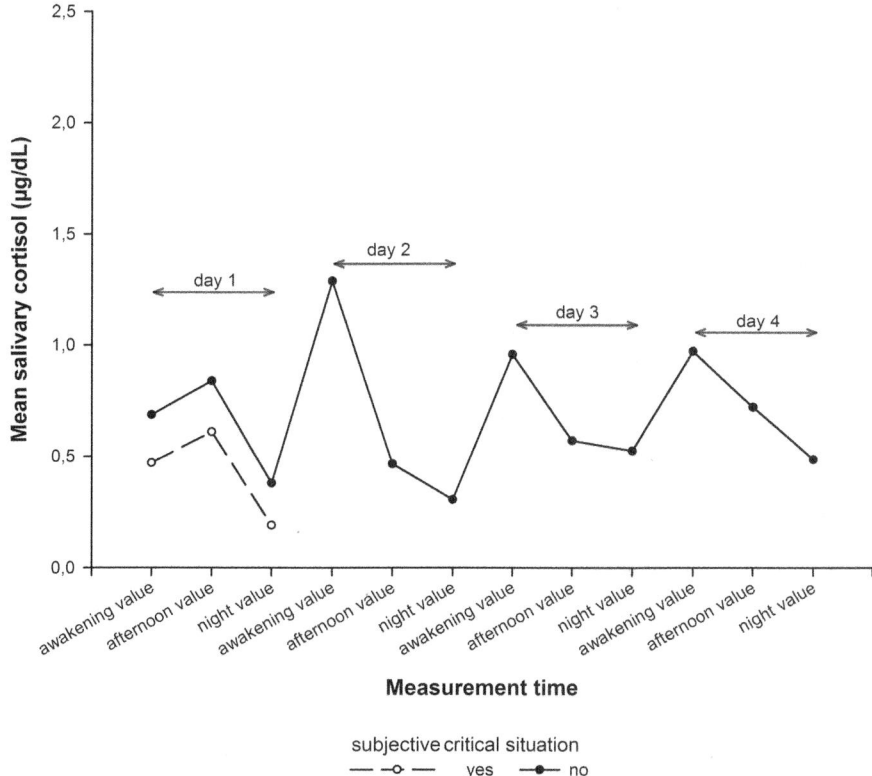

FIGURE 16.3 Mean salivary cortisol concentration [μg/dL], for the groups subjective critical situation yes/no during four days (Vienna Change & Transition Study; $N = 32$ air traffic controllers, Kallus, Hoffmann, & Winkler, 2008).

on a 50-point scale; $N = 7$) drastically increased awaking values were observed (group SCS 'yes' in Figure 16.3). The increased values declined on the consecutive days, but without reaching day 1 baselines on day 4 (Figure 16.3). These observations indicate that subjective critical situations might cause longer lasting stress reactions. Of course, these small sample observations should soon be validated with larger samples.

Critical situations and stress

The high impact of SCS-scores could also be shown in a sample of military personnel ($N = 39$; most of them working in military air traffic management; Kallus et al., 2014). High correlations ($r = .58$) between SCS and cortisol awakening levels could be shown (Figure 16.4).

Due to the skewed distributions a 2x2 Fisher Test was computed with the groups in Table 16.1.

Fisher's exact test shows an association between SCS and the cortisol awakening level on the subsequent morning with a p-value of $p = .04$.

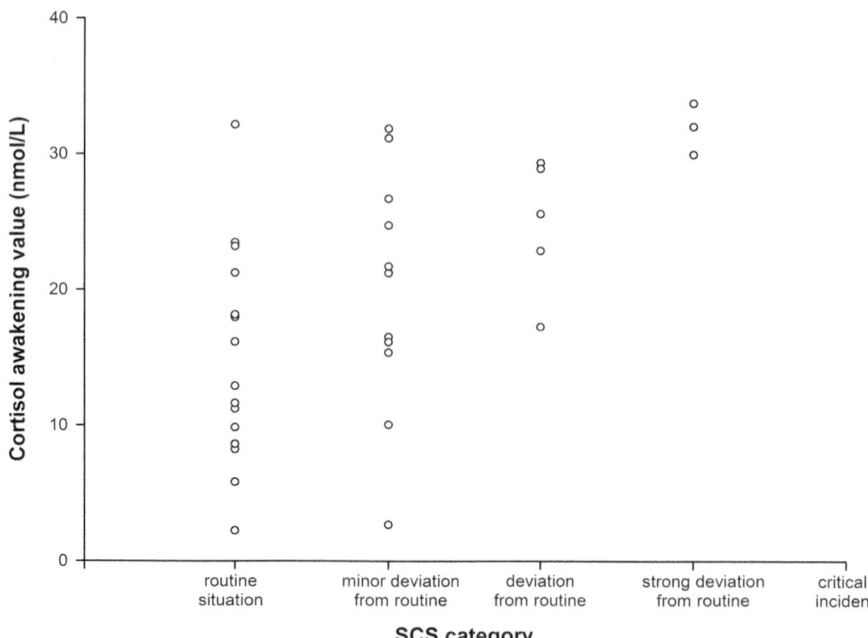

FIGURE 16.4 Subjective Critical Situations and cortisol awakening values on the subsequent day.

TABLE 16.1 Fisher's exact test between Subjective Critical Situations and cortisol.

	SCS low	SCS high	
Cortisol high	11	9	20
Cortisol low	16	3	19

For the sample above clear differences occur for subjects with high and low SCS ratings of the preceding working day and could also be obtained on the subjective level with the German Beanspruchungs-Mess-Skalen (BMS; Debitz, Plath, & Richter, 2016). This questionnaire assesses four basic work-stress dimensions (*Fatigue, Monotony, Stress,* and *Satiation*). Highly significant differences could be shown (Figure 16.5).

Our results on long working hours and subjective critical situations indicate that:
- Long working hours disrupt the recovery-stress balance
- Long working hours affect psychophysiological functions (stress-cortisol, stress-thyroid-functions)
- Subjective critical situations disturb psychophysiological functions
- Subjective critical situations can disturb the recovery-stress balance

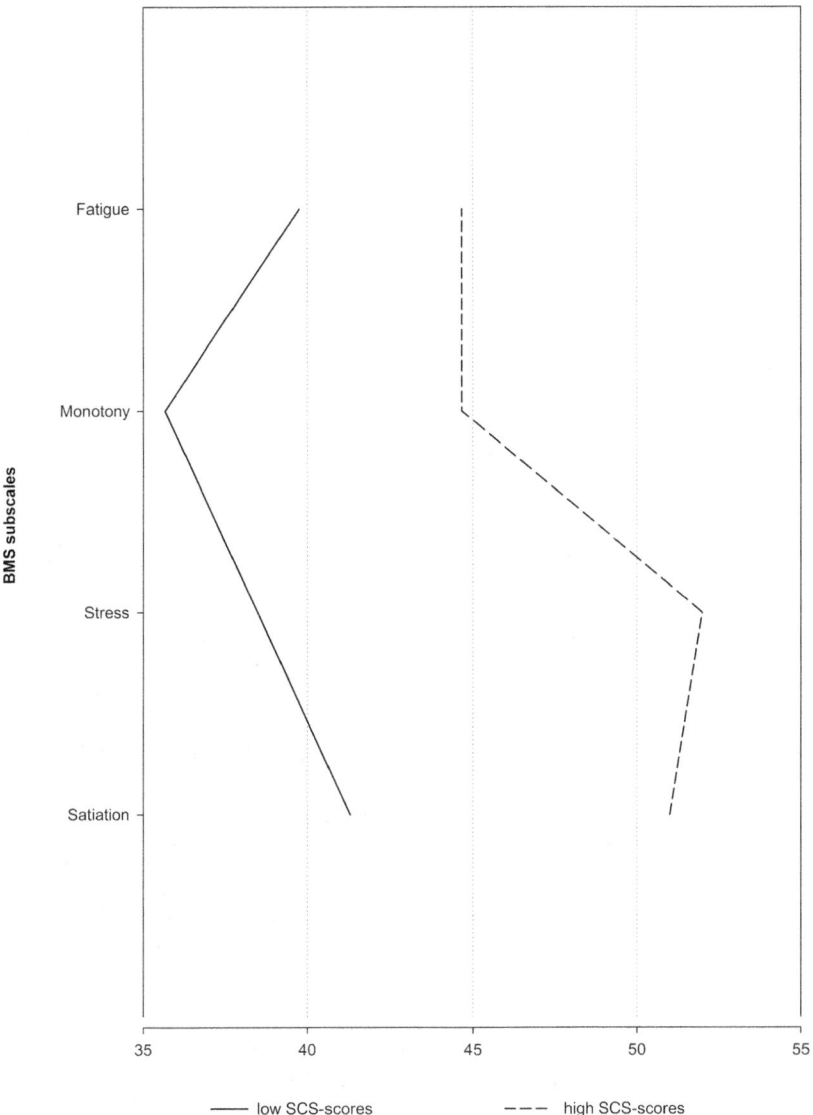

FIGURE 16.5 Subjective Critical Situations (SCS) rating and *Fatigue, Monotony, Stress,* and *Satiation* (sub-dimensions of the BMS) for groups without (straight line) and with high SCS-scores (dotted line).

Thus, long working hours and subjective critical situations might be interesting aspects for training-monitoring in high-performance athletes. Long working hours are of high relevance for those amateurs, who do a regular job in addition to their high-performance sports. Maybe the critical value of 60h/

week from the work area can be extended a bit, as sports and work consume partly different resources. However, time budget monitoring should include the working hours. The method of subjective critical situations might prove useful in sports as they are highly sensitive to detect stressful events from the athletes' perspective.

Breaks as options to cope with the effects of long working hours and subjective critical situations

Subjective critical situations call for systematic debriefing and coping, which can be derived from more intensive situations. However, there is still an unresolved debate on how to optimise the benefits of critical incident stress debriefings.

More data are available for the topic of breaks, which received some attention in the old studies of the Kraepelin group (Graf, 1922), indicating that early and repeated breaks result in a netto performance increase (better performance despite a 'loss' of working time) in a 3-hour work period of short cyclic easy mental activities (Graf, 1922, 1926).

High task load in sports (e.g., during training) is primarily antagonised by intelligent breaks and intelligent training schedules (Schmidt & Lee, 2005). Some recent results from our studies on breaks support the importance of intelligent schedules. A study on shift duration in rail traffic controllers (Kallus et al., 2009) compared two shift models. Nine rail traffic controllers worked an eight-hour shift schedule in blocks of five shifts with irregular recovery breaks, while nine controllers worked 12-hour shifts in blocks of four, resulting in a regular block with 24 hours of recovery between shifts. Measurements of fatigue with the BMS, which were taken at the end of shift 1 and the final two shifts are depicted in Figure 16.6. Those working 12 h report higher fatigue than those working eight hours after the first shift ('start' in Figure 16.6), which had to be expected. However, the picture changes for the final two shifts. For the 8-hour shift system a marked increase of fatigue is visible, which does not occur for the 12-hour shift system. Note that total hours worked is lower at the end of the final shift for the 8-hour system ($5 \star 8\ h = 40\ h$) than for the 12-hour system ($4 \star 12\ h = 48\ h$). These results show that not only total working time is relevant but also the rostering schedule (and maybe the attitude of the workers, who preferred the old 12-hour system). Furthermore, the results are in line with those of an independent study of Kirchler and Schmidl (2000) with performance measures.

Finally, data from a laboratory study again indicate that not only breaks are necessary in prolonged working situations, but also intelligent schedules are needed. The study with $N = 61$ working employees was conducted in the late afternoon to simulate a working day with overtime. Age was included as a factor in the analysis of performance data. The expected result of a study, with aging subjects was found in simple reaction time assessed by the Vienna Test System (Schuhfried, 2014). Older workers had significant prolonged reaction times and reaction time was shorter after a break. However, errors in a selective attention

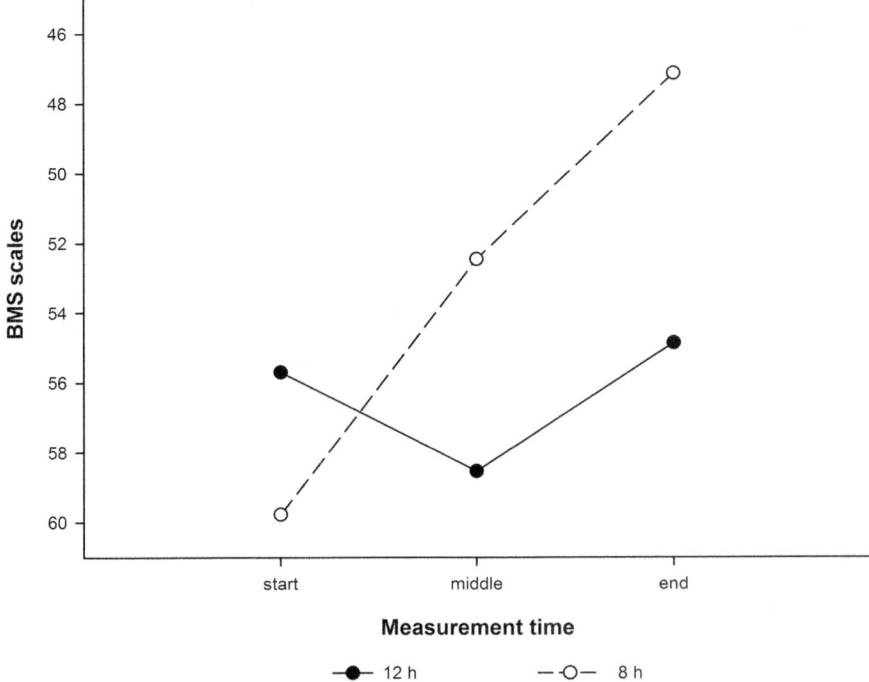

FIGURE 16.6 Fatigue (end of shift) of 12-hour and 8-hour systems of railway workers.

test (also assessed with the Vienna Test System) shows that errors decrease during performance of the test [start to end of work-block1 (WB1) and WB3]. A paradox effect of breaks occurred as errors increase after the breaks (end of WB1 and WB3). Both effects are more pronounced for the older employees (Figure 16.7).

The results indicate an interruption effect due to the breaks, which might be similar to interrupting an athlete during flow. In work settings breaks always bear the risk of interrupting an ongoing activity, with high costs of reestablishing a smooth action. This can also be the case in sports e.g., during training.

Conclusion and recommendations for practise

Breaks are not just 'time' and work-rest-schedules need intelligent solutions (timing, spacing, change of activity, 'interpunction'). Timing of breaks with respect to onset, duration, and content needs much more attention in research and in different areas of application. In sports, it is trivial not to interrupt a flow by an unwanted break. Breaks should not be interruptions but a tool to create activity rhythms. Activity rhythms play a central role to obtain a good recovery-stress balance, work

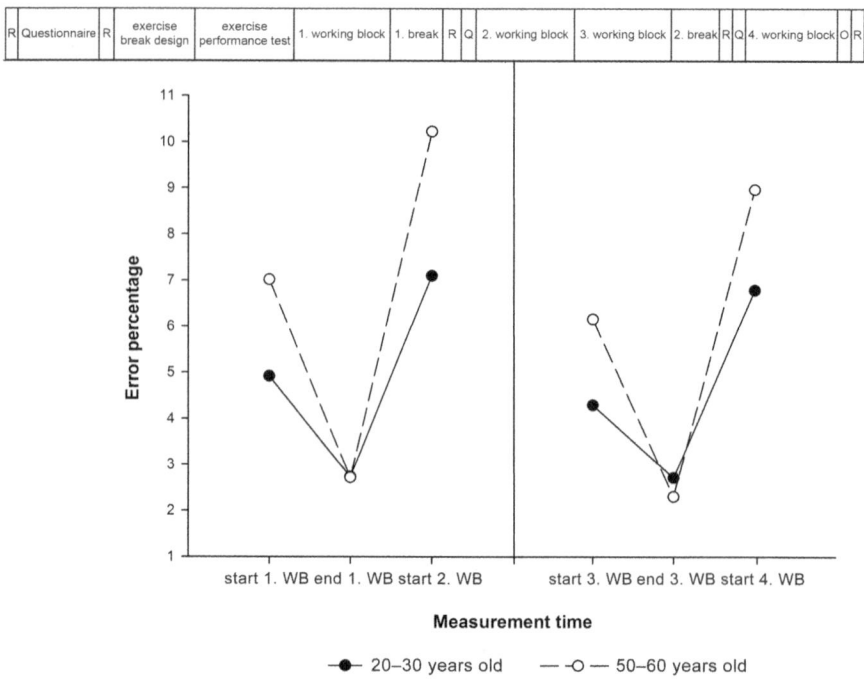

FIGURE 16.7 Attention performance changes over working blocks (time x age; $F[4,2;378,6] = 8.27, p < .001$).

rest schedules need much more attention, as time alone is not the only variable which has to be considered in high-performance sports and in a high-performance society.

The SCS scaling and systematic debriefing of critical situations might be new useful tools to reduce strain from top performance. This was repeatedly agreed on in the symposium and can empirically be substantiated from research in critical incident stress management. However, short, easy-to-use guidelines must be developed, together with clear indication and contraindication of debriefings, especially, when non-psychologists use the approach. Results from Work Psychology on the issue of long working hours indicate that the time budget of athletes especially when working with young amateurs might need some more attention. Recovery needs time and maybe should be in accordance with biological rhythms, which can easily be disrupted by excessive training requirements. The risk, that extensive training times might have similar effects to long working hours at least constitutes a risk for health problems and burnout in high-performance amateurs.

References

Allmer, H. (1996). *Erholung und Gesundheit* [Recovery and health]. Göttingen: Hogrefe.
Bettendorf, M., Binder, G., Hauffa, B. P., Pohlenz, J., Rohrer, R., Schöfl, C., & Dörr, G. (2016). Wachstum bei Störungen der Schilddrüsenfunktion im Kindes und Jugendalter: Störungen

der Schilddrüsenfunktion und Wachstum [Growth in thyroid dysfunction in children and adolescents: Disorders of thyroid function and growth]. *Monatsschrift Kinderheilkunde, 164*(8), 689–696.

Buchegger, C. (2017). *Eine empirische Untersuchung zum Einfluss des aktuellen Erholungs-Beanspruchungs-Zustands auf den Kurerfolg* [An empirical study on the influence of the current recovery-stress state on the treatment outcome]. Unpublished doctoral dissertation, University of Graz, Austria.

Caruso, C., Hitchcock, E., Dick, R., Russo, J., & Schmit, J. (2004). *Overtime and extended work shifts: Recent findings on illnesses, injuries, and health behaviors.* Cincinnati: NIOSH Publications Dissemination.

Council of the European Union. (1993). *Council Directive 93/104/EC of 23 November 1993 concerning certain aspects of the organization of working time.* Brussels: Council of the European Union.

Council of the European Union. (2000). *Directive 2000/34/EC of the European Parliament and of the Council of 22 June 2000 amending Council Directive 93/104/EC concerning certain aspects of the organisation of working time to cover sectors and activities excluded from that Directive.* Brussels: Council of the European Union.

Council of the European Union. (2003). *Directive 2003/88/EC of the European Parliament and of the Council of 4 November 2003 concerning certain aspects of the organisation of working time.* Brussels: European Parliament, Council of the European Union.

Debitz, U., Plath, H. E., & Richter, P. (2016). *Beanspruchungs-Mess-Skalen: Verfahren zur Erfassung erlebter Beanspruchungsfolgen: Psychische Ermüdung – Montononie – Psychische Sättigung – Stress. Manual* [Methods for assessing experienced consequences of stress: Psychological fatigue – monotony – psychic saturation – stress: Manual]. Göttingen: Hogrefe.

Dex, S., Clark, A., & Taylor, M. (1995). *Household labour supply. Department of Employment Research Series: Vol. 43.* University of Essex, Colchester: ESCR Research Centre on Micro-social change.

Eberspächer, H., Hermann, H.-D., & Kallus, K. W. (1993). Psychische Regeneration und Erholung zwischen Beanspruchungen [Mental recovery and recovery between stress]. In J. R. Nitsch & R. Seiler (Eds.), *Bewegung und Sport: Psychologische Grundlagen und Wirkungen* [Movement and sport: Psychological basics and effects] (Vol. 1, pp. 237–241). Sankt Augustin: Academia.

Eurofound (European Foundation for the improvement of living and working conditions). (2007). *European industrial relations dictionary.* Retrieved October 17, 2016, from www.eurofound.europa.eu/observatories/eurwork/industrial-relations-dictionary/overtime

Gaisbachgrabner, K. (2014). *Empirische Untersuchungen zu langen Arbeitszeiten und dem Hypothalamus-Hypophysen-Schilddrüsen-System im Mehrebenenansatz* [Empirical studies on the effects of long working hours on the hypothalamus-pituitary-thyroid-system]. Unpublished doctoral dissertation, University of Graz, Austria.

Graf, O. (1922). Über lohnenste Arbeitspausen bei geistiger Arbeit [Optimal restpauses and mental work]. *Psychologische Arbeit, 7,* 548–611.

Graf, O. (1926). Über Pausenwirkung bei Arbeit mit verschiedener Willensanspannung [The impact of restpauses in work with various levels of effort investment]. *Psychologische Arbeit, 9,* 228–243.

Iwasaki, K., Takahashi, M., & Nakata, A. (2006). Health problems due to long working hours in Japan: Working hours, workers' compensation (Karoshi), and preventive measures. *Industrial Health, 44*(4), 537–540.

Jiménez, P., Dunkl, A., & Kallus, K. W. (2016). Recovery-Stress Questionnaire for Work. In K. W. Kallus & M. Kellmann (Eds.), *The Recovery-Stress Questionnaires: User manual* (pp. 158–187). Frankfurt am Main: Pearson Assessment.

Kallus, K. W., Boucsein, W., & Spanner, N. (2009). Eight- and twelve-hour shifts in Austrian rail traffic controllers: A psychophysiological comparison. *Psychology Science Quarterly*, *51*(3), 283–297.

Kallus, K. W., Hoffmann, P., & Winkler, H. (2008). The concept of individual critical situations (SCS). In A. Droog (Ed.), *Proceedings of the 28th Conference of the European Association for Aviation Psychology from 22. to 31. October 2008 in Valencia, Spain* (pp. 27–31). Amsterdam: European Association for Aviation Psychology.

Kallus, K. W., & Kellmann, M. (Eds.). (2016). *The Recovery-Stress Questionnaires: User manual*. Frankfurt am Main: Pearson Assessment.

Kallus, K. W., Schwarz, M., Langer, C., Moser, G., Könczöl, C., & Gaisbachgrabner, K. (2014). Assessment of stress in aviation personnel. In A. Droog (Ed.), *Proceedings of the 31st Conference of the European Association for Aviation Psychology from 22. to 26. September 2014 in Valletta, Malta* (pp. 360–367). Amsterdam: European Association for Aviation Psychology.

Kellmann, M. (2010). Preventing overtraining in athletes in high-intensity sports and stress/recovery monitoring. *Scandinavian Journal of Medicine & Science in Sports*, *20*(Suppl. 2), 95–102.

Kirchler, E., & Schmidl, D. (2000). Schichtarbeit im Vergleich: Befindensunterschiede und Aufmerksamkeitsvariation während der 8-Stunden- versus 12-Stunden-Schichtarbeit [Comparison of shifts: Differences in health and attention during the 8-hour versus 12-hour shifts]. *Zeitschrift für Arbeits- und Organisationspsychologie*, *44*(1), 2–18.

Kirschbaum, C. (1991). *Cortisolmessung im Speichel – Eine Methode der Biologischen Psychologie* [Cortisol measurement in saliva – a method of Biological Psychology]. Göttingen: Huber.

Knauth, P. (2007). Extended work periods. *Industrial Health*, *45*, 125–136.

Nachreiner, F., Rädiker, B., Janßen, D., & Schomann, C. (2005). *Untersuchungen zum Zusammenhang zwischen der Dauer der Arbeitszeit und gesundheitlichen Beeinträchtigungen – Ergebnisse einer Machbarkeitsstudie* [Studies on the link between the duration of working hours and health impairments – results of a feasibility study]. Final Report Hans-Böckler-Stiftung. Oldenburg: GAWO.

Schmidt, R. A., & Lee, T. D. (2005). *Motor control and learning: A behavioral emphasis* (4th ed). Champaign, IL: Human Kinetics.

Schuhfried, G. (2014). *Daueraufmerksamkeit – DAUF.* Version 27 [Continuous attention: Version 27]. Mödling: Schuhfried.

Spurgeon, A., Harrington, J. M., & Cooper, C. L. (1997). Health and safety problems associated with long working hours: A review of the current position. *Occupational and Environmental Medicine*, *54*, 167–375.

Tucker, P., & Folkard, S. (2012). *Working time, health and safety: A research synthesis paper*. Geneva: International Labour Organization.

17
PSYCHOLOGICAL RELAXATION TECHNIQUES TO ENHANCE RECOVERY IN SPORTS

Michael Kellmann, Maximilian Pelka, and Jürgen Beckmann

Introduction

Stress and recovery have been discussed extensively in the context of sport performance settings. The term stress is used to describe a process, caused by a load or demand beyond the level of normal functioning characterised by homeostatic dysregulation (Kellmann & Kallus, 2016). It has long been recognised that exposure to severe bio-psycho-social stressors (i.e., noise, pain, family, finances, social relationships, etc.) negatively affects a person's health status (Tennant, Langeluddecke, & Byrne, 1985). Even short-term imbalances between stress and recovery could already lead to critical disadvantages (Bengtsson, Ekstrand, & Hägglund, 2013). Consequences of these imbalances such as increased fatigue, poor concentration, disturbed mood, and altered eating and sleeping patterns are often associated with short-term decrements of performance. Additionally, muscular tension, anxiety, and subsequent heightened arousal impair athletic performance. Learning self-regulation skills to improve recovery is therefore paramount for sustaining or improving well-being and athletic performance.

To mobilise performance reserves during competition, an athlete needs to be sufficiently activated. However, arousal levels can develop too quickly and become dysfunctional. Through specific psycho-regulative procedures from sport psychological training, athletes can be taught self-regulation skills, which enable them to achieve an optimal state of activation in training and competition, i.e., appropriate levels of mental and/or physical excitement. Self-regulation training is not only aimed at changing performance-impairing physical activation, but also at eliminating irrelevant thoughts, which could cause confusion and affect concentration negatively (Seers & Carroll, 1998). Furthermore, it is aimed at eliminating a motor performance-impairing self-focus (Beckmann, Gröpel, & Ehrlenspiel, 2013; Mesagno & Beckmann, 2017). Irrelevant thoughts can also result from the perception of increased physical activation ('I am nervous'). In sports performance, it is essential that the athlete can avoid the occurrence of such potentially performance-reducing reactions. If such reactions still occur, he/she should be able to deal with them. Systematic relaxation techniques can play a central role in those processes.

A prerequisite for optimal performance in sports is, in addition to relaxing, being able to systematically activate oneself or being able to modify activation/arousal states. For many years it has been assumed that optimal performance is expected at a moderate activation/arousal state of athletes (Andreassi, 2007; Yerkes & Dodson, 1908). If the activation level is too low, performance-relevant components cannot be retrieved, possibly due to the lack of competition activation. If levels are too high, optimal performance is not to be expected due to the accompanying muscular tension and tightness. The decisive factor in that process is not the physical arousal itself, but the cognitive processes triggered by it (Beckmann & Rolstad, 1997), such as irrelevant thoughts.

Since the optimal arousal for performance can vary inter-individually from one sport to another (Beckmann & Elbe, 2015) there are individual characteristics of optimal activation. This is also referred to as the zone of individually optimal functioning (IZOF; Hanin, 1997). To achieve an optimal level of competition activation, athletes should be able to relax or to activate themselves dependent on the context. In many psychological techniques, the ability to relax is a prerequisite for their successful execution (Birrer & Morgan, 2010), e.g., imagery requires a relaxed state. In addition, relaxation is an important basis for many other sport psychological intervention and training programs (Beckmann & Elbe, 2015).

Altogether, there are three general fields of application for relaxation training: (1) recovery, (2) self-regulation for optimal activation, (3) pre-requisite for psychological skills training. Derived from the title of the book, this chapter will primarily deal with the function of relaxation as a recovery tool to support performance and well-being.

Relaxation as a recovery tool

Relaxation serves many different functions in managing a variety of health conditions. In clinical practise, the value of relaxation as a supportive method has been shown repeatedly (Petermann & Vaitl, 2014). In sports, relaxation techniques are primarily used with the following four aims:

> Firstly, in the long-term, a greater serenity with regard to the onerous training and competition situation should be established. This should be combined with building up expectations to be able to regulate oneself effectively in these situations. The second, short-term aim points towards disturbing thoughts that are to be removed in the immediate preparation for competition and during it in order to achieve and keep full focus on it. However, the necessary competition activation must not be reduced. Thirdly, relaxation

supports regeneration after training and competition, especially in the case of injuries. Finally, relaxation is the basis for the training of further self-regulation skills, such as imagery, similar to systematic desensitization in behavioral therapy.

From these aims it can be derived that the function of relaxation techniques as a recovery tool in sport is threefold: Being (a) a strategy to develop inner balance; (b) a regeneration accelerator; and (c) a self-regulation tool. Recent research found that the most used techniques are progressive muscle relaxation, systematic breathing, hypnosis, eastern meditation, and imagery (Kudlackova, Eccles, & Dieffenbach, 2013; Pelka et al., 2016).

Relaxation as a means of developing inner balance

Looking at long-term effects of training, relaxation techniques can be used to develop the personality of an athlete in the sense of increasing his/her inner balance. The athlete learns to focus on and at the same time solve problems of his/her specific sport. Practising relaxation techniques should start at the beginning of the preparation for a season and then should be taken over the entire preparation period.

In addition to the elimination of tension and the support of regeneration, direct body-related goals are the sensitisation for and focus on one's own body and the physical processes. Being aware of one's body can support the movement sequences, which are practised. In addition, a feeling for tensed and relaxed muscles should be developed. The acquisition of relaxation skills should lead towards the ability to self-regulate one's own physical and psychological state.

At the same time, athletes should develop greater serenity, which allows them to accept unexpected – in particular, unfavourable – conditions. In golf, for example, it is said that the golfer should develop humility. This is connected with the fact that perceptual thresholds increase against disturbing internal and external stimuli. There should also be an affective equilibrium, so athletes are no longer sitting in an emotional 'rollercoaster', i.e., the feeling of excitement after a success is no longer acknowledged with absolute dejection in a subsequent failure/loss. This should also increase the ability to concentrate.

Last but not least, the serenity that develops through relaxation training also contributes to the improvement of general well-being. The positive overall feeling with a lack of negative affect reduces a defensive attitude and creates access to one's own strengths and own resources (Kuhl, 2001).

Relaxation as a regeneration accelerator

Recovery processes in elite sports also serve to restore the individual operational conditions and well-being after training and competition (Kellmann, 2002; Meyer, Kellmann, Ferrauti, Pfeiffer, & Faude, 2013). In today's high-performance sport environments training is scheduled twice or three times a day (training camp).

Outside of training camps, demands from school, university, and/or work as well as personal relationships affect an athlete and all of which must be paid tribute within a limited overall time budget. With systematically practised relaxation techniques, the probability of successfully using the scarce resource 'time' after training or in short breaks within a day is increased. Therefore, the somatotropic and psychotropic effects of relaxation can have the function of a 'regeneration accelerator'. The relaxation between training sessions accelerates the natural recovery process and allows for more intensive and increased training loads (Pelka et al., 2017). The authors furthermore argue that recovery after stress is more rapid with the aid of relaxation techniques compared to passive recovery. Regeneration processes play a decisive role in the event of rising fatigue, with regard to restore the ability to act after stress.

If regeneration is not possible and stress (physical and psychological) accumulates, underrecovery or overtraining are possible consequences. However, if recovery is used appropriately, high stress levels can be tolerated and it does not have to be negative to be highly stressed. In the context of this chapter, relaxation is thus classified as a purposeful recovery strategy.

Relaxation as a method of self-regulation

Prior to competition, relaxation has two important functions that can be actively controlled by the athlete. On the one hand, many – sometimes even experienced – athletes report that they cannot sleep properly two to three nights before an important competition (Erlacher, Ehrlenspiel, Adegbesan, & Galal El-Din, 2011). This reduced sleep quality and quantity can be detrimental to physical performance. This happens either directly through lack of recovery or indirectly through the fact that an athlete, after bad sleep, doubts whether he is still able to perform at all (Ehrlenspiel, Erlacher, & Ziegler, in press). In these situations, the deliberate creation of a relaxation state could lead to a stop of rumination. Using relaxation as 'sleep assistance' is a functional aid to react to disturbing cognitions and support overnight recovery.

On the other hand, on the day of the competition, athletes experience different levels of activation, depending on their experience and self-regulation ability. As stated earlier, a certain level of activation is necessary to provide athletic performance. Therefore, in the sense of a contraindication, there should be no relaxation training on the competition day, as otherwise the necessary activation could be lost. The use of systematic relaxation techniques (e.g., progressive muscle relaxation, or autogenic training) is only possible and useful if athletes have learned to reactivate themselves properly. For some athletes however, relaxation as a strategy is a prerequisite to build up the concentration necessary for performing in competition.

If athletes do not possess relaxation and/or mobilisation skills, the relaxation response could be triggered through imagery, especially on competition days. At first, it is possible to initiate the elicitation of the relaxation response through systematic breathing. Besides that, and as a matter of principle, athletes should always try to relax briefly while preparing for competition so that 'uncontrollable' activation tips could be prevented. The same also applies to the time period right before competition. For example, in rowing, boats usually lie at the start at least ten minutes before competition. During these ten minutes, most athletes try to build up concentration for the race through a ritualised process with smaller tasks to avoid irrelevant cognitions. If these still occur, a relaxation response should be triggered through visualizing a relaxing image, which then should lead to concentration and focus on the competition.

Recently, self-regulation has also been increasingly discussed in the context of embodied cognition (MacIntyre, Madan, Brick, Beckmann, & Moran, in press). It is assumed that cognition, emotion, and physical processes are closely related. Linked to that, a very simple technique has proven to be effective. Squeezing the left hand for a few seconds causes so-called 'high alpha' (10–12 Hz) waves in the brain, which relaxes and inhibits disturbing thoughts (Cross-Villasana, Gröpel, Doppelmayr, & Beckmann, 2015). Because of the higher connectivity of the right hemisphere, this self-relaxing technique only works when the left hand is pressed. Several studies have shown that this technique can prevent choking under pressure (Beckmann et al., 2013; Gröpel & Beckmann, 2017).

Procedure

In sport psychological consultation, relaxation is an important topic (Sherman & Poczwardowski, 2000). Primarily, the focus lies on the current concern of the athlete and how to stabilise or optimise performance in the specific context. However, it is frequently the case that a missing key variable is relaxation. Thus, further tests, e.g., questionnaires, or (semi-) structured interviews, are carried out to assess how the athlete is usually using relaxation and whether a relaxation response can be elicited in a targeted manner. In recent years, the interest in systematic relaxation techniques has increased (Kudlackova et al., 2013). Responses to the various techniques (e.g., systematic breathing, progressive muscle relaxation, autogenic training, hypnosis) are individually different and have different areas of application in sports. Therefore, together with the athlete, the sports psychologist should define the procedure to be learned and explain the background information and possible effects. The selection of the appropriate technique is then based on previous experience, type of sport, and the specific problem in combination with the clients' preference.

The structure of relaxation training in sports is derived from Vaitl (2014) and consists of an introductory phase, which is followed by the relaxation induction and the actual development of the relaxation response. In addition, imagery can be integrated at the end of the development of the relaxation response. In this specific situation, the athlete puts herself/himself into a relaxing and positive situation and links this relaxing state to a self-selected image. Linking a relaxation state and an image is intended to create a firm 'connection', so that optimally an athletes' image elicits a relaxation response (Martin, Moritz, & Hall, 1999). The procedure is completed by bringing participants back from the relaxation state to a conscious, wakeful, and relaxed state. After every session, a debriefing should be scheduled to assess whether there were difficulties or if modifications should be made. The ultimate goal is that athletes use relaxation techniques independently.

Techniques

Relaxation techniques used in sports are manifold and include amongst others, autogenic training, biofeedback, progressive muscle relaxation, systematic breathing, and hypnosis (e.g., Kudlackova et al., 2013; Pelka et al., 2016; Weinberg & Gould, 2010; Williams, 2009). Other widely used strategies in recovery settings are music and power naps (Jones, Tiller, & Karageorghis, 2017; Pelka et al., 2017). The following paragraphs exemplarily display three strategies which support the recovery process.

Hypnosis

Basically, hypnosis induces a state of trance that does not greatly differ from the trance brought about by autogenic training. Thus, hypnotic inductions are primarily associated with relaxation, sedation, and well-being. The hypnotherapist will address the person: 'As you sit here, and as you, despite the environment or just because of the noise you hear, focus more and more on the words you hear, you perhaps notice that you would like to close your eyes...'. This is a way of inducing a state of trance, which might be deepened by saying, 'With each exhalation you become more relaxed, with each breath you get deeper into trance'. Ligget (2000) advocates self-hypnosis in sports. This can only be recommended after several sessions with a professional hypnotherapist because in trance, psychological problems that were well suppressed until now might enter consciousness and the athlete might not be able to handle this. However, if after a number of sessions with a hypnotherapist, the likelihood of those problems turning up is considerably low, self-hypnosis may be an option. One trance induction technique that could be used is the '5, 4, 3, 2, 1 technique' (Dolan, 1991). It is a type of meditative technique. The client is told to fix focus on a specific point. Then five things that can be seen in the client's peripheral vision are stated. Next five things that can be heard are addressed. Then five things that can be sensed are stated. In a next round, four things that can be seen, heard, and sensed are stated. With every round the number of things perceived is reduced by one. After having addressed only one thing that is seen, one thing that is heard and one thing that is felt usually a state of trance is reached. The client may now close his/her eyes. After arriving at a stage of mild trance (deep trance is not required) forms of imagination can be used such as 'safe place', 'improving concentration' etc. The client can be asked to imagine a safe place in which he/she felt relaxed and stable on a somatic level, a situation in which the body felt vital, resilient, and fully comfortable. The client is instructed to indulge completely in this situation, to feel it in every cell of his body, and to fully revive the positive feelings. When basking in the situation the hypnotherapist asks the client to give a name for his/her safe place. The client is told that he/she can go to this place whenever he/she needs to go there to relax and build confidence. Many of the objectives to be achieved through imagery can also be addressed through hypnosis. The difference to mental skill training lies in the induction of a state of trance in hypnosis that attempts to arrive at changes on the level of unconsciousness.

Music

Almost every athlete spends some time before, between, and/or after competition or training with self-selected music from portable devices. In addition to the widespread use, there is no strategy which is as tailor-made to one's preferences as music. Recent studies have shown that music affects attention, emotions, and regulation of emotions, and has an influence on increased work readiness and performance, as well as on reducing inhibitions. Compared to systematic relaxation techniques, music is often regarded as a naive strategy, but in the end it is, as already indicated, one of the most popular and attractive strategies. Many findings also show effects of music on a variety of performance-related parameters (Loizou & Karageorghis, 2015). According to Karageorghis and Priest (2012), music can be regarded as a legal stimulant or sedative.

In physiological terms, increases or decreases of the respiratory rate or heart rate, are potential responses to rhythmic components of music. Research so far has mainly dealt with the preparation for and the time during performance (Terry & Karageorghis, 2006). The physiological processes, however, are the same regarding recovery. It was postulated that music induces relaxation through the influence on automatic and central nervous processes (Gillen, Biley, & Allen, 2008). On one hand, the anxiolytic effect of music is manifested through the suppressive effect on the sympathetic nervous system, i.e., reducing adrenergic activity and neuromuscular arousal. On the other hand, music triggers the limbic system to release endorphins, which play a decisive role in the enhancement of well-being. It has already been shown that music can attract attention from incriminating events to more pleasant and soothing thoughts, and thereby reducing symptoms of anxiety and pain (MacDonald et al., 2003; Nilsson, 2008). Among the few researchers who have assessed the efficacy of music as recovery from exercise, Jones and colleagues (2017) found that fast-tempo, positively-valanced music (applied during recovery periods) induces a more pleasant experience in a high-intensity interval training setting. Summarising, relaxation and music are both associated with decreased heart rate, systolic blood pressure and norepinephrine production (Szmedra & Bacharach, 1998). A further similarity is the reduction of muscle tension followed by an increased blood flow and faster lactate decomposition.

Progressive muscle relaxation

One of the most used techniques in sports is progressive muscle relaxation (Kudlackova et al., 2013). A reason could be that athletes are already familiar with relaxing and activating their muscles during the training process. Therefore, this technique is supposed to be the most 'physical' of the relaxation procedures. The change of tension and relaxation during the exercise is so familiar to the athletes that they usually have no difficulties to relax while following the instructions (see Table 17.1 for modified instructions). Consequently, progressive muscle relaxation is usually preferred over other procedures. However, it should also be taken into account that

TABLE 17.1 A procedure for relaxation induction with progressive muscle relaxation and subsequent imagination (based on Bernstein, Carlson, & Schmidt, 2007).

Initiation: Reduction of exaggerated expectations and fears
- Background information about mechanisms and effects of progressive muscle relaxation
- Practise effects
- Aim: Highly concentrated execution without falling asleep

Relaxation induction: Shifting attention to a (passive) receptive, inwardly-directed orientation; reduction of sensory input
- Taking a seat (cabman's relaxing position) or laying on the floor (mat)
- Instruction to rest, starting to focus (setting up concentration)

Developing relaxation: Staying in an intermediate state between wakefulness and sleep

order	muscles	instruction	frequency (session number)		
			1–3	4–6	7–9
(1)	forehead	frowning	3×	2×	1×
(2)	around nose, cheeks, and chin	pull a face	3×	2×	1×
(3)	shoulders and neck	raise shoulders	3×	2×	1×
(4)	arms	tense upper arm and forearm (right and left)	3×	2×	1×
(5)	fingers	make a fist (right and left)	3×	2×	1×
(6)	focus on breathing	inhale (4s), hold breath (1–2s) and exhale slowly (6–8s)	3×	3×	3×

Instruction: 'The entire upper body is relaxed now, let the relaxation flow into your legs'.

(7)	thighs	tense both thighs	3×	2×	1×
(8)	calves	pull your toes towards your head (while your legs remain on the floor)	3×	2×	1×
(9)	toes	roll your toes	3×	2×	1×

Linking relaxation to a self-selected picture (imagery)
- Instruction: 'The whole body is relaxed [...] head, upper body and legs. Now imagine a situation in which you feel comfortable. [...] For some it is staying at the beach, for others a clearing in the forest, or a completely different situation. [...] Take such a situation and try to imagine everything as detailed as possible. [...] Feel the warmth on your skin, hear the voices around you, and experience relaxation. [...] Imagine the colours and experience your environment precisely. [...] Devote yourself fully to the situation... [...]'.

Retrieval
- Instruction: 'Please follow my instruction while I will soon count backwards from ten to one. [...] 10, 9, 8, 7, 6 (move your muscles slowly), 5, 4, 3 (stretch and move a little bit more), 2, 1 (open your eyes, you are awake now, focused and relaxed)'.

Debriefing
- Ask if and how the relaxation has worked, if and if yes which disturbances have occurred, and which sensations have been encountered.

not all athletes react similarly to each technique. Regular feedback loops are an important feature for the learning process during the relaxation process, if necessary, to: (a) modify the procedure; or (b) select another technique. A detailed description of a progressive muscle relaxation session is provided in the following section.

Modification of a standard procedure

If learning of relaxation techniques in a systematic way is not possible, e.g., for time-related reasons, we recommend the use of progressive muscle relaxation with subsequent imagery. Essentially, progressive muscle relaxation, which is predominantly used in sport, follows the structure of a standard procedure (Bernstein & Borkovec, 1973; Hamm, 2014). For athletes, it is useful to use a shortened form as they are already familiarised with the change between relaxed and tensed muscles through their physical training. A progressive muscle relaxation version, preferred by us, is aimed at eight muscle groups and systematic breathing. From our applied experience it seems to be helpful that after an introductory concentration phase, the program starts with the facial muscles. This order supports building up concentration for the entire phase in the beginning of the procedure (see Table 17.1).

In the first three sessions the muscle groups are repeatedly tensed and relaxed (three times). In order to be economic, some muscle groups are grouped together during sessions four to six, i.e., muscle groups are then activated simultaneously. These groups are then tensed and relaxed twice. In the seventh to ninth sessions, the grouped muscles are tensed and relaxed only once. In addition, the instruction is shortened from the seventh session on, i.e., only the muscle groups are announced and the athlete controls tension and relaxation time himself/herself.

In the beginning, the sport psychologist informs the athlete about the course, mechanisms, and possible effects of the progressive muscle relaxation. In addition, attention is drawn to practise effects, i.e., time to elicit a relaxation response is reduced following repeated execution. Furthermore, the athletes receive the instruction that they should execute the relaxation technique highly concentrated and should not fall asleep (which still happens to many during the first sessions).

Conclusion and recommendations for practise

Relaxation techniques should be integrated as an essential part of an athletes' training regimen. They should be practised before or between training sessions, so that athletes are still able to engage in them in a concentrated state. Essentially, an efficient provision of relaxation competence requires a long-term perspective. Adopting such a long-term systematic practise approach (Beckmann & Elbe, 2015) is accompanied by various positive side effects. Relaxation could serve as a regeneration accelerator and is particularly helpful in case athletes tend to be nervous prior to competition ('starting fever') and/or cannot sleep or sleep badly in the night before competition. Additionally, relaxation marks a prerequisite for the execution of mental training (e.g., imagery). However, practising relaxation techniques in their detailed version on the competition day is contraindicated, because it could jeopardise the necessary activation for competition.

In the beginning of a long-term approach, systematic breathing should be introduced and practised. Systematic breathing is administered at this point, as it is one of the simplest approaches to relaxation and additionally an integral part of every other relaxation technique. Thereby, the exhalation should be deliberately prolonged compared to the inhalation (Pelka et al., 2017). After exhaling, a short pause follows, after which the inhalation automatically starts again. If an understanding of the actual physiological mechanisms of relaxation is necessary, it can be conveyed via biofeedback in this phase. Through the use of biofeedback (as technical support) ordinarily unavailable internal physiological processes can be made visible for the athlete in a meaningful, rapid, precise, and consistent form (Zaichkowsky & Fuchs, 1988). This is followed by the introduction of progressive muscle relaxation (about eight to ten sessions) with the goal of achieving sensitisation for the body/muscles. The last episode of the training program would consist of autogenic training with a focus on three basic exercises (heaviness, warmth, respiration) aiming at long-term psychotropic effects. Thereafter, autogenic training and progressive muscle relaxation may remain an integral part of the training regimen. The composition and development of the training schedule strongly depend on previous experiences and individual preferences. Additionally, like practising their physical skills, it is important that athletes practise their psychological skills such as relaxation techniques and routines daily.

References

Andreassi, J. L. (2007). Concepts in psychophysiology. In J. L. Andreassi (Ed.), *Psychophysiology – human behavior and physiological response* (pp. 16–42). New York, NY: Psychology Press.

Beckmann, J., & Elbe, A.-M. (2015). *Sport psychological interventions in competitive sports*. Newcastle, UK: Cambridge Scholars Publishing.

Beckmann, J., Gröpel, P., & Ehrlenspiel, F. (2013). Preventing motor skill failure through hemisphere-specific priming: Cases from choking under pressure. *Journal of Experimental Psychology: General, 142*, 679–691.

Beckmann, J., & Rolstad, K. (1997). Aktivierung, Selbstregulation und Leistung: Gibt es so etwas wie Übermotivation? [Activation, self-regulation and performance: Is there anything like over-motivation?]. *Sportwissenschaft, 27*(1), 23–37.

Bengtsson, H., Ekstrand, J., & Hägglund, M. (2013). Muscle injury rates in professional football increase with fixture congestion: An 11-year follow-up of the UEFA Champions League injury study. *British Journal of Sports Medicine, 47*(12), 743–747.

Bernstein, D. A., & Borkovec, T. D. (1973). *Progressive relaxation training. A manual for the helping professions*. Champaign, IL: Research Press Company.

Bernstein, D. A., Carlson, C. R., & Schmidt, J. F. (2007). Progressive relaxation. In P. M. Lehrer, R. L. Woolfolk, & W. E. Sime (Eds.), *Principles and practice of stress management* (pp. 88–124). New York, NY: The Guilford Press.

Birrer, D., & Morgan, G. (2010). Psychological skills training as a way to enhance an athlete's performance in high-intensity sports. *Scandinavian Journal of Medicine and Science in Sports, 20*, 78–87.

Cross-Villasana, F., Gröpel, P., Doppelmayr, M., & Beckmann, J. (2015). Unilateral left-hand contractions produce widespread depression of cortical activity after their execution. *PloS One*, *10*(12), e0145867.

Dolan, Y. (1991). *Resolving sexual abuse: Solution-focused therapy and Ericksonian hypnosis for adult survivors*. New York, NY: W.W. Norton.

Ehrlenspiel, F., Erlacher, D., & Ziegler, M. (in press). Changes in subjective sleep quality before a competition and their relation to competitive anxiety. *Behavioral Sleep Medicine*. doi:10.1080/15402002.2016.1253012

Erlacher, D., Ehrlenspiel, F., Adegbesan, O. A., & Galal El-Din, H. (2011). Sleep habits in German athletes before important competitions or games. *Journal of Sports Sciences*, *29*(8), 859–866.

Gillen, E., Biley, F., & Allen, D. (2008). Effects of music listening on adult patients' pre-procedural state anxiety in hospital. *International Journal of Evidence-Based Healthcare*, *6*(1), 24–49.

Gröpel, P., & Beckmann, J. (2017). A pre-performance routine to optimize competition performance in artistic gymnastics. *The Sport Psychologist*, *31*, 199–207.

Hamm, A. (2014). Progressive Muskelentspannung [Progressive muscle relaxation]. In F. Petermann & D. Vaitl (Eds.), *Entspannungsverfahren* [Relaxation techniques] (5th ed., pp. 154–172). Weinheim: Beltz.

Hanin, Y. L. (1997). Emotions and athletic performance: Individual zones of optimal functioning model. *European Yearbook of Sport Psychology*, *1*, 29–72.

Jones, L., Tiller, N. B., & Karageorghis, C. I. (2017). Psychophysiological effects of music on acute recovery from high-intensity interval training. *Physiology and Behavior*, *170*, 106–114.

Karageorghis, C. I., & Priest, D.-L. (2012). Music in the exercise domain: A review and synthesis (Part I). *International Review of Sport and Exercise Psychology*, *5*(1), 44–66.

Kellmann, M. (2002). Psychological assessment of underrecovery. In M. Kellmann (Ed.), *Enhancing recovery: Preventing underperformance in athletes* (pp. 37–56). Champaign, IL: Human Kinetics.

Kellmann, M., & Kallus, K. W. (2016). The Recovery-Stress Questionnaire for Athletes. In K. W. Kallus & M. Kellmann (Eds.), *The Recovery-Stress Questionnaires: User manual* (pp. 86–131). Frankfurt am Main: Pearson Assessment.

Kudlackova, K., Eccles, D. W., & Dieffenbach, K. (2013). Use of relaxation skills in differentially skilled athletes. *Psychology of Sport and Exercise*, *14*(4), 468–475.

Kuhl, J. (2001). *Motivation und Persönlichkeit: Interaktionen psychischer Systeme* [Motivation and personality: Interactions of psychological systems]. Göttingen: Hogrefe.

Ligget, D. R. (2000). *Sport hypnosis*. Champaign, IL: Human Kinetics.

Loizou, G., & Karageorghis, C. I. (2015). Effects of psychological priming, video, and music on anaerobic exercise performance. *Scandinavian Journal of Medicine and Science in Sports*, *25*(6), 909–920.

MacDonald, R. A., Mitchell, L. A., Dillon, T., Serpell, M. G., Davies, J. B., & Ashley, E. A. (2003). An empirical investigation of the anxiolytic and pain reducing effects of music. *Psychology of Music*, *31*(2), 187–203.

MacIntyre, T. E., Madan, C. R., Brick, N. E., Beckmann, J., & Moran, A. P. (in press). Imagery, expertise, and action: A window into embodiment. In M. L. Cappuccio (Ed.), *The MIT Press handbook of embodied cognition and sport psychology*. Cambridge MA: MIT Press.

Martin, K. A., Moritz, S. E., & Hall, C. R. (1999). Imagery use in sport: A literature review and applied model. *The Sport Psychologist*, *13*, 245–368.

Mesagno, C., & Beckmann, J. (2017). Choking under pressure: Theoretical models and interventions. *Current Opinion in Psychology*, *16*, 170–175.

Meyer, T., Kellmann, M., Ferrauti, A., Pfeiffer, M., & Faude, O. (2013). Die Messung von Erholtheit und Regenerationsbedarf im Fußball [The measurement of recovery and regeneration requirements in football]. *Deutsche Zeitschrift für Sportmedizin, 64*, 28–34.

Nilsson, U. (2008). The anxiety-and pain-reducing effects of music interventions: A systematic review. *AORN Journal, 87*(4), 780–807.

Pelka, M., Heidari, J., Ferrauti, A., Meyer, T., Pfeiffer, M., & Kellmann, M. (2016). Relaxation techniques in sports: A systematic review on acute effects on performance. *Performance Enhancement and Health, 5*(2), 47–59.

Pelka, M., Kölling, S., Ferrauti, A., Meyer, T., Pfeiffer, M., & Kellmann, M. (2017). Acute effects of psychological relaxation techniques between two physical tasks. *Journal of Sports Sciences, 35*(3), 216–223.

Petermann, F., & Vaitl, D. (2014). Entspannungsverfahren. In F. Petermann & D. Vaitl (Eds.), *Entspannungsverfahren* [Relaxation techniques] (5th ed., pp. 77–172). Weinheim: Beltz.

Seers, K., & Carroll, D. (1998). Relaxation techniques for acute pain management: A systematic review. *Journal of Advanced Nursing, 27*, 466–475.

Sherman, C. P., & Poczwardowski, A. (2000). Relax! . . . It ain't easy (or is it?). In M. B. Andersen (Ed.), *Doing sport psychology* (pp. 47–60). Champaign, IL: Human Kinetics.

Szmedra, L., & Bacharach, D. W. (1998). Effect of music on perceived exertion, plasma lactate, norepinephrine and cardiovascular hemodynamics during treadmill running. *International Journal of Sports Medicine, 19*(1), 32–37.

Tennant, C., Langeluddecke, P., & Byrne, D. (1985). The concept of stress. *Australian and New Zealand Journal of Psychiatry, 19*(2), 113–118.

Terry, P. C., & Karageorghis, C. I. (2006). Psychophysical effects of music in sport and exercise: An update on theory, research and application. In M. Katsikitis (Ed.), *Psychology bridging the Tasman: Science, culture and practice – proceedings of the 2006 Joint Conference of the Australian Psychological Society and New Zealand Psychological Society* (pp. 415–419). Melbourne, VIC: Australian Psychological Society.

Vaitl, D. (2014). Neurobiologische Grundlagen der Entspannungsverfahren. In F. Petermann & D. Vaitel (Eds.), *Entspannungsverfahren* [Relaxation techniques] (5th ed, pp. 18–35). Weinheim: Beltz.

Weinberg, R., & Gould, D. (2010). *Foundations of sport and exercise psychology*. Champaign, IL: Human Kinetics.

Williams, J. M. (2009). *Applied sport psychology*. Mountain View, CA: Mayfield.

Yerkes, R. M., & Dodson, J. D. (1908). The relationship of strength of stimulus to rapidity of habit formation. *Journal of Comprehensive Neurology and Psychology, 18*, 459–482.

Zaichkowsky, L. D., & Fuchs, C. Z. (1988). Biofeedback applications in exercise and athletic performance. *Exercise and Sport Sciences Reviews, 16*(1), 381–422.

18
SPORT, RECOVERY, AND PERFORMANCE

A concluding summary

Michael Kellmann and Jürgen Beckmann

Appreciation of recovery

In the last chapter of the book *Enhancing recovery: Preventing underperformance in athletes*, Kellmann (2002) expressed his hope that "... in the future more publications will deal with enhancing recovery to prevent underperformance in sport" (p. 310). About 15 years later we can conclude that the term 'recovery' has become well accepted and appreciated in applied sport science. Meanwhile, a majority of coaches realises the potential of recovery activities to have a positive impact on performance. Also, outside of sport science recovery has increasingly been considered (see Kallus & Gaisbachgrabner, this volume; Nicolas, Gaudino, & Vacher, this volume). Recent milestones in this development were the conference *Monitoring Athlete Training Loads – The Hows and the Whys* in March 2016 which was convened in Doha (Qatar), and the symposium on *Recovery and Performance* which was held in September 2016 in Burghausen (Germany).

Part of this positive development is due to changes in the recognition and acceptance of recovery in coaches and sporting organisations (see Nash & Sproule, this volume; Venter & Grobbelaar, this volume). For example, in 2012 the German Federal Institute of Sport Science funded the project *Optimization of Training and Competition: Management of Regeneration in Elite Sports* (REGman; Meyer, Ferrauti, Kellmann, & Pfeiffer, 2016) which investigates the impact of various regeneration techniques and strategies in athletes. The extension of this project by four additional years shows how well it was received and appreciated. Its impact on research was acknowledged as well as the consequences for sport practise because it provides evidence for the successful integration of recovery activities during and after training/competition. The tools developed in the REGman project increase the quality of monitoring systems which are integrated in teams, clubs, and sporting organisations.

Monitoring tools

The application of such systems/tools monitoring stress and recovery is strongly recommended for sports (Bertollo, Nakamura, Bortoli, & Robazza, this volume; Brink & Lemmink, this volume; Heidari, Kölling, Pelka, & Kellmann, this volume; Robazza, Forzini, di Fronso, & Bertollo, this volume), health (Frank, Nixdorf, & Beckmann, this volume), for the work context (Kallus & Gaisbachgrabner, this volume), and extreme situations like polar stations and space flights (Nicolas et al., this volume). Because in many of these areas 'time' is a scarce resource shorter monitoring tools are frequently asked for. Often, self-developed single item measures are used to monitor training load and recovery (Saw, Kellmann, Main, & Gastin, 2017). However, the development of short monitoring tools is limited by the necessary length to provide reliable and valid assessment tools. This dilemma limits the interpretation and generalisation of the results. The theory based development of the *Acute and Short Recovery and Stress Scales* (Kellmann, Kölling, & Hitzschke, 2016; Nässi, Ferrauti, Meyer, Pfeiffer, & Kellmann, 2017) is hopefully a milestone to start a new generation of short assessment tools. In this context, Saw and colleagues (2017) propose a framework for steps to be taken in a selection process to identify the right measure. Heidari et al. (this volume) discuss currently available instruments and provide an overview for which purpose the instruments can be used best. In addition, it will be very important to use and apply these tools online to enable a worldwide assessment and feedback when athletes are travelling.

When instruments are developed in one language the validation process of the translated version is often not realised as detailed as for the original version impacting the quality of the outcome. Certainly the validation process can be shorter to some degree – because the structure of the instrument and the items have already been developed in the original. However, different results in reliability and validity can also be due to cultural differences and a slightly different understanding of the language. Even within the same language there are sometimes differences in the interpretation of British, North-American, and Australian/New Zealand English. We came across that issue translating the *Acute and Short Recovery and Stress Scales* into English (Nässi et al., 2017), where we use adjectives to assess recovery and stress states and had to rely on experts from these three regions realising the back-to-back translation. So, it is important to be aware of the problems arising from instruments which have been adapted from a different language or context.

Individualisation

The common theme throughout the book is the emphasis on the individual athlete and the importance of individualisation to prevent underrecovery and underperformance (e.g., Bosquet, Berryman, & Mujika, this volume; Coutts, Crowcroft, & Kempton, this volume; Meeusen & De Pauw, this volume; Sharma & Mujika, this volume). This includes the relatively new area of mental health issues in athletes (Frank et al., this volume). Athletes' responses to training are affected by the current health, training load, social life etc. which explains that responses to training are different across individuals (Bourdon et al., 2017). Therefore, individual differences may limit the diagnostic accuracy of group-based reference ranges. That also refers to the responses to research on recovery activities and strategies. Hecksteden and colleagues (in press) address this by introducing a new attempt to develop individualised reference ranges using a Bayesian approach comparable to that developed for the athlete biological passport. In the case of fatigue assessment, two physiological states have to be discriminated and interindividual variation seems to be present with regard to the general 'level' of indicators (between-subject variation) as well as concerning the magnitude of fatigue induced changes (fatigue-by-person interaction). Therefore, decisions should likely be based on two reference ranges (fatigued and recovered) instead of simply detecting deviations from the recovered state.

Sleep

Fatigue in athletes frequently results from extensive travelling which sometimes is associated with sleep deficits especially when travelling across time zones. Sleep is the most natural and important recovery strategy for humans. Disturbed sleep, however, will affect performance in sport and in general life as well as athletes' health (Fullagar et al., 2015; Hirshkowitz et al., 2015). Duffield and Fowler (this volume) summarise the effects of travel on sleep and the resulted impact on the organism. Short flights affect our sleep quality less than a long-haul flight. Regarding the long flights across time zones travelling westbound or eastbound strongly affects sleep and sleep quality (e.g., Kölling et al., 2017). Erlacher and Ehrlenspiel (this volume) also refer to the importance of dreams during sleep and the functional importance it has on the quality of life. They offer a special focus on lucid dreaming – dreams in which the dreamer is aware of the dream state and the possible application of this phenomenon in sports (e.g., motor learning or psychophysiological correlates of dreaming). However, before you start dreaming you must go to bed, and if you are in bed you need to fall asleep. What sounds easy is often difficult for the travelling athlete. The own bed is different compared to a bed in hotels or training camps; rooms often are shared and individuals have different routines going through the nights which may disturb others. In those cases, the use of relaxation techniques is helpful to fall asleep quicker and sleep better (Kellmann,

Pelka, & Beckmann, this volume). Also, the use of electronic devices seems to take its toll on individual athletes who are not able/willing to turn off the smartphone at a certain point at night staying connected to friends and family. The exposure to bright light (like that emitted by a smartphone or computer screen) can disrupt circadian rhythms, and suppress melatonin production, leading to an increase in alertness and disturbed sleep. In consequence it leads to disturbances in regular sleep patterns, poorer sleep quality, sleep loss, and increased daytime fatigue (Exelmans & Van den Bulck, 2016). Caia, Kelly, and Halson (this volume) also report that elite athletes frequently obtain less than the 8 hours of sleep recommended for the general population. This is not surprising considering that a lot of sports (e.g., rowing, swimming) involve early morning (before school) training/practise sessions with opportunities to nap during daytime being restricted to school and university life.

Mental fatigue and mental recovery

So far physical fatigue and recovery strategies have been emphasised in research. Recently the element of mental fatigue and consequently the need for mental recovery embrace the spotlight of research. Prolonged periods of demanding cognitive activity lead to mental fatigue (Marcora, Staiano, & Manning, 2009), which is reflected by an increased tiredness or even exhaustion, an aversion to continue with the present activity, and a decrease in the level of commitment to the task at hand (Boksem & Tops, 2008). In sports with high cognitive challenges combined with physical tasks this can lead to a substantial performance decrement (Coutts, 2016; Duncan, Fowler, George, Joyce, & Hankey, 2015; Smith et al., 2016). In a systematic review Van Cutsem et al. (2017) analysed the effects of mental fatigue on physical performance, focusing on eleven articles, of which six were of strong and five of moderate quality. The duration and intensity of the physical task seem to be important factors in the decrease in physical performance due to mental fatigue; the key factor appears to be the level of perceived exertion. However, the basis of the review with eleven studies needs to be extended; further research is needed to broaden the basis for intervention for mental recovery strategies in sport.

Final remarks

We have come a long way but there is still some distance to cover in recovery research in sport and other areas. The beauty of research in sport is that the relation to performance is obvious, regardless of how this is measured in a specific sport. Accordingly, most research results on recovery are from the area of sports and hence, this book mainly focuses on recovery and performance in sport. Nevertheless, some of the findings can be transferred to the non-sport context and vice versa. Examples are given for life at polar stations and space flights. Performance measurement is much more complex in the work context and it may have more impact on society if a wrong decision is made being a pilot or a traffic controller compared to winning or losing a game of football. Learning about the different performance conditions in other areas of life and how they are affected by recovery respective a lack of recovery will broaden our understanding of the concept. Having started the interdisciplinary dialogue across different domains will further advance theoretical and applied perspectives on recovery and performance.

References

Boksem, M. A., & Tops, M. (2008). Mental fatigue: Costs and benefits. *Brain Research Reviews*, *59*(1), 125–139.

Bourdon, P. C., Cardinale, M., Murray, A., Gastin, P., Kellmann, M., . . . Cable, N. T. (2017). Monitoring athlete training loads: Consensus statement. *International Journal of Sports Physiology and Performance*, *12*(Suppl. 2), S2161–S2170.

Coutts, A. J. (2016). Fatigue in football: It's not a brainless task! *Journal of Sports Sciences*, *34*, 1296.

Duncan, M. J., Fowler, N., George, O., Joyce, S., & Hankey, J. (2015). Mental fatigue negatively influences manual dexterity and anticipation timing but not repeated high-intensity exercise performance in trained adults. *Research in Sports Medicine*, *23*(1), 1–13.

Exelmans, L., & Van den Bulck, J. (2016). Bedtime mobile phone use and sleep in adults. *Social Science & Medicine*, *148*(1), 93–101.

Fullagar, H., Skorski, S., Duffield, R., Hammes, D., Coutts, A. J., & Meyer, T. (2015). Sleep and athletic performance: The effects of sleep loss on exercise performance, and physiological and cognitive responses to exercise. *Sports Medicine*, *45*(2), 161–186.

Hecksteden, A., Pitsch, W., Julian, R. A., Pfeiffer, M., Kellmann, M., Ferrauti, A., & Meyer, T. (in press). A new method to individualize monitoring of muscle recovery in athletes. *International Journal of Sports Physiology and Performance*. doi:10.1123/ijspp.2016-0120

Hirshkowitz, M., Whiton, K., Albert, S. M., Alessi, C. A., Bruni, O., DonCarlos, L., . . . Katz, E. S. (2015). National Sleep Foundation's sleep time duration recommendations: Methodology and results summary. *Journal of the National Sleep Foundation*, *1*(3), 40–43.

Kellmann, M. (2002). Current status and directions of recovery research. In M. Kellmann (Ed.), *Enhancing recovery: Preventing underperformance in athletes* (pp. 301–311). Champaign, IL: Human Kinetics.

Kellmann, M., Kölling, S., & Hitzschke, B. (2016). *Das Akutmaß und die Kurzskala zur Erfassung von Erholung und Beanspruchung im Sport – Manual* [The Acute Measure and the Short Scale of Recovery and Stress for Sports – Manual]. Hellenthal: Sportverlag Strauß.

Kölling, S., Treff, G., Winkert, K., Ferrauti, A., Meyer, T., Pfeiffer, M., & Kellmann, M. (2017). The effect of westward travel across five time-zones on sleep and subjective jet-lag ratings in athletes before and during the 2015's World Rowing Junior Championships. *Journal of Sports Sciences*, *35*, 2240–2248.

Marcora, S. M., Staiano, W., & Manning, V. (2009). Mental fatigue impairs physical performance in humans. *Journal of Applied Physiology*, *106*(3), 857–864.

Meyer, T., Ferrauti, A., Kellmann, M., & Pfeiffer, M. (2016). *Regenerationsmanagement im Spitzensport* [Management of regeneration in elite sports]. Köln: Sportverlag Strauß.

Nässi, A., Ferrauti, A., Meyer, T., Pfeiffer, M., & Kellmann, M. (2017). Development of two short measures for recovery and stress in sport. *European Journal of Sport Science*, *17*(7), 894–903.

Saw, A. E., Kellmann, M., Main, L. C., & Gastin, P. B. (2017). Athlete self-report measures in research and practice: Recommendations for the discerning reader and fastidious practitioner. *International Journal of Sports Physiology and Performance, 12*(Suppl. 2), S2127–S2135.

Smith, M. R., Zeuwts, L., Lenoir, M., Hens, N., De Jong, L. M., & Coutts, A. J. (2016). Mental fatigue impairs soccer-specific decision-making skill. *Journal of Sports Sciences, 34*(14), 1297–1304.

Van Cutsem, J., Marcoram, S., De Pauw, K., Bailey, S., Meeusen, R., & Roelands, B. (2017). The effects of mental fatigue on physical performance: A systematic review. *Sports Medicine, 47*, 1569–1588.

INDEX

Acute Recovery and Stress Scale (ARSS) 11–13, 24
acute-to-chronic workload ratio (ACWR) 26
aerobic 22, 97, 133, 158
aerobic endurance (AE) 88–91
altitude 53, 133–141, 183–190, 221
anaerobic 22, 133, 159
autogenic training 40, 250–252

blood volume 88–102
breathing exercise 40
burnout 6–8, 60, 79, 124–127, 216, 244

cardiorespiratory fitness 76, 78
career 87, 121, 171
choking under pressure 251
circadian rhythms 10, 157–163, 184–192, 263
cold water immersion (CWI) 37–43
compression garments 38–43, 214, 215
contrast water therapy (CWT) 37–42
cool down 6, 35, 36, 208, 209
cortisol 53, 58, 75–80, 112, 140, 153, 237–240
cyclists 63–70, 88, 133, 140, 172
cryotherapy 37–39

Daily Analysis of Life Demands for Athletes (DALDA) 24, 137, 138
debriefing 40, 242, 244, 251, 255
Delayed Onset Muscle Soreness (DOMS) 37, 38, 209, 214, 215

depression 11, 13, 55–57, 66, 122–127
detraining 87–91, 97, 101, 132
dose-response relationship 19–26, 55, 99, 133
dream 152, 168–178, 262
dream, lucid 168–178, 262
dropout 123–127
dysfunctional attitude 127

eastern meditation 249
electroencephalography (EEG) 75–79, 170
electromyography (EMG) 75, 170
electrooculogram (EOG) 170
embodied cognition 251
endurance sports 63, 64, 132–142
energy 22, 52, 63–67, 90–97, 133, 202, 214, 226
energy cost of locomotion (Cr) 88, 91
exertion/velocity ratio 141
exponentially weighted moving average (EWMA) 26
extreme situation 221–228, 261
extreme sports 221, 226

fatigue, chronic 34, 60, 74, 223
fatigue, mental 112, 138, 263
fitness 23
fitness-fatigue model 19, 20, 26
force, maximal 92–97
functional overreaching (FOR) 51–57, 101

group-based reference 262

health 5–9, 25, 41, 43, 59, 63, 119–127, 140, 151, 168, 191, 201–211, 226, 247, 261, 262
health, mental 124, 127, 262
health, problems 119–127, 235, 244
health, somatic 122, 127
heart rate (HR) 8, 22–28, 56–63, 75–89, 111, 136–142, 190, 253
heart rate, resting 8, 23, 56, 79
heart rate recovery 23
heart rate response to exercise 23
heart rate variability (HRV) 56, 75–79, 227
home advantage 187, 194
hormones 54
hypnosis 252
hypoxia 140, 185, 188

iceberg-profile 11, 56
illness 26–28, 52–59, 123, 192, 193
imagery 40, 176, 215, 248–256
imagination 176, 252
immune function 123, 185
immune measures 25
immune system 57, 77, 119, 123, 191, 210
immunity 57, 160
individualisation 101, 102, 262
individual zones of optimal functioning (IZOF) 67, 248
infection 8, 57, 123, 193
inflammation 36, 160
injury 7–9, 13, 70, 74, 78, 108–116, 119–125, 137, 160, 214, 249
injury, prevention of 4, 78, 108–113, 134
injury, vulnerability to 119

jet lag 59, 156, 184–192
junior athletes 121, 122

lactate 23, 36, 56, 57, 91, 133–141, 215
Lamberts and Lambert Submaximal Cycle Test (LSCT) 9, 136
load: Acute and chronic training 10, 24, 63; competition 9, 132, 135; external 21–23, 74–81, 111, 133–141; injury relationship 110, 111; internal 22, 23, 76–79, 111, 113, 133–142; parameter 98; reduction 97, 102
long working hours 233–244

Management of Regeneration in Elite Sports (REGman) 260
marker, biochemical 25, 76, 77, 112
mars 222–229
massage 37, 39, 71, 209
meditation 40, 155, 216, 249
monitoring instrument 9, 11, 13

monitoring system 19–29, 87, 111, 115, 142
mood disturbances 10, 11, 56, 66
mood state 10–13, 52, 55, 66, 67, 157, 163, 185–190
muscle damage 25, 36, 38, 60, 163, 211–215
muscle lipoprotein 91
music 40, 41, 253

nap 35, 155, 160–164, 178, 193, 263
neuromuscular system 92, 95
non-protein respiratory exchange ratio (RER) 90
nutrition 52, 58, 210

overreaching 11, 24, 25, 51, 65, 74–79, 87–102, 133
overreaching, nonfunctional (NFOR) 51
overtime 234, 235, 242
overtraining syndrome (OTS): Assessment of 53; diagnosis 51–59; hormones 54, 57; marker 53–60; performance 55; prevention 51–57, 65, 78, 79, 108–116
oxygen consumption 63, 77, 136
oxygen saturation 185, 188
oxygen uptake 9, 24, 56, 88–92, 138

perfectionism 121, 127
performance: Cognitive 159, 185, 186; jump 189; maximising 151, 163, 168; memory 159; motivation 7; peak 5, 34, 97, 132–138, 168, 212
periodisation 6, 135, 212, 213
personality 8, 14, 60, 121, 123, 224–229, 249
physiological adaptation 135, 139
physiological and biochemical indicators 137
polar station 221–224
polysomnography 153, 154, 169, 170, 176
power, maximal 92–97
prayer 40, 41
principle of converging evidence 76, 78
Profile of Mood States (POMS) 10–13, 55, 66, 70, 137, 138
progressive muscle relaxation (PMR) 40, 249–257
psychobiosocial state 63–70, 75–80

rapid eye movement sleep (REM) 152–163, 176, 178
Rating of Perceived Exertion (RPE) 10, 13, 22–28, 57, 76–80, 111, 115, 137, 139–141
recovery: Active 6, 34–43, 208, 209; activity 5, 8, 56, 65, 120, 228, 260–262; intervention 7, 42, 44, 205–217;

knowledge of 42, 120–127, 201–217; lack of 69, 119–125, 250, 264; mental 4, 263; modality 33–44, 126, 153, 202–214; natural strategies 34; passive 5, 6, 38, 39, 58, 64, 121, 213, 233, 250, 254; physical and physiological strategies 34, 37; proactive 6, 8, 65, 75, 121, 127; psychological strategies 40, 66, 70, 215, 216; psychosociological modalities 39; quality and quantity of 125; strategy 6–14, 33–44, 114–121, 207–218, 227, 250, 262, 263
recovery-injury relationship 112
recovery-stress balance 6, 9, 63–70, 74–83, 108–115, 132–142, 228, 229, 237–244
recovery-stress factors 64, 67
recovery-stress imbalance 6, 121
Recovery-Stress Questionnaire for Athletes (RESTQ-Sport) 11, 13, 24, 56, 65–70, 75–83, 101, 114, 120, 123, 138, 202, 204, 224–227, 231, 235
recovery-stress state 3–12, 235
regeneration accelerator 249–256
relaxation response 250–256
relaxation techniques 215, 216, 247–257, 262
relaxation training 248–251
resilience 64, 66, 126, 127
respiratory rate 253

salivary cortisol concentration 239
scissor model 7, 125, 126
self-hypnosis 252
self-regulation 11, 65–69, 75, 120–127, 204, 247–251
session-RPE 13, 22, 23, 57, 78, 111, 115, 137, 139
Short Recovery and Stress Scale (SRSS) 11–13, 24, 237, 261
sleep: Deprivation 35, 158–161; disruption 121, 155, 192, 193; disturbed 35, 155–157, 172, 263; efficiency 153–161, 171; extension 161, 164; fragmentation 158; function 153; hygiene 155–164, 192; loss 53, 58, 59, 157–164, 179, 263; measuring 168, 171; non-rapid eye movement (NREM) 152; objective measures 169, 170; onset latency 154–161, 169, 186–193; patterns 35, 155–163, 187, 188, 263; quality 11, 35, 65, 67, 120, 151, 157, 169–173, 206, 234, 235, 250, 262, 263; rapid eye movement (REM) 152–163, 176, 178; recording 168, 170; slow-wave (SWS) 152–163, 171; subjective measures 169, 170
sleep/wake behaviour 171
sleep-wake cycle 35, 186, 191
smallest meaningful change 27
social support 40, 110, 123, 225
spaceflights 221–226
specificity 27, 135, 170
stress load 120, 121, 139
stress-related problems 126
stretching 4, 6, 34–43, 64, 207, 208, 213
stroke volume 88, 89, 97
subjective critical situations 238–242
submaximal strength 95–97
systematic breathing 40, 249–257

taper 99–101
thyroid function 235, 237, 240
time zone 156, 157, 184–192, 262
Total Quality of Recovery (TQR) 24, 112, 113
training: Cessation 88–97, 102; impulse (TRIMP) 76, 137, 140; intensity 8, 10, 22–25, 59, 88–100, 134–140; quantification of 132
training/recovery ratio 57
travel: Conditions and effects of air 185; duration 184; during 188–192; eastward and westward 186–193; fatigue 158, 184–194; long-haul 156, 164, 183–194, 206; pre- and post 186, 190–193; short-haul 157, 183–194; transmeridian air 185–192

underperformance 34, 58–60, 65–70, 121, 201, 215, 260, 262
underrecovery 6–11, 49, 58, 119–127, 138, 139, 234, 250, 262
upper-respiratory tract infection (URTI) 52, 57, 59, 190

water immersion 37, 39, 208, 211, 212
well-being 6, 29, 35, 41, 58, 63, 77, 114, 133, 137, 151, 168, 190, 201, 210, 221–228, 248–253
workload 26
work/rest ratios 141
wrist actigraphy 153, 154, 170

young athlete 121, 122, 237

zeitgeber 185, 191